Kirkus Reviews:

An acupuncturist and Eastern health expert offers alternative medicine wisdom.

In this debut book about salubrious "Secrets," Senogles, one of the first graduates in acupuncture and "Oriental Medicine" in the United States, shares his wealth of disease prevention knowledge. In openly believing that "health, happiness, and enthusiasm are our birthright, and that they are attainable," the author parlays over 40 years of private medical practice into a manual that promotes fitness through root-cause determination rather than ascribing to a symptom-driven state of perceived wellness. Readers need to first understand and be open to the origins of his methodology; Senogles touts traditional Eastern medicine as a supremely effective alternative health system for the human body.

Split into two sections, the first aims to demystify the integral, vital, and interlocking organic functionalities of the human body and make this often complicated information comprehensible to the average person. Many of the chapters spotlight a hypothetical case at a clinic and the tecÚiques used to alleviate the issue. "Tired Tom" complains of low energy, and the author adroitly describes the complex inner mechanisms of cellular metabolism, but in layperson's terms. This explanatory simplicity creates an appealingly relatable quality to the narrative and has the potential to quell the squeamisÚess some readers experience when perusing medical texts for help. The same can be said for segments on blood's life-sustaining capacity, stress treatments, acupuncture benefits, digestion processes, and some important guidance about how to preserve kidney function well into advanced age.

Even more accessible is the book's second section, which delves into the numerous, intricate biological systems that operate the body and the most common maladies that can plague these areas. Senogles delivers strategies for optimal bone health, sound ways to avoid everyday toxins, and the building blocks of proper, non-genetically modified nutrition ("Shelf Defense"). Though some segments are overly short and only scratch the topic's surface, others provide more in-depth discourse.

The volume is attractively embellished by debut illustrator Cauker's line drawings, which demarcate chapters in a creative fashion.

Overall, the author coaches readers on the benefits of using safe, natural methods to fix ordinary problems except, of course, for what he calls "The Big C." The grave seriousness of a cancer diagnosis is outside the scope of this manual, although he suggests that his tips might stave off the development of that disease. The book's disclaimer smartly states that Senogles' advice should not be considered a definitive or conclusive diagnosis or treatment for illnesses. He counsels readers with serious conditions or symptoms to consult a medical professional.

Still, whether or not readers ascribe to Eastern medicine, this sage volume remains a timely, neighborly nudge to regularly examine their diets, exercise levels, and general sense of well-being. And the work serves as a reminder to prioritize the cultivation of optimum health and wellness by becoming an active monitor.

Achieving the natural state of health remains the goal of this practical, beneficial guide heavily influenced by Eastern medicine.

—Kirkus Reviews

Indie Reader:

[*Body Wisdom*]… is a beginner's guide to the physical self an the alternative healing methods of Eastern Medicine in order to help readers understand their bodies… and put down the book "a lot more knowledgeable" than when they picked it up. [Senogles]… doesn't rush through his information or assume that the reader has medical knowledge. He starts with the basics of how the body works and from there builds a picture of an entire person.

The chapters in *Body Wisdom* are well-ordered by topic… citing examples of [Dr. Senogles'] practice. The author writes with a conversational and accessible tone, so even when he delves into more tecÚical definitions, such as of the autonomic nervous system, they are easy to follow and understand.

Body Wisdom is a useful read that teaches the reader many facts and gives practical tips about living healthier. The black and white artwork [by Katy Caulker] peppered throughout the book is stirring and well worth look.

—Indie Reader

Body Wisdom

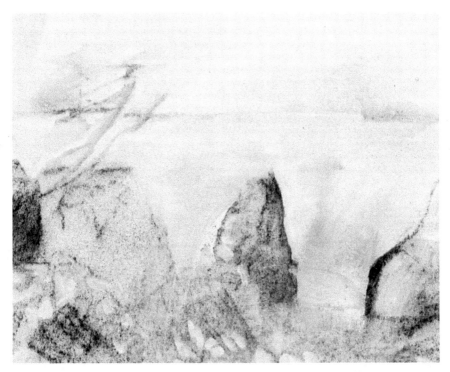

Wishing you... Health
and Happiness !!

Dr G.J. Senogles
DOM, L.Ac.

Body Wisdom

*Secrets for Achieving Health,
Happiness & Longevity*

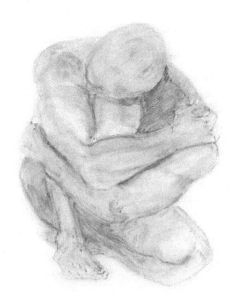

Dr. Gerald Senogles

D.O.M., L.Ac.

Illustrations by Katy Cauker

Fire & Water Publishing

DISCLAIMER

Nothing in this book should be construed as specific medical advice for any particular patient. If someone is suffering from a symptom or malady, it is advised they consult with a medical professional.

Contents

ACKNOWLEDGMENTS

When one studies a medical system with thousands of years of an unbroken accumulation of knowledge and wisdom, many of the doctors to thank are not only long dead but also completely unknown and unknowable, and yet one must pay homage to these unseen benefactors none the less, and I do.

I acknowledge my principle teacher as well: Dr. Cheung Wai Tak, who not only shared his medical and life wisdom with me, but showed me how caring and generous a doctor can be.

And finally, I thank my friend and co-practitioner Kristopher Kokay, who took over much responsibility at the clinic allowing me time to complete *Body Wisdom*.

DEDICATION

Body Wisdom is dedicated to my wonderful family:
my son Sean and my wife Katy Cauker.
They are the ground on which I walk.

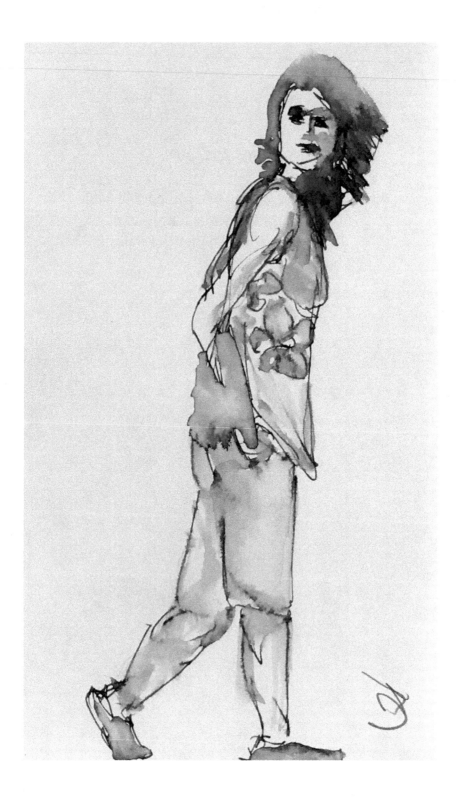

Introduction

The Case of "Poor Jane"

There was no polite way to say it—Jane was a medical disaster! She suffered from insomnia, depression, acid reflux, headaches, low back pain, and terrible menstrual cramping.

Jane consulted six different medical "specialists" for her six different symptoms: a psychiatrist for depression, an Ob-Gyn for menstrual cramping, a GP for insomnia, a gastroenterologist for acid reflux, a neurologist for headaches, and an orthopedist for back pain. Each one prescribed a different drug, but she still felt lousy, and afraid all those drugs were going to harm her in the long haul, and I certainly had to agree!

Fortunately it was relatively easy for me to solve her problems, and within a few months she was drug free and feeling the way she wanted to feel.

You will meet Jane again later in this book, only by then you will understand how the human body works well enough to know exactly why she had all of her problems and why they proved so easy to fix. (Hint: we only had to fix one thing for all of Jane's seemingly unrelated symptoms to go away).

Body Wisdom

An alternative working title was *How The Human Body Works*, and you will see this referred to repeatedly, because helping you understand this important subject is one of the goals of *Body Wisdom*.

Body Wisdom is written with the knowledge that more and more, people want to be active participants in their own health maintenance and, when necessary, their own healing.

Body Wisdom is for those who don't think their problems are brought on by not enough drugs and that all they need are more drugs to make them healthy.

It's for those who believe (as I do) that health, happiness, and enthusiasm are our birthright, and that they are attainable!

Perhaps you feel these statements describe you, and if that is true, *Body Wisdom* was written for You!

In more than 40 years (as of this writing) of private medical practice, I have seen that the people who do the best and make the wisest decisions for their health are those who understand how their bodies work and therefore, are most likely to follow good sound medical advice. When necessary they ask their doctors the tough questions and even seek a second or third opinion before submitting to the potentially dangerous regimens of drugs or surgery.

Health

How do you feel about health?

Do you want to be well?

Really well?

I'll say at the outset that of the thousands of patients I treated over the years more than 95% didn't have good health as their primary goal! Surprising?

It was to me at first, and more than a little discouraging.

I don't mean to imply they didn't have a symptom or two they wanted me to fix, but really vibrant good health was not something they were willing to work to attain.

I've come to the conclusion that this is because people (and the medical system in which they were raised) are almost exclusively "symptom driven." Symptom driven means they only care how they feel Right Now! If they don't experience their symptoms Right Now, then they think they are healthy. And it doesn't matter how many drugs they take to achieve this feeling, or how much damage those drugs will do in the long haul, and make no mistake, all drugs do damage in the long haul! It seems we have lost sight of what it means to be truly well and healthy; maybe we have become so discouraged from watching our friends and loved ones suffering from long intractable diseases, we don't believe anymore that true health is even possible.

A Better Way

Body Wisdom grew out of a series of articles first appearing in the pages of Aikido Today, a magazine of Oriental philosophy and martial arts in which I had a medical column for six years, until it ceased publication in 2005.

For *Body Wisdom*, I have used many of the original article titles as chapter headers. Many have "clever" turns-of-phrase, employed to attract the attention of the passing reader. You may find some of the chapter headers a bit whimsical but I can assure you the information contained within is the real meat and potatoes stuff you can use to keep yourself healthier, and to better your understanding of how your body works and how to take better care of it.

Oriental Medicine

Traditional **Oriental Medicine (OM)** is one of the most knowledgeable and effective medical systems on earth and has been the medical system of choice for a quarter of the world's population for well over 3,000 years. It treats the full range of human medical problems, from the common cold to cancer. It is also the fastest growing alternative medical system in the United States, with millions of patient visits to OM practitioners every year. It's growing because it works! And it works because it understands how the human body functions!

When I first started medical practice full time in 1979, patients asked if I treated some particular condition or another (asthma, colitis, arthritis, etc.) and, being a new practitioner, I thought I would do well to learn more about these conditions than I had learned in Oriental medical school. My strategy, at first, was to look them up in *The Merck Manual*, the so-called "Bible" of Western medical thought and treatment. Diseases are couched in Western medical terminology and put into Western diagnostic categories, so I thought I could learn something more by seeing what Western medical science knew about the causes and treatment of these diseases. But as I looked up one condition after another I was given the same answer (or non-answer, as the case may be), to wit: "We don't know what causes this condition and we don't know how to cure it." I had never asked a question of my OM teachers without being given a concise answer to help solve my patients' problems. It was in Oriental Medicine where I would really understand where disease and pain come from, and how to truly solve medical problems.

A medical system can have a lot of facts and/or data, but if it doesn't have a theoretical framework, provided by an understanding of how the body truly works to plug those facts into, then you cannot use that system to solve the root cause of a patient's medical difficulties. In Oriental Medicine, covering up symptoms with drugs is not good enough.

So it is to the Oriental Medical system with its knowledge and understanding we shall turn to learn why we develop disease conditions and how to treat the root causes of those conditions so the body can return to the natural state of health to which we are all entitled.

Section One of *Body Wisdom* covers the basics of how your body works: the parts of your body that *run* your body, and for the most part, determine your current state of health. We will look at some symptoms that can arise if there are malfunctions in these basic components.

Section Two looks at some particular diseases or conditions common and important enough to warrant their own chapters, plus some other issues that can impact your health and happiness. This is a more fun and freewheeling section that includes chapters on everything from back pain to menopause; from bone strength to diet and nutrition; from arthritis to sinusitis; from the common cold to cancer; and many points in between.

Even though the chapters in **Section Two** deal with a broad range of subjects, they consistently refer back to the information given in **Section One**. In this sense these two sections (and all of *Body Wisdom*) are of a single fabric and as you read the chapters in **Section Two**, your understanding of the basic workings of your body, as presented in **Section One**, will grow!

Part of my purpose in writing *Body Wisdom* is to demystify the workings of the human body, to make it understandable to the average person in plain simple English. It is my firm belief that you don't have to memorize 2,000 Latin words in order to understand how the body works, as some might have you believe.

Good News

All of the medical conditions discussed in *Body Wisdom* are potentially fixable using safe natural methods. In fact, many of them are relatively easy to resolve with the exception of cancer, which all medical systems consider a challenge to control, to say the least. This is why **Chapter 15 – The Big C** is so heavily weighted toward things you can do right now to significantly reduce your chances of developing this potentially deadly disease in the first place.

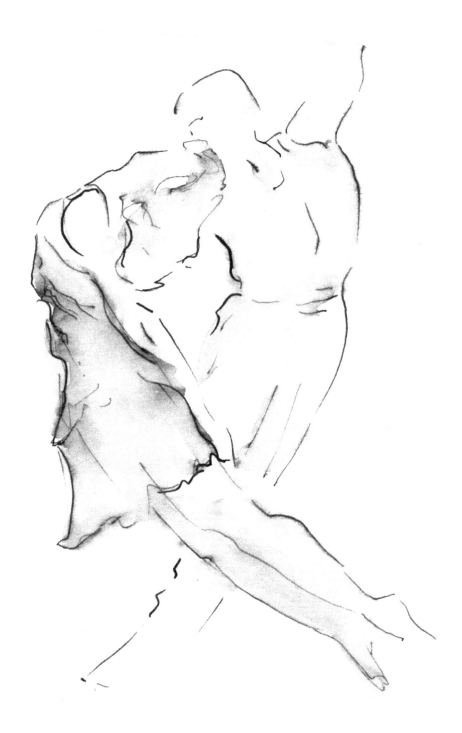

SECTION ONE

THE BASIS OF HEALTH

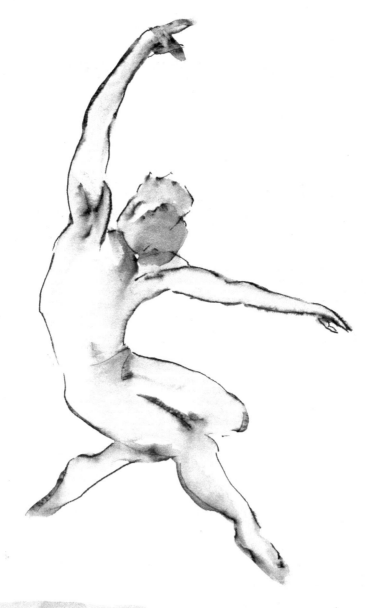

Chapter 1

The Ways of Energy: What Is it and What Does It Do for You?

The Case of "Tired Tom"

Tom came to the clinic complaining of low energy. Using diagnostic procedures particular to Oriental Medicine, his body was found to have plenty of energy. So, what can possibly account for this disparity?

Energy is like money. If you make $10,000 a week (wow!) but your bills are $11,000 a week, you would say you are "broke," meaning you don't have any discretionary money to spend on the things you want.

This is equivalent to what was happening to Tom. Even though his body possessed enough energy, too much of it was tied up in destructive and contradictory processes (he had many medical problems, and any one serious medical issue can cause you to lose energy). Because Tom didn't have enough discretionary energy to spend, he felt "exhausted all the time." It just required solving his medical problems to free up his abundant energy!

Energy

Webster's Dictionary defines energy as "the unifying concept of all physical sciences that associates with any system a capacity for work..."

Energy exists throughout the entire universe. It causes the earth to spin around on its axis and to orbit around the sun. It is responsible for the sun's light and heat and is the motive force behind the universe's expansion.

It is also essential to life. In fact it is so essential to life that we even have a name for a body that doesn't have any; we call it a "corpse."

Energy serves several major functions in your body: most notably it keeps you warm, holds things up, moves things around, is responsible for the functioning of organs and glands (plus the nervous and circulatory systems), performs trillions of metabolic functions every second, and also gives you the ability to do the things you want to do.

Your Source of Energy

Your basic energy comes from something called Cellular Metabolism. Cellular Metabolism is a complex process, but for the purpose of this work we can define it as the "burning of fuel" (provided by the digestive system) in the presence of oxygen (O_2) provided by the lungs.

Trillions of microscopic living organisms (cells) make up your physical body, doing all the things that living organisms do, like being born, taking in nutrients, eliminating waste products, reproducing, and dying. In the process they are generating minute amounts of energy (and heat). It is the sum total of these energy/heat units added together that keeps your body 98.6° Fahrenheit regardless of the ambient temperature in which you happen to find yourself. In fact, one of the ways to tell if a body has been vacated by energy (has died!) is that it becomes cold (assumes room temperature—usually about 70° Fahrenheit).

The amount of metabolically generated energy, over and above that which is needed to heat your body, is the energy available to your system to perform its myriad functions; any energy left over after these needs are met is the amount you have to spend doing what you want to do. I call this usable energy "discretionary energy."

Besides keeping you warm your basic energy also holds things up. Not only does it help you stand upright but it also helps the structures of your body stay in place. This function, like any other, can fail; in fact there is even a special medical name for problems that develop when this malfunctions. If things in your body fall or sag out of place they are said to "prolapse." To prolapse, according to the dictionary, means, "the slipping out of an organ of the body from its normal position, such as, a prolapse of the uterus."

Energy also moves things around in your body. It is responsible for the circulation of blood and electricity, the movement of substances through the gastrointestinal tract (esophagus, stomach, intestines, rectum, etc.), the expansion and contraction of the lungs, and much more.

In fact, all of the actions of all of the cells, as well as all the organs and glands (plus the nervous and circulatory systems) are reliant on the presence and actions of energy. The Chinese word for energy is "chi." You will see this word used in *Body Wisdom* and elsewhere.

In Oriental Medicine we concentrate on functional disorders, and proper body functioning relies on energy, so first we examine the status and amount of energy in each patient's body.

Energy Pathologies

We assess three main conditions of energy in our patients: the amount of energy, the circulation of energy, and the distribution of energy. Each of these can malfunction and, in so doing, create its own special set of difficulties.

Amount of Energy. If something doesn't have enough energy, we say it is "energy deficient"—it is weak or under functioning. As an example, a weak digestive system means you don't digest your food well and, therefore, don't get the energy and raw materials from your food that you should, which is a common occurrence, especially as people get older!

If we find a weakness (diminished function) in any system in a patient's body we use the methods and substances of Oriental Medicine to add energy to that component, thereby returning it to its correct functional strength. In some instances however, people may not have enough energy in general. In that case, we must strengthen the body's ability to produce more energy or, as with "Tired Tom," correct any underlying medical problems that may deny access to their discretionary energy. We discuss low energy issues over and over again throughout *Body Wisdom* so you will be certain to understand it thoroughly before we are finished.

The Circulation of Energy

Energy, like blood, circulates throughout your whole body. Energy (as measurable electricity) circulates in the nervous system and circulates in the meridian system: this is the system utilized by acupuncture to solve problems (more on this later). Every cell in your body, and every structure composed of cells, must have energy brought to it. Anything restricting this circulation creates problems of function in that particular component.

Energy circulation problems can also create pain. One of the most commonly seen examples is sciatic nerve pain down the back of the leg. The sciatic nerve is the largest nerve in your body—it is about as big around as your thumb. It begins in the lower back, where a series of individual smaller nerves, which exit from between the vertebrae, combine to form one large nerve going down the back of the leg. If anything impinges on this nerve strongly enough it will retard its energy circulation and cause pain to radiate down the leg. Chances are you have experienced this or know someone who has. It is a common problem!

The Distribution of Energy

The tendency of energy is to rise, like the air nearer the ceiling is warmer than the air nearer the floor. If you studied physics you learned that heat is just a measure of molecular activity and, as we saw earlier, activity levels are a function of energy levels. So, we can say that the air by the ceiling is warmer (has more molecular activity) than the air by the floor because it has more energy. Energy's proclivity to rise is just part of the way it naturally behaves.

Since your body is an energy containing system, and since the laws of physics apply, this tendency toward the unequal distribution of energy (more at the top than the bottom) must exist in your body just like in your rooms at home. And it does! This will usually manifest as some kind of excess activity or "commotion" in the upper body; headaches, ringing in the ears, hay fever symptoms, or upper body/neck tension or stiffness.

You can use fans and other air redistributing devices in your rooms at home, and your body has its own set of mechanisms to counter this tendency, but it is still possible for your body to develop symptoms as a result of the unequal distribution of energy. Thankfully, there are things that can be done to correct this and other energy pathologies.

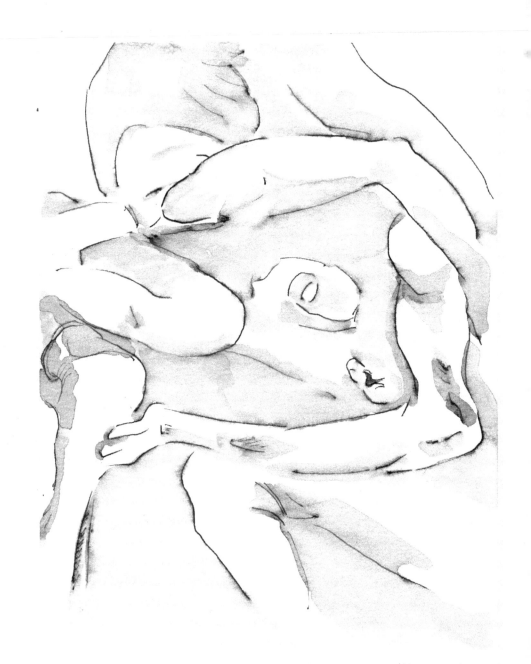

Chapter 2

Blood: The Precious Liquid

Two principle things circulate in the body: *blood and energy*. Unlike energy (considered "mysterious" in Western Medicine) blood is known to everyone. You have seen it many times, and can see it again any time you like simply by poking a hole somewhere in your body. Blood, because it can be seen (and analyzed by machines), is accorded more "reality" status than energy, which cannot be seen but must be inferred or deduced by its behavior. Even though we all know of the existence of blood, we might justifiably ask, "What is blood and just what does it do for us?"

The Functions of Blood

Blood performs four primary functions in your body. I have assigned each function a number but not in order of importance. All are equally important.

1. Blood Distributes and Delivers necessary substances throughout your body. Your body is a colony of trillions of living cells, all of which must be provided with key components in order to stay alive and function properly. Blood delivers oxygen and the fuel necessary for cellular metabolism, plus myriad other substances essential to proper functioning and repair on the cellular level.

2. Blood Gathers and Collects waste products from around your body and delivers them to various sites where they can be either chemically neutralized (i.e., by the liver), or removed from your body (i.e., by your kidneys, skin, and lungs).

3. Blood Helps Cool your body and maintain a constant and correct temperature. Think of the cooling system in your car and you have a picture of what the blood does with this aspect of its function. Like many of the "inventions" of humankind, cooling systems in our cars are just copies of things that already exist in nature.

4. Blood Moistens cells and tissues to help maintain their proper moisture content, thereby keeping their necessary suppleness and flexibility. Think of the difference between a fresh juicy steak bought at the market and a piece of beef jerky. The steak is moist and supple because it still has the approximate moisture content it did while the animal lived, but the moisture has been removed from the jerky. The steak bends and stretches while the jerky cracks and breaks.

How Blood Goes Wrong

Blood pathologies fall under three main categories: problems of quality, quantity, and circulation. Let's look at these separately.

Problems of Quality would include anemia, leukemia and other structural pathologies. Most of these are problems of the cells (some of the solid materials) floating in the fluid (serum) of the blood. Quality problems are often detectable by the methods and machines of Western Medicine because they are problems of matter and can usually be seen by a microscope.

Understanding why one or another of these problems may have developed in a patient in the first place, and how to treat it without harmful drugs, is another thing entirely. It is worth pointing out that most structural problems, like these blood quality issues, begin as a result of functional disorders and need to be solved ultimately at the functional level in order to achieve real long-term solutions.

Problems of Quantity means the right amount of blood in your body in general, or at a particular site at a particular time, to ensure that the blood's functions (and certain organ and gland functions) are performed properly. These problems are so common and potentially serious that all of **Chapter 13-The Blood Speech** is devoted to them.

Problems of Circulation can be from annoying to deadly. Blood needs to have a free and unimpeded flow to every cell and system in your body or difficulties can ensue. Some of the more common circulation problems include: angina pectoris, myocardial infarction, and phlebitis.

Angina Pectoris is pain in the chest brought on by a restriction in the flow of blood in one or more of the blood vessels of the heart. The body of the heart is made up of muscle tissue and like all muscle tissue it is supplied with blood by a system of arteries; and just as with retarded energy flow in the nerves or meridians, a restriction of blood flow can cause pain. Note that not all chest pains are caused by this problem; but if someone has chest pain severe or recurrent enough, they should be checked out for this condition. If it is severe enough an emergency room visit might even be necessary.

Phlebitis is a restriction of the blood flow elsewhere in the body, which can also be painful. This often occurs in peripheral appendages: arms and, especially, the legs.

Myocardial Infarction is a potentially lethal type of heart event. It is caused by blockage(s) in the blood vessels of the heart; in this case the blockages are complete enough so a part of the heart muscle is denied its blood supply and therefore suffers structural death. This condition can be mildly debilitating to deadly. They say that for one third of heart attack victims the first sign of a problem is death.

Notice that, as with energy circulation, blood circulation problems can be painful.

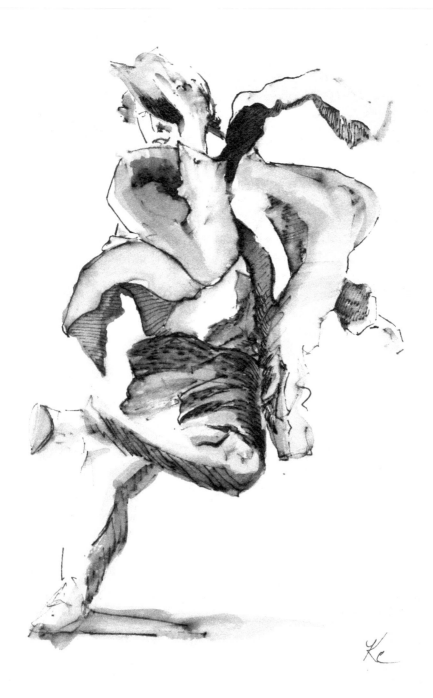

Chapter 3

Systems: Where Would You Be Without Them?

Betty's Knee Pain

"**B**etty" came in complaining of knee pain so severe, she walked with a pronounced limp. As we worked on Betty her knee pain began to improve so much, she was walking almost normally. Then something unexpected happened. Betty started to complain of a pain in her hip which she didn't remember ever having before. Truthfully, we were not surprised and I'll tell you why.

Wandering Pain:

There are three principle reasons why pain can shift from one place in the body to another.

1. Some arthritis or fibromyalgia-like pains do naturally *wander* around the body. First you feel them one place and the next day you may feel *the same pain* in a totally different location. This didn't explain Betty's circumstance, because this type of *wandering pain* moves around before the patient begins treatment, but Betty's pain had been concentrated in her knee.

2. When a natural practitioner begins to work on a painful area (knee, hip, back, etc.) we often find only a small number of *sore, inflamed spots* creating the bulk of the trouble. As these *worst spots* begin to heal, the patient may feel the next worst spots, maybe in a slightly different location in the affected area, so the patient feels that the pain has moved. These secondary painful places were there all along but weren't being noticed because the original worst painful spots overshadowed them. This doesn't explain Betty either. If it were this circumstance, the pain would have just shifted to another aspect of her knee.

3. Here's what happened in Betty's case. The body is a system, and in a system every part is somehow connected to every other part. Because

Betty walked incorrectly for years all of her other muscles and joints, including her hip, adopted somewhat unnatural postures to compensate. Now that she was starting to walk more correctly again, her hip muscles were adjusting themselves to the new, more correct reality and were temporarily sore in the process. In fact, we never had to work on her new hip pain because it went away on its own as her muscles and joints adapted to her newly improved knee and more normal gait.

Systems

Webster's dictionary defines a system as "an orderly, interconnected, complex arrangement of parts." For our purposes, let's say that a system means an assemblage of parts working together to perform a common set of functions, and that share a common purpose, outcome, and destiny.

There are many systems you interact with every day. Some examples are your car, TV, computer, dishwasher, your body, etc. Let's discuss some characteristics of systems using your car as an example.

Your car is a collection of parts that must all work properly, and all must work together (two separate but related requirements of systems). If these parts all work properly and all work together then you get from your car what you want: you slide in, turn on the key and drive where you want to go. Another characteristic of systems is that some parts are more important than others; you can drive your car without a back seat or rearview mirror, but not without an engine or transmission. A third characteristic of a system is that a change in any part will impact, to some degree, every other part and cause them to change in order to adjust and form a new equilibrium. Pluck Mars out of the solar system and you can bet there will be consequences here on Earth!

The human body is a system as well, and the important parts (that run your body) are the organs and glands. As I say in my classes: "Organs and glands run your body, including your nervous and circulatory systems. Any medical problem or disease you develop spontaneously (not from an accident or injury) is the result of the breakdown of function of one or more of your organs or glands."

This is the key statement to understand as you begin to take responsibility for your own health.

Organs or glands can malfunction for myriad reasons – many of which are discussed in depth elsewhere in *Body Wisdom*. Either way, their functional status will go a long way toward determining your health and longevity.

Vital Organs

In Oriental Medicine we concentrate our efforts on ensuring the proper functioning of the five most important organ and gland groups: the heart and circulatory system, the lungs and respiratory system, the stomach and digestive system, the kidney and adrenal gland complex, and the liver and gall bladder pair. These are the "vital organs," necessary to life—you can't live without them!

Because these particular organ and gland systems (for convenience sake let's just call them "organs") are so vital, it turns out that many of the symptoms or disease conditions that can develop are a result of a breakdown in the functioning of one of these.

Structure vs. Function

This is a good place for two very important concepts relating powerfully to health and your body, namely: structure and function.

Structure means what something is made of, how it is configured, and its location. In the study of medicine this is called "anatomy."

Function means how something works or what it does. In medicine this is "physiology."

Most medical problems are either structural or functional. There are many more disease conditions brought on by functional failures than structural ones. Let's discuss the difference between the two as it applies to the body, using the heart as an example.

Heart Events

There is a type of traumatic heart event called a "myocardial infarction." In this condition there is a blockage in one or more of the arteries of the heart; this prevents the blood from reaching one or more sections of the heart, and as a result the part of the heart usually served by that blood supply dies. This is a structural problem: the structure of the artery is blocked, and the cells of the heart beyond that point suffer structural death.

Compare this to a heart that is just beating irregularly. There is no structural damage, it just isn't working right. This is a functional problem.

Don't get me wrong, functional problems of the heart (and other organs) can be medically serious as well, but they are of a different quality than structural problems.

Another important difference between structural and functional problems is that you can "see" structural problems. This is why Western Medicine with its concentration on structure has so many ways (using machines) to "look" at things. There are X-rays, MRIs, Microscopes, CT scans, GI scopes, angiograms, ultrasound, and, if all else fails, exploratory surgery, to name a few. Most problems that develop as a result of an injury or accident, like a broken bone, are structural issues as well.

Function

Functional problems, by far the most common, include most degenerative diseases such as diabetes, fibromyalgia, asthma, hypertension, Parkinson's disease, colitis, most headaches, acid reflux, insomnia, PMS, clinical depression, anxiety, etc. Functional problems cannot be seen but instead must be deduced or intuited from the various signs and symptoms the body presents. It is here where Oriental Medicine, with its exceptional depth of understanding of how the body works, really shines.

Functional problems, unlike many structural problems, tend to develop over much longer periods of time, and are often the result of years of gradual deterioration. It is worth noting that most structural problems (that do not result from an accident or injury) are a result of functional problems allowed to linger untreated, or that have had their symptoms suppressed by medications while the real cause remained unchanged or, most likely, gotten worse.

Oriental Medicine

Generally speaking, Western Medicine concentrates on structural problems and Oriental Medicine concentrates on functional problems. In Oriental Medicine we specialize in the diagnosis and treatment of functional diseases and have spent thousands of years studying the way to utilize and direct the energy circulating in the Autonomic Nervous System to adjust the functional status of your organs and glands (see **Chapter 28 – Ying and Yang**). After all, it takes energy to make structure function. Let's look at this phenomenon.

If you had a fan (structure) in your room and you wanted it to spin around (function) to cool you off, you would have to get energy to it (in the form of electricity). You must plug it in and turn it on to get what you want from that fan.

There is no structure, inside or outside of the body, that functions without energy. Energy is a necessary component of function: no energy = no function!

Now to the five organ systems most vital to your health and well-being.

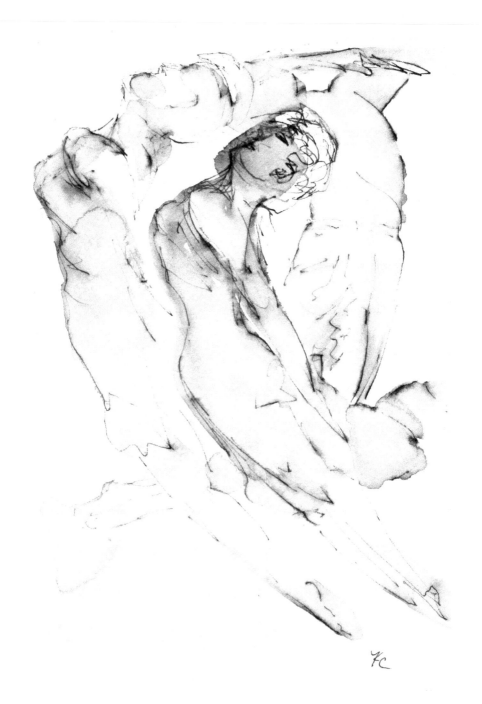

Chapter 4

The Heart and Circulatory System

Palpitating Patty

Patty's heart would sometimes beat in unusual ways and when it did she felt anxious and uneasy. There are three principle ways to experience the heart beating incorrectly.

Too Fast: Here, the heart may just suddenly shift into a very rapid beat for no apparent reason. A normal heart rate is 72 beats per minute (BPM), even though we pretty much accept 60-80 BPM as the normal range. Strenuous exercise will naturally cause the heart to beat well above the normal range, but if it spontaneously jumps to well above 100 BPM, this clearly represents a problem.

Irregular Beats: The heart can also have some beats crowded too closely together while others are so far apart as to represent some beats missing altogether. This is not good either.

Too Strong: the heart will suddenly start beating so strongly that someone might say, "My heart was beating so hard I was afraid it would burst out of my chest."

What troubled Patty was the sudden irregularity of the beats, but once we straightened that out with acupuncture and the Chinese herbal formula Tien Wang Bu Hsin Wan, she was OK both physically and emotionally.

Heart Function

Your heart's principle function is the circulation of blood throughout your body, facilitated by the circulatory system (blood vessels). Every living cell in your body needs its own supply of blood to work properly and, indeed, survive.

There are two branches of the circulatory system: the arterial (arteries) system which carries the newly oxygenated blood away from your heart to the rest of your body, and the venous (veins) system which returns the blood to your heart which then sends it to the lungs to have the carbon dioxide removed and be re-oxygenated. Arteries have a palpable pulse and measurable blood pressure, veins do not.

Hearts, like all organs or glands, can develop either structural or functional problems. And, as always, the number and variety of symptoms is greater with functional problems than with structural ones.

Functional problems can be harder to trace to their origins, for two reasons: one, because they cannot be "seen" in the same way structural problems can (but must rather be deduced or intuited); and two, issues don't always take place at the site of the organ or gland causing them.

Symptoms of functional problems of the heart can vary from the more obvious issue of irregular heartbeats (palpitations, fibrillation, tachycardia, etc.), to less obvious issues like insomnia, anxiety (and panic attacks), concentration and memory problems, and other issues of emotional health or mental ability/stability. This latter set of symptoms are not (yet) known in Western Medicine to be connected to heart malfunctions, but they are!

A common cause of heart functional disorders is an inadequate supply of blood in the chambers of the heart. This was the case with Patty. This is such a widespread problem that all of **Chapter 13 - The Blood Speech** is devoted to it.

Because the heart is so important to us (it can be a matter of life or death) it pays to be proactive when it comes to its health. "An ounce of prevention is worth a pound of cure." Oriental Medicine has a lot to offer here. Both acupuncture and Oriental herbal formulas work to ensure that the heart and circulatory system continue to function correctly, supporting us (hopefully) into a ripe old age.

STRESS: ITS MEANING AND TREATMENT

For the purposes of discussing the influence of stress on a symptom or disease process, let's define stress as "...a physical, mental, or emotional factor causing bodily or mental tension. Stress can be external (from the environment, or social or psychological situations) or internal (from illness or a medical procedure)."

Patients often say their symptoms are "caused by stress." What I point out is that stress is not so much a cause as a catalyst. Stress puts a load on the system such that it breaks down at its weakest point. For example: under stress, a person with asthma may have difficulty breathing, while someone suffering from colitis could experience an increase in diarrhea and cramping, and a third person who tends to get migraine headaches might see an increase in the frequency and severity of their headaches when stressed. We might legitimately ask if stress causes breathing difficulties, diarrhea, or perhaps headaches. Of course, it doesn't cause any of these but it does put a load on your system, and then you find out where your body doesn't work well enough.

It's like if we wanted to tow one car with another and we hooked up a chain between the two. As soon as we put tension on that chain, it is under stress, and if it has a weak link anywhere, it will break (have symptoms), but if it is strong throughout then it can successfully tow your car.

While we certainly say stress is not particularly good for your health, we still have the possibility of solving your health problems even if we can't remove the stress from your life. This brings up another truth: stress is not just what happens in our lives but more a function of how we or our bodies react or respond to those circumstances.

By using the tecÚiques of Oriental Medicine to calm down and relax our patients, we can actually reduce the consequences of stressful circumstances to their peace of mind, and in that way reduce the stress in their lives.

Some people benefit from counseling (or other forms of talk therapy), but it is also true that by treating the heart (the seat of all emotions), and the liver (which influences and is influenced by anger and frustration) with a combination of acupuncture and herbal formulas, we can return a patient to a more calm and peaceful state of mind.

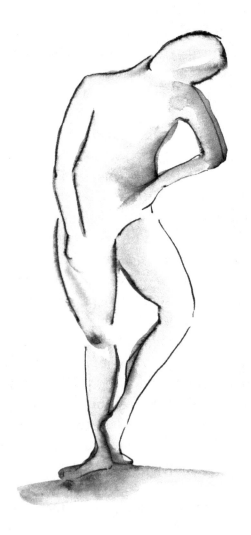

Chapter 5

The Digestive System: You Aren't What You Don't Eat (or Digest!)

A Case of "IBS"

A female patient aged 45 came in diagnosed with **"Irritable Bowel Syndrome" (IBS)**. Her problem was diarrhea, often accompanied by severe abdominal cramps. Each morning she had multiple, urgent, loose stools, and sometimes she couldn't leave the house until the afternoon, definitely disrupting her life as well as being darned uncomfortable.

To me, "Irritable Bowel Syndrome" is a consistent misdiagnosis in Western Medicine, or at least a mislabeling. By referring to the bowel (colon, large intestine) it appears that the colon is the source of the problem, that the colon is at fault—this is almost always not true!

Raw materials enter our mouths as food and are acted upon in various ways by the organs and glands of digestion until the unwanted components ultimately exit our bodies as fecal material. The colon (and rectum) are the last places that act upon this material, but they are by no means the only (or even the primary) ones that determine the frequency and consistency of bowel movements. In the case of "IBS" the colon is more often the victim of improper processing higher up in the gastrointestinal (GI) tract, rather than the perpetrator.

The colon is not designed to process too many bowel movements in a given day, so if there are malfunctions in some other digestive components that cause frequent, caustic and inflammatory movements, the colon will get irritated—to put things in a more proper light, **IBS** should be called *Irritated* (not irritable) Bowel Syndrome.

In Oriental Medicine we know we must often correct the functions of some combination of the other digestive organs so the frequency and consistency of bowel movements will be normalized; in this way the irritation to the bowel will be naturally corrected. In this particular case, it proved to be the liver/gall bladder functional group at fault, and once that was brought into line using acupuncture, the "IBS" became a thing of the past.

Nutrition

The purpose of digestion is to be able to extract nutrients from our food and drink. Here's how it works.

A tube runs through the body called the gastrointestinal **(GI) Tract.** It starts at the mouth and ends at the anus, and it is in this tube that the principle activities of digestion take place. Digestion happens in this tube through the agency of the organs and glands that make up the tube, aided by some other components lying just outside of it.

Digestion starts in the mouth and is continued in the esophagus, stomach, duodenum, small intestine, and large intestine (colon). Some of the organs lying outside the GI tract that contribute to this process are the pancreas, liver and gall bladder. These latter three organs are attached to the GI tract by small tubes delivering substances necessary to the digestive process.

Digestion

Digestion is the process by which large things (foods) are broken up into smaller and smaller bits until small enough to enter your bloodstream through the walls of the small intestine.

Digestion isn't just about what you swallow. You could swallow a small pebble today and it would just end up in the toilet tomorrow. Digestion is about the nutrients made available to your bloodstream so they can be distributed to the rest of your body through the bloodstream's delivery function.

In this way our bodies are provided with the thousands of chemical compounds available in foods—especially the more complex foods like fruits and vegetables. These compounds are the building materials needed for growth and the repair and replacement of the estimated 50 trillion cells that make up our bodies. It is also through digestion that we get the fuel (glucose) needed for cellular metabolism; so in this way it is also intimately tied to our basic energy. To put it another way: problems of digestion can reduce our available energy.

DR. GERALD SENOGLES

The Process

Digestion is accomplished by a series of mechanical and chemical processes provided by organs and glands. The first step in the breaking down of foods is chewing, which accomplishes two things: it physically crushes the food and simultaneously mixes it with saliva to moisten it and begin the chemical breakdown. This slurry of food and saliva goes down the esophagus to the stomach where it is further acted upon mechanically (churning), and chemically by gastric juices like hydrochloric acid and enzymes. This, by now, very liquid medium moves on to the small intestine where it is further acted upon by intestinal and pancreatic enzymes and liver bile secreted by the gall bladder. It is in the small intestine that the process is completed; most nutrients now enter the bloodstream through the walls of the small intestine, and to some degree the large intestine as well.

Digestive Disorders

These can be far ranging; a partial list includes heartburn, colitis, IBS, GERD, excess phlegm (**Chapter 18 - Phlegm Fatale**), acid reflux, diarrhea, mucus colitis, low energy, anemia, blood deficiency (**Chapter 13 - The Blood Speech**), belching, indigestion, vomiting, motion sickness, morning sickness, constipation and more. To better understand these disorders it is worth discussing two specific characteristics of the GI tract: motility and directionality.

Motility simply put means movement. We put things in at the top and they are supposed to move toward the bottom. Like every function, motility can perform less than optimally, contributing to such symptoms as constipation, diarrhea (things can move too quickly as well as too slowly), or the feeling that food just sits in the stomach too long after eating—perhaps for many hours.

Directionality means there is only one correct direction of movement, and that is from the top down. Symptoms can include vomiting, heartburn (stomach acid backing up into the esophagus), **GERD**, acid reflux, and even belching.

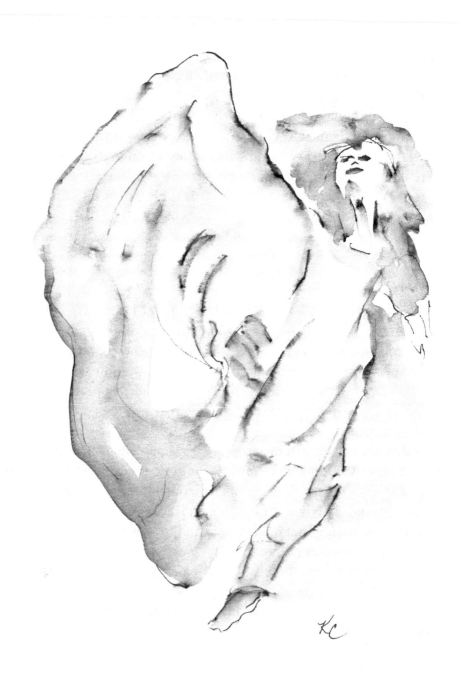

Chapter 6
The Lungs and Respiratory System

The principle function of your lungs is, of course, breathing, or to be a little more tecÚical, providing Oxygen (O_2) to your bloodstream. In fact, this function is so important that your heart (which pumps the blood) and your lungs (which oxygenate the blood) share their own private circulatory loop. Your lungs also remove waste products (like carbon dioxide) from the bloodstream and eliminate them from the body through the breath.

Energy

Oxygen is very important to your overall energy picture. In order for the cells of your body to metabolize fuel (glucose provided by what you ingest—your food and drink) they must have an ample supply of oxygen. As was pointed out in **Chapter 1 - The Way of Energy**, it is the sum total of energy generated by each cell during metabolism that adds up to the basic energy your body has and makes available for your use. So, even though it is true that any problem (a cold, diarrhea, headache, back or joint pain, etc.) anywhere in the body can be serious enough to lower your energy, it is also true that anyone who has a serious lung problem (asthma, emphysema, COPD, etc.) is pretty much guaranteed to have an energy problem.

Immune Function: Defensive Energy

Another important function of the lungs is to administer *defensive energy* (in Chinese "wei chi"). One way to think of *defensive energy* is as a component of your immune system: the ability of your body to ward off or fight disease. How many people reading *Body Wisdom* are old enough to remember when we didn't have an immune system? I have been a serious student of medicine and how the body works, since the early 1970s and I can tell you that it wasn't until later in the 70s, with the advent of AIDS, that medical professionals, let alone lay people, began to speak of the immune system at all. So, you had an immune system before that, but I am willing to bet you never heard anything about it until then.

The concept of the immune system is merely the recognition that your body has the ability to protect itself from disease, or we could say, from harmful microorganisms like bacteria, funguses, and viruses. You don't get sick every time you come in contact with "germs" or you wouldn't last very long, as they are everywhere. Nor could you visit your friends if they landed in the hospital, which has the highest concentration of germs in town. Did you know that 1.7 million people pick up infections in American hospitals every year, and that a minimum of 99,000 of them die as a result? And remember, these are conditions they didn't have when they went into the hospital! According to the December 2014 issue of the *International Journal of Nursing Sciences*, "*Hospital acquired infections are a serious global health issue and pose risks to staff, patients and the broader community (1).(2). In fact, hospital acquired infections are the fourth most frequent cause of death in the United States behind heart disease, cancer and stroke.*" [emphasis added]

Whether you get sick or not has less to do with the germs you come in contact with, and more to do with how your body's defense mechanisms are working. After all, even people with **AIDS (Acquired Immune Deficiency Syndrome)** don't die of **AIDS**, they die from the opportunistic diseases that take advantage of their compromised immune systems. Thankfully, new substances and procedures have been developed that allow many **HIV Positive** people to live long and normal lives.

In Oriental Medicine we know that if someone is especially prone to colds, flus or respiratory infections, it represents a weakness in the lung's performance of its immune function. I have seen numerous patients over the years who sought medical help because they were getting four or five 3–4 week long colds a year. If you do the math you will see that some of these people were suffering with a cold thirty percent of the time! The solution for this is to strengthen lung function so it can assist their bodies in fighting off these infectious conditions. For more on the lungs see the story about "Asthmatic Andy" in **Chapter 10 – It's All One.**

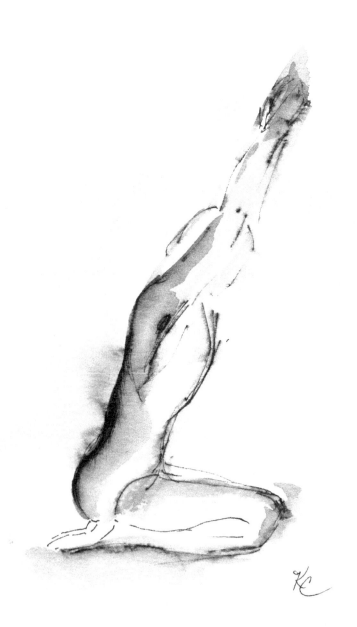

Chapter 7

The Kidneys: Old Age and Death

"Old Ed"

An elderly gentleman came into the office complaining of back pain which was better in the morning after a good night's rest but got worse as the day went on, especially if he had been particularly active that day. As I asked him a series of questions I was surprised to find out that "Old Ed" was only 61 years old. He looked and moved like he was 80!

Ed also had a virtually nonexistent sex drive and was diagnosed with "prostate" problems, as he had to get up 4–5 times a night to urinate which was negatively impacting his sleep, and consequently his energy level the next day.

Everything about Ed told me his problems were caused by his kidneys being prematurely weak. By strengthening his kidneys we not only solved his back problem but his night urination as well. Needless to say he had more energy now that he was sleeping through the night and his pain was gone; in many ways he felt better and, in a way, younger.

Let's look at Ed's prostate diagnosis for a moment. Yes, his prostate was enlarged, and yes, he had to go to the bathroom frequently at night, but it can be a mistake to automatically assume that if two things change at the same time one must be causing the other. In this case a third thing had changed (his kidney function had weakened), and this third factor was what caused his enlarged prostate, his need to urinate so frequently at night, and his back pain.

The Kidney/Adrenal Complex

When we say kidneys in Oriental Medicine we are actually referring to the kidney/adrenal gland complex; a structural and functional grouping residing in the lower back. For simplicity sake, we just call this functional pair "kidneys."

Kidney Functions

There are a number of kidney functions very important to your health. Here's a list of some of the things your kidneys do for you. They are not numbered by order of importance (they're all important!) but rather because I will refer to these numbers later in this chapter.

The Kidneys:

1. **Set the Fluid Balance in the Body** by removing excess fluid from the bloodstream and sending it down to the urinary bladder, where it is stored to be periodically released from the body at (hopefully) our discretion. They also provide the energy for the urinary bladder and control its functioning.

2. **Remove Waste Materials from the Bloodstream**, including the normal substances generated as a byproduct of metabolism, and toxins introduced into the body from our increasingly toxic environment.

3. **Provide the Energy for and Control the Lower Back.** As a result of a breakdown in this function, many of the low back problems/pains people experience are really a result of kidney functional disorders. Since these are a result of functional issues, rather than structural ones, they are not detectable by Western medical tests. An OM practitioner should be able to deduce them, however, as well as correct the symptom of low back pain. In the typical Oriental medical practice back pain is relieved 80–90% of the time.

4. **Determine and Control the Basic Cycles of Life and Stages of Development** including birth, childhood development, puberty, sexual development, adulthood, **old age, and death.**

5. **Act as a Storehouse for the Basic Energy of the Body** in much the same way that a battery does for your car.

6. **Store Our "Essence"** ("jing" in Chinese). As this implies, this is very foundational to our health and well-being.

7. **Store the Basic Yin and Yang of the Body.** Please consult **Chapter 28 - Yin & Yang** for a simple and understandable explanation of this concept and how it relates to your health.

For Students of Oriental Philosophy or Martial Arts I also point out that our "Hara" lines up with the kidney chakra and some very important kidney energy acupuncture points on the lower abdomen.

DR. GERALD SENOGLES

Kidney Weakness

The basic pathology of the kidneys is that they weaken over time. This is just part of their nature and is inevitable; virtually all kidney symptoms come as a result of this weakening. The kidneys are like a storage battery of energy that resides in our lower back. When you buy that 36 month Diehard battery at Sears you can be sure it won't last more than 36 months. It only has so much energy built into it and therefore the seeds of its own demise are built right into it as well. The same is true for your body in the sense of how much energy the kidneys are storing, which is a function of how much they were given in the first place and how judiciously you have used it.

Kidney Symptoms

Here is a partial list of problems that can be caused by weakening kidneys. The numbers in parentheses refer back to the numbers we assigned on the opposite page, and show which aspect of the kidneys is not performing adequately and therefore creating each symptom.

Edema/Fluid Retention (1) Fluid retention will usually manifest as swelling. This can be at particular sites, like the ankles or hands, or more generalized throughout the body. As an example of kidney generated fluid retention we have a condition referred to in Western Medicine as "congestive heart failure," a symptom of which is edema (fluid buildup) around the heart. Even though it may not usually be recognized as such in the West, this is definitely tied to kidney weakness; which is why one of the Western treatments is to give diuretics ("water pills") that force the kidneys to put out more fluid through increased urination, thereby relieving pressure on the heart and enabling it to function more correctly.

Also, the weight gain that tends to come with age is often just a generalized fluid retention that occurs as a result of our kidneys weakening.

Urinary Dysfunction (1) This is a large category of symptoms including (but not limited to) frequent urination, night urination, inability to completely empty the bladder, incontinence or leaking urine, infrequent urination, urinary urgency (not enough notice of the need to void which can sometimes lead to "accidents"), as well as too frequent bladder/urinary tract/kidney infections. An excellent Chinese Herb formula, Jin Suo Gu Jing Wan, helps with incontinence or control/urgency issues.

Incidentally, the functional and structural status of the prostate gland in men is under the control of the kidneys.

Arthritis (2)(5) If the kidneys fail to remove enough waste material from the bloodstream, these caustic and inflammatory materials will build up and be constantly re-circulated throughout the body. If these materials build up to dangerous levels in the blood stream (an intolerable condition that can kill you if allowed to go too far) then the body, in an act of self-protection, will remove them. These inflammatory materials from the bloodstream can be deposited in various sites around the body; especially the joints. This can and will often lead to swelling, redness, and pain. In other words, "Arthritis!"

It is worth noting that these same symptoms can occur with an injury, like a sprained ankle or knee, in which case they are not related to the kidneys at all.

American actress and singer Selena Gomez is quoted in USA today (Oct. 31, 2017) as saying "...as soon as I got my kidney transplant my arthritis went away, (and) my lupus...(my) blood pressure is better, my energy, my life has been better."

Low Back Pain (3)(5)(7) This could include some involvement of the hip, or even pain radiating down the leg—especially the back of the leg. Kidney weakness is a common cause of this problem, especially when the pain gets worse with increased activity, or as the day goes on (in the afternoon or evening). It isn't necessary that someone has any other kidney symptoms; sometimes the only symptom of kidney involvement is the back or leg pain. You may also see these same symptoms brought on by liver malfunction; most symptoms have more than one possible cause. This is where the skill and expertise of a medical professional is necessary to determine exactly which organ or gland is responsible for a given symptom in a particular patient at a particular time. This is necessary in order to solve it at the causal (organ or gland) level.

Impotence, Frigidity, and Infertility (5)(6)(7) The energy of the kidneys provides the motive force for human sexuality and to a large degree, sexual desire. Like virtually all symptoms, any of the four symptom groups listed above can have other possible causes as well, so if you have symptoms, get checked out by a competent medical professional. (I am reminded of a patient with such horrifically painful and pathological periods that a side effect of normalizing her periods was that she almost immediately got pregnant. She never worried about birth control before as her "internal workings" hadn't functioned well enough to support a pregnancy.

Development/Stages of Life Problems (4) In young children these include problems with bone or tooth development, proper growth rates, or any mental or physical characteristic not developing properly.

In teenagers it could be a problem with the development of secondary sexual characteristics. In adults it includes premature aging.

There are such wide ranging symptoms that they all cannot be listed here! Developmental problems can be difficult to decipher and likely necessitate consulting with an Oriental medical practitioner, as well as other health professionals.

Old Age and Death

Many of the indications and problems we think of as signs of old age are really signs of kidney weakness and deterioration, which is why they can happen to people at any age. Here's a list, again in no particular order of importance.

Hearing Loss: The kidneys provide the energy for, and control of, your sense of hearing. As kidneys diminish so can the sense of hearing. That is why you see so many hearing aids at the retirement home or convalescent hospital.

Head Hair Turning Gray: This is a reflection of the status of your kidneys and indicates they are weakening. Incidentally, the loss of head hair is not a reflection on the strength of the kidneys, nor is the status of body and facial hair a reflection of the kidneys, but rather the lungs.

Bone and Tooth Deterioration: The health, strength, and density of your skeletal system is a reflection of kidney health. Problems here include osteoporosis, tooth loss, and bones that fracture too easily. You may have noticed some of your older friends and relatives are not as tall as they used to be. This is usually a result of bone loss and even compression fractures of the spinal vertebrae, where the vertebrae fracture vertically by essentially collapsing (kind of like crushing a soda can), thereby making the person shorter. Bone density problems can be so serious, even deadly, that all of **Chapter 19 - Don't Need a Break** is devoted to ways you can improve the density and strength of your bones.

Urinary and/or Bowel Incontinence: The energy for the control of these two lower orifices is provided by the kidneys and as they weaken, control can start to be lost. This is not the issue of diarrhea so urgent one does not get enough advance warning and therefore has an "accident" on their way to the bathroom. Rather, it is the lack of control that requires someone to wear pads or adult diapers to maintain minimal cleanliness. Adult diapers are delivered by the truckload to the nursing homes.

Aging: As an experienced medical practitioner I separate someone's chronological age from their physiological age: I determine the status of the principle working parts of a patient's body and how much functional life is left in them. I see people at 70 years of age who have 15–20 good years left in them, and I see people at 50 who don't. We might reasonably ask the question, "Which one is older?"

Death

There are certainly many things from which to die, but if you don't die from something else first, then eventually your kidneys will get too weak to perform (and support life) and you will die from some malady connected to kidney malfunction. As I have said many times in my classes, "If nothing else kills you first then your kidneys will." To an Oriental medical practitioner this is the only "death from natural causes" there is.

Good News and Bad News

If kidneys are really this important to your health (and they are!), then you might reasonably ask two questions:

Are there things one can avoid that might weaken them prematurely? and

Are there ways to strengthen them, thereby adding to their (and your) life spans? Fortunately the answer to both questions is, Yes!

Good News: What to avoid: many of these are obvious because we all recognize them as bad for our health anyway. A *partial* list includes: smoking, excess alcohol, illegal drugs, prescription and over the counter medications, inadequate exercise, too much exercise (yes there is such a thing!), not enough rest/sleep, not resting/sleeping at the right time (it is especially important to be resting/sleeping between 11 PM and 3 AM, when the liver works the hardest to prepare your body for the next day), poor diet, and excess use of stimulants, covered in depth in **Chapter 24 - Getting Up Again**.

Bad News: Another area of activity with a profound effect on kidney health: sexual activity. Excess sexual activity (an idea that doesn't even exist in our culture) will also weaken the kidneys. For men the sex act itself is draining to the energy and essence stored in the kidneys. Some overt signs of excess include: lightheadedness, ringing in the ears, fatigue, and aching back or joints after sex.

For women it isn't so much the sex act itself but more about how many pregnancies and babies, what age they are when they have them, how much they rest after birthing, and how much time for recovery between each birthing. Have you known a woman whose body changed dramatically or whose health was impacted significantly from delivering a child? I certainly have!

Please keep in mind that for both men and women this is about the idea of excess. What is an excessive amount of sex for a man, or birthing for a woman? The short answer is, "It is different in every case." I would suggest you consult an Oriental medical practitioner for the answer in your case.

Strengthening the Kidneys

The three proactive steps I know to strengthen your kidneys are acupuncture, herbs, and certain specific foods. Some of the helpful foods are: parsley, cinnamon, chestnut, mussels, yams, chicken, beef, walnut, dill, fennel, millet, string beans, adzuki beans, lotus seed, and grapes. Some are not the most common foods we eat but we would do well to work them into our diets.

Acupuncture and Chinese herbal formulas (the two pillars of Oriental Medicine) are also very useful in this regard. Because we in Oriental Medicine are aware of the importance of kidney strength to your health and longevity, we have paid attention over the last several thousand years, to methods and substances that strengthen your kidney/adrenal complex.

I have been taking kidney strengthening herbal formulas since I was 40 and as of this writing, at age 77, still don't manifest any overt signs of kidney weakness.

So, yes you can do things to increase your kidneys' energy and therefore your longevity. This doesn't mean, of course, that we can keep someone alive forever; but it does mean we can push back that fateful day when you must move on. And, of course, people can't be made to live longer without making them healthier and happier at the same time; so it's a win-win!

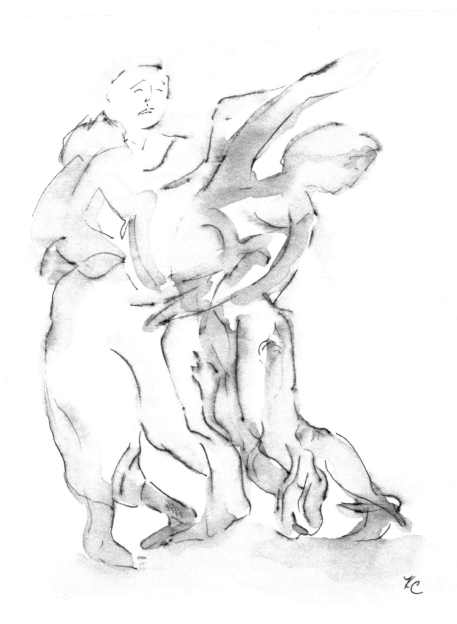

Chapter 8

The Vectors of Dying

As has been determined in Oriental Medicine, the Kidneys store our Basic Energy (BE). Our body's storehouse of **Basic Energy** is used up as we go through life until such time as it becomes so depleted it will no longer support the necessary processes of life, and at that point our bodies die.

This process is represented here in a series of graphs showing our diminishing energy moving us toward our terminal event. These graphic representations are what I call, "The Vectors of Dying." For the purposes of *Body Wisdom*, we can define a vector as a graphic representation of movement in a direction.

Basic Energy

The genesis of our Basic Energy (BE) comes from the combination of two sources.

Original Energy (OE) is the energy we are given at birth—after all a newborn baby has not done anything on its own to generate energy: it has been given its initial store of energy by its parents. This amount of energy would be somewhat different for each individual, just like we can buy a 36 month car battery or a 90 month battery, the more **OE** one is given, the more potential one has for a longer life. To this is added **"Acquired Energy" (AE)** to determine our **Basic Energy (BE)**. The equation looks like this: **OE + AE=BE.**

Acquired Energy (AE) is that which we generate throughout our life. This comes from cellular metabolism—the process by which our trillions of individual cells "burn" blood sugar (glucose: extracted from what we eat and drink by our digestive system), in the presence of **Oxygen (O_2)** provided by our lungs (respiratory system).

As was shown earlier our **Basic Energy** is stored in the Kidney/Adrenal Complex in the lower back. On the following pages are graphs that symbolize how our **Basic Energy** can diminish until the point of our death.

VECTOR TYPES

Ideal type

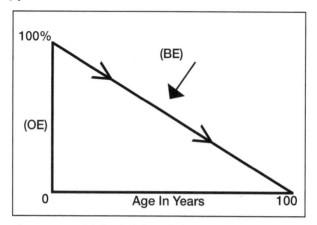

This is what it would look like if there were no outside forces negatively impacting our health. Here I posit 100 years as the maximum age potential for a human. A nice ideal, not one likely to happen to the vast majority in the real world. Let's look at some other, more common types.

Lower Original Energy type

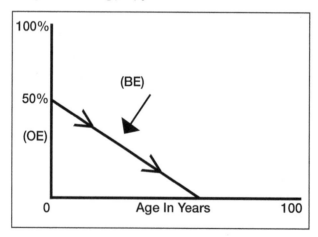

Most of us are not likely to be given the maximum amount of OE possible for a human. In this case I'll choose a 50% allotment—this person has definitely been shortchanged at birth, as most of us will receive more than this. The angle of the descending vector is the same as in the Ideal Type but this person will necessarily have a significantly shorter life.

Dr. Gerald Senogles

Traumatic Event Type

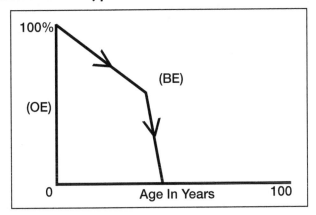

Here we see a life cut short by any one of a series of possible life ending events, i.e. serious illness, fatal accident, suicide, homicide, etc.

The vector for this body is trending for a naturally long life but is unfortunately interrupted by a terminal circumstance, possibly a fatal accident or disease.

Negative Lifestyle Choices Type

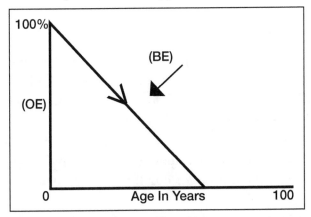

This person's initial allotment of Original Energy (OE) has not been sufficiently augmented by the right amount of Acquired Energy (AE) to achieve the length of life we would project for this individual. In order to more closely approach our Ideal Type life span we need to lead a pretty clean life—this person didn't.

The list of poor lifestyle choices is practically endless but would include: poor or inadequate diet (overly processed junky foods come to mind), smoking, excess alcohol, too many legal or illegal drugs, staying too long in bad or abusive situations (work place, marriage, family or "friend-ships," etc.).

Representative Type

This is how most of our own lives will likely graph.

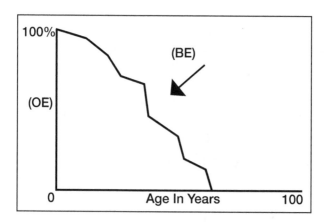

As we go through life we will experience negative events that, in the long run, shorten our lives. These could include non-terminal illnesses, accidents, emotional traumas, etc. For most of us we start with the angle of an Ideal Vector, but the consequences of these periodically occurring negative events will graph as occasional downturns that shorten our lives, causing our graphs to look somewhat like a set of stairs.

It is worth pointing out that if these life-shortening events occur in our earlier lives they are not as life threatening as they would be if they occurred as we approach the ending of our lives; a time when we cannot afford a sharp downturn.

These five graphs represent "pure" types that could combine to show possible permutations.

LONGEVITY HERBS

Naturally there are many negative lifestyle choices we can make that can reduce our lifespan, and many positive ones that can extend it. Here are three particular Oriental herbs considered as especially conducive to a longer, healthier life.

Reishi Mushroom (*ganoderma lucidum*)
One of the most powerful immune system boosters on earth. Known in the Orient to reduce the risk of cancer, as well as assist in the treatment of cancer and other major diseases.

Astragalus
This is also referred to in **Chapter 15 – Reducing the Risk**. A powerful immune booster we also recommend to reduce the deleterious effects of radiation and chemotherapy on the healthy cells in your body. A major disease fighter!

He Shu Wu
(Sometimes mistakenly referred to in the West as Fo Ti Tien). There are many stories in the Orient about this herb aiding people to achieve very advanced ages. It is said to supplement "Essence" (Jing in Chinese); as this word implies, this will contribute to our health, well being and longevity.

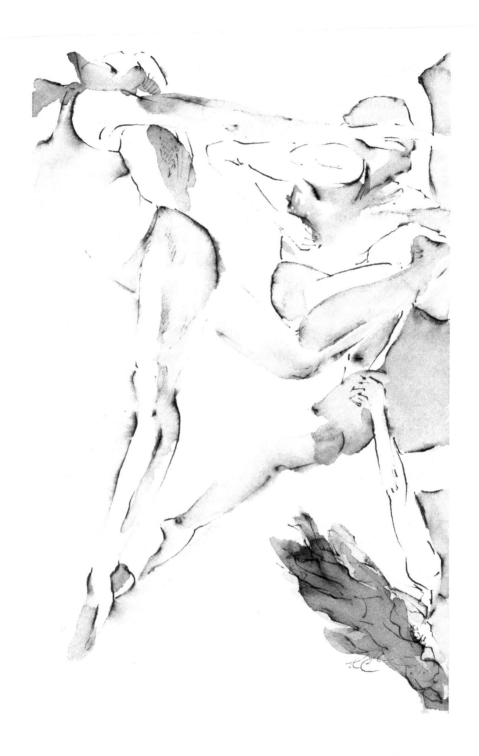

Chapter 9.

The Liver: Organ of Overreaction

Poor Jane (Again)

You remember Jane from the **Introduction**, but let's recap her list of symptoms. Jane suffered with headaches, insomnia, depression, back pain, acid reflux, and menstrual cramping. A formidable list, to be sure!

Now that you know the primacy of organ and gland function to your health, and you know that a given organ malfunction can cause multiple symptoms, it may come as no surprise that every one of Jane's problems was brought on by only one organ malfunction: her liver!

To correct all of her problems we really only had to fix one thing!

Structure

The liver is the largest organ in your body. In an average adult, it is the size of a shoe box and accounts for about 2% of your body's weight. It centers on the right side of your body, tucked in just under the rib cage, but it is so large it crosses the midline of the body and some of it is on your left side as well.

When we speak of the liver in Oriental Medicine, we also include the gall bladder; a small gland attached to the liver to form a structural/functional pair.

Physiology/Functions

The liver is the most complex organ in your body. It is literally a chemical factory working night and day to maintain the correct chemical makeup of your body. It does more separate things for you than any other organ or gland, therefore there are more different things it can do incorrectly. As a consequence, it can cause a wider range of symptoms than any other organ when it malfunctions. When I first started studying medicine in the early 1970s, Western Medicine had identified over 300 separate functions that the liver performed. Last time 1 heard (late 1990s) that number was up to over 500, and we have just scratched the surface. We may never know all that is done there, but we can make a list of some general categories of its functions.

1. It is a virtual chemical factory that neutralizes and detoxifies harmful chemicals, while at the same time deconstructs and reconstructs other usable chemical compounds and distributes them for use around your body.

2. It produces liver bile for the digestion of fats and oils in the small intestine.

3. It is the storehouse for a large quantity of blood.

4. It is responsible for the circulation of energy throughout your body.

Symptoms of Liver Pathology

It's hard to go through life without acquiring some liver malfunctions. I've said in my classes, "I never see an adult American without some degree of liver functional pathology." It is not possible to list all of the things it does, but we can list some areas where symptoms of liver malfunction are likely to show up.

Digestion: The liver, through its agent the gall bladder, can have many consequences throughout the gastrointestinal tract. A partial list of symptoms include: heartburn, nausea, vomiting, acid reflux, constipation, diarrhea, or any of the other symptoms listed in **Chapter 5 - The Digestive System**.

Emotions: Lots of issues here, anything from clinical depression to impatience, irritability, being judgmental and difficulty making decisions. Of course we all have problems with these issues from time to time as circumstances dictate, but the question becomes, "Are they too frequent or too severe, or do the circumstances not warrant them?" If the answer to any or all of these questions is "Yes," then liver functional pathology is indicated.

Menstrual Problems: The liver is profoundly tied to a woman's periodic cycle. The most common menstrual symptoms associated with the liver are menstrual cramping and **PMS (premenstrual syndrome). PMS** symptoms tied to the liver include depression, irritability, headache, back/hip pain and breast tenderness.

Body Aches and Pains: Some of the pains diagnosed as arthritis come from here, but certainly every patient I have ever seen whose pains have been diagnosed as "fibromyalgia" have liver functional pathology as the ultimate cause of their painful condition. The liver can be responsible for pains anywhere from the top of the head to the bottom of the feet!

Headaches: First, headaches don't always have their ultimate origins in the head. When they do, the cause is often detectable by Western tests, as with a brain tumor or a concussion, both of which can cause a headache and would be detectable by an MRI or possibly a CT scan.

Most headaches, however, are just a "pain in the head" symptom telling us something, somewhere in the body is not working right. A good example is a recurring headache during a woman's periodic cycle. In this case the headaches would be 'hormonal," though they would have their origin in the liver, as the liver controls so much of the hormonal actions of the menstrual cycle.

Either way, this points out that headaches can have complex causes ultimately not located at the site of the pain. The liver is implicated in many other headaches besides those triggered by the hormonal cycle, and certainly when we see someone with headaches diagnosed as "migraine" headaches, the liver is always involved.

Low Back/Hip/Leg Pain: You may have noticed that we discussed this same set of symptoms under the kidneys; many symptoms can have more than one possible cause. Since in Oriental Medicine we want to correct the cause of a problem so it doesn't readily recur, not just cover up the symptoms with drugs while the underlying cause may in fact be getting worse, it is up to the practitioner to determine which organ is responsible for a given symptom in any particular case.

Back/hip/leg problems are so common that for many practitioners it is the number one complaint of their patients.

Insomnia: Insomnia can have more than one possible cause also, and the liver is implicated particularly where one can get to sleep easily enough but wakes in the middle of the night and has difficulty getting back to sleep. This as opposed to someone who can't get to sleep in the first place, but when they finally do they can usually stay asleep (this usually comes from a heart functional pathology).

Allergies: By allergies we mean overreacting to ordinary substances. If you vomit or have diarrhea (or both) after eating tainted seafood, that is your body's natural protective mechanism for removing toxic substances from your body, hopefully before they can do you much harm. As unpleasant as this may be it is in your own best interest. This is not an allergic reaction! I'm fond of saying everyone is "allergic" to enough strychnine (a deadly poison); but if, as with one of my patients, your throat swells shut from a few drops of tomato juice, you are having a potentially deadly overreaction unrelated to any inherent toxicity in the tomato itself. This, then, fits the definition of an allergic reaction.

It doesn't matter what you overreact to, or what your symptom is. If pollen makes you sneeze, or cats make your eyes swell shut, or cheese gives you diarrhea, or peanut butter puts you in bed for days (I had a patient with this), or whatever, then you are overreacting, and the liver is implicated.

Cancer: This falls within the general category of what I call "accumulations." By this I mean things appearing, forming, or growing where they don't belong. This would include cysts, tumors (benign or malignant), lumps, fibrous masses, and even the bone spurs of osteoarthritis. Liver pathology is involved in all accumulations because things don't form or grow where they don't belong if the circulation of energy in the area is good; and the circulation of energy is the responsibility of the liver. The liver is to the circulation of energy as the heart is to the circulation of blood. If energy circulation is retarded/blocked in an area long enough then blood circulation will become retarded as well, and visa-versa.

The liver, therefore, is implicated in all tumor-based cancers. Not all cancers are tumor-based however; leukemia, a cancer that shows up as changes in the composition of the bloodstream, is not tumor-based.

It is very easy to trace breast and uterine cancer back to the liver because of its connection to the hormonal system.

Because cancer is such a serious problem, and is beginning to reach epidemic proportions in the US, I have devoted all of **Chapter 15 – The Big C -Reducing the Risk** to ways to reduce your risk of developing this potentially deadly disease. All of these recommended procedures can be applied to reduce the risks for your family and loved ones as well.

So, now you have a partial list of symptom areas relating to the liver (and remember it is only partial). I should also point out that you can pass your liver function test from your family doctor and still have lots of liver functional disorders. Remember, they can test only a very few of the known (and none of the, as yet, unknown) liver functions.

Prevention (Jane Redux)

As we work to eliminate Jane's list of problems (and they are all correctable by the methods and substances of Oriental Medicine) you can see we help to prevent, or at least reduce the risk of, the development of all the other liver based diseases; up to and including cancer.

This is the way medicine should be done!

THE TREATMENT OF ALLERGIES
WITH ACUPUNCTURE

By an allergy we mean overreacting to ordinary substances. Everybody has a bad reaction to strycÚine—a deadly poison. But, if you can't walk through a field of wildflowers on a beautiful spring day without a runny nose, sneezing, runny itchy eyes, etc., but everyone else can, then the problem is not the grasses, or the pollen, but in your body. It doesn't matter what the substance or the reaction is; if pollen makes you sneeze, or tomatoes make your throat swell shut, you are overreacting to ordinary substances. In other words if everyone else is fine, then there is something malfunctioning in your body.

There are generally two categories of allergens (substances that cause allergic reactions), "environmental" and "food."

Environmental includes grasses, hay, trees, pollen, dust and dust mites, animals and animal dander, fabrics, soaps, body products, chemicals, perfumes, and others.

Allergies to Food are much more common than most people realize. Some of the most common are: milk and dairy products, wheat, gluten, corn products, (if you think you don't eat much corn read the labels on every packaged, baked, frozen or canned food you consider buying—you may be surprised!), soy (another food scattered throughout prepared products), peanuts, yeast, caffeine, alcohol.

(I once had a 24 year old patient who could eat only eight different foods without severe cramping and diarrhea. Imagine 60 more years of living like that!)

The list of possible allergic reactions is practically endless, but certainly include: hay fever, rashes, hives, asthma, Irritable Bowel Syndrome, palpitations, migraine headaches, dizziness, reduced energy, acid reflux. One of the more unusual characteristics of allergies is that the reaction can occur only infrequently while the offending allergen can be something you are ingesting virtually every day. If you were allergic to watermelon you would undoubtedly figure that out in a few seasons—you would go 10 months without eating any and then go on a picnic and eat some, and then when you reacted, you would say, "I think I'm allergic to that" and stop eating it.

But some allergies are not so easy to detect, which is why patients need to be tested. Migraine headaches always have a food allergy component to their causation. I had a patient who experienced one three-day migraine every month. Upon testing her for allergens I discovered a severe corn intolerance (she happened to be eating a taco in her car just before coming in for her first appointment). People are often allergic to the foods they like or to which they are most attracted! When we turned around her allergic reaction to corn, the headaches went away.

All allergies/sensitivities are related to the liver, so as we fix your allergy problem we are making your liver function more correctly—an added bonus as far as your current and future health are concerned.

There is a great allergy elimination tecÚique called NAET which I use to solve these problems. If you know someone, or suspect you have symptoms brought on by allergies, look for a local practitioner who uses this tecÚique.

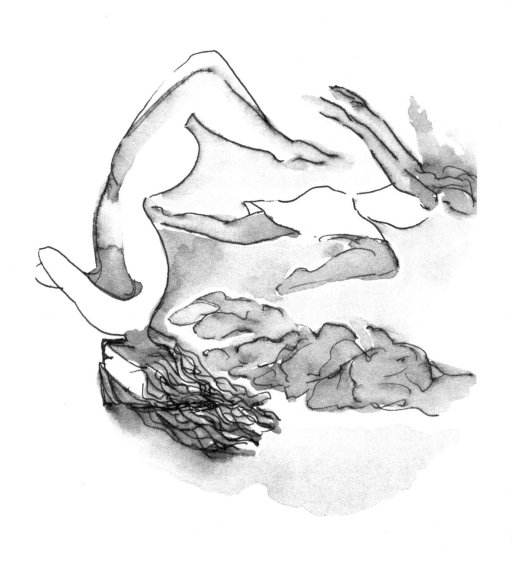

Chapter 10

It's All One: The Interactions of Organs and Glands

The Case of "Asthmatic Andy"

A ndy had severe asthma. Asthma is defined in *Taber's Medical Dictionary* as "a set of conditions characterized by difficulty breathing."

Andy would get a tight constricted feeling in his chest and then have difficulty breathing and a need to cough. He used inhalers for several years and they helped him breath immediately after using them, but he found he needed them more and more frequently and was just not getting any better, in fact he was getting worse!

To help determine what was responsible for his condition, we asked him a simple question. We asked if he'd noticed difficulty breathing in one direction more than the other? To clarify, if he had clearly more difficulty taking a breath in, letting his breath out, or if he experienced equal difficulty in both directions. All of these are possible; and the answer helps us determine which other organs, if any, besides the lungs might be causative or contributory to a particular person's asthma.

In Andy's case he'd noticed he could breathe out easily enough but breathing in was difficult.

In Oriental Medicine we know that if someone has more trouble breathing out, it is usually just the lungs at fault; if it is more difficult to breathe in, malfunctions in either the kidneys, the liver, or both, are contributing to the problem. This was the case with Andy.

By working to strengthen Andy's lungs and kidneys, plus assisting his liver to function correctly, we got him off the inhalers and breathing much better on his own than he had in years.

Systems

Since the body is a system and in a system all the parts are tied together, it shouldn't be too surprising to learn that the malfunction of one or more organs can adversely affect the functioning of an entirely different organ or gland system in the body.

To put it another way: a symptom can show up in one organ or gland system while the ultimate cause of that organ's problem can come from a malfunction in a completely different organ or gland; which is why in Oriental Medicine we don't just treat symptoms but work to determine and treat the cause where ever it may be. Here's an example.

Lung Symptoms

Of the five vital organs discussed so far in **Section One** (heart, lungs, digestion, kidneys and liver) the lungs and respiratory system are the most likely organs to develop symptoms as a result of malfunctions in an organ or gland system elsewhere in the body.

Almost all lung diseases involve the symptoms of difficulty breathing and/or coughing, with the possible complication of phlegm congestion. All of these (and more) can be brought on by malfunctions in either the liver, kidneys or digestive system, as well as the lungs.

In the language of the legal system, the lungs are not necessarily the guilty party (perpetrator) but may be, in fact, the victims of misbehavior elsewhere. Since we want to treat the cause of a medical problem (being a Doctor of Oriental Medicine is not unlike being a detective), we want to find out "who done it?" and direct our attentions there.

This brings up another problem with the Western approach of artificially and arbitrarily controlling symptoms with drugs. Not only do drugs have dangerous side effects but they don't often work to correct the underlying cause of the symptoms they control. Therefore these untreated causes are allowed to languish, and in most cases, get worse.

The lungs again will provide us with a good example: in my considerable experience working with lung diseases (asthma, emphysema, chronic obstructive pulmonary disease (COPD) patients on bronchial inhalers just use more and more in higher and higher doses.

Treating the Cause

From the Oriental Medicine perspective, if you do not treat the cause at the same time you treat the symptoms (and yes, in Oriental Medicine we do want to give relief of symptoms as quickly as possible), then you are not working to effect a real cure.

Nine Different Doctors

If you recall from **Chapter 9 - The Liver:** when it malfunctions, the liver creates the broadest range of symptoms of all the organs and glands, and because most of the symptoms do not occur at the site of the liver itself, it is not often recognized as causative and treated as such by Western doctors. As you can imagine, this leads to a major missing component in the treatment strategy, and little hope of effecting a permanent solution.

Compounding this, each category of liver symptoms are treated by a different Western medical "specialist"—none of whom would recognize the liver's involvement and treat it.

Here is a list of symptoms brought on by liver malfunctions and in parentheses the different types of specialists; the sheer size of this list illustrates how much trouble a malfunctioning organ can cause to other systems in the body.

Digestive symptoms (Gastroenterologist); depression (Psychiatrist); menstrual cramps (Ob-Gyn); insomnia (Internist); headaches (Neurologist); allergies (Allergist); cancer (Oncologist); fibromyalgia (Rheumatologist); back/hip pain (Orthopedist). The liver can also create lung symptoms like coughing or shortness of breath, so we can add a Pulmonologist to the list for a grand total of ten different doctors, none of whom would treat the ultimate cause in the liver!

Is this any way to do medicine?

Prevention

The ideal medical system should not only be able to influence a particular disease's symptoms, it should also be able to help prevent the recurrence of that disease, or the emergence of some other disease/symptom, by truly correcting its underlying cause.

Oriental Medicine does that!

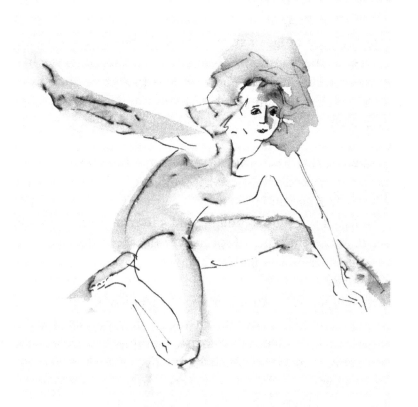

SECTION TWO

OTHER HEALTH-RELATED PROBLEMS AND SOLUTIONS

N ow that we have identified the basic components, let's look at some different problems, conditions and other health related subjects (diet, nutrition, GMOs, injuries, acupuncture, stimulant abuse, menopause, PMS, etc.) that can make a difference in how you feel.

You will also see that for many of the problems brought up, a solution will be offered. I believe that anyone in the healing professions is not doing you a favor by pointing out potential problems if they don't offer solutions.

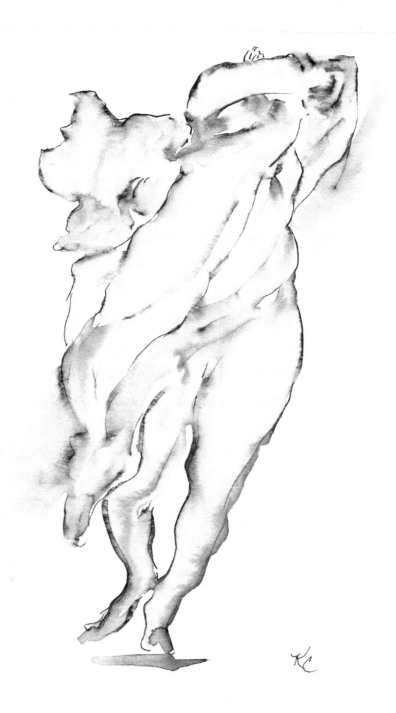

Chapter 11

How Acupuncture Works

The Importance of Acupuncture

Acupuncture is one of the most powerful and effective tecÚiques on earth for maintaining the human body in a correct state of health, or for correcting health problems, if that is what is needed.

The origins of acupuncture are unknown as it predates writing in the Orient. In fact, one of the first Chinese books ever written, the *Huang Chi Nei Ching*, refers to it as being part of medicine in "ancient times," and it was written more than two thousand years ago!

It is also one of the fastest ways to improve health and especially to relieve pain regardless of the cause of the pain, whether from an accident, injury, or a disease process such as arthritis or fibromyalgia.

Modalities of Oriental Medicine

Before explaining how acupuncture works let's discuss the two principle modalities (groups of tecÚiques used to facilitate healing) of Oriental Medicine and compare them to the two principle modalities of Western Medicine. The modalities of Oriental Medicine are acupuncture and medicinal herbal substances and formulas, while the modalities of Western Medicine are drugs and surgery.

Drugs or surgery are what I call "crisis level medicine:" you don't resort to them because they are good for you, but only if you get in so much distress you feel you have to, but you hope you don't have to!

Drugs

It's not like the doctor says, "Well, the average American is taking three drugs and you're only taking one so we better see if we can't find two more for you to take. You want to be like everyone else don't you?"

Or how about, "We know certain antibiotics can be used to treat pneumonia so why don't you take them all the time on the chance they will stop you from getting pneumonia in the first place."

We hope neither of these scenarios would take place, even though it happens too often. I have frequently seen something like this in the U.S., where people take far too many drugs.

The reason you shouldn't take drugs unless it is absolutely necessary is because all drugs have "side-effects;" they may have the effect you want, but they all have unwanted effects that are damaging, disruptive, or even deadly to the normal working mechanisms of your body. Almost 1/3 of all hospital admissions in the U.S. are brought on by the side-effects of prescription drugs, and that's not because the doctor prescribed the wrong drug for a particular condition, or even the wrong dosage, but from the correct drug at the correct dosage.

According to a September 27, 2016 article in US News, prescribed medications kill more than 128,000 Americans a year (a conservative estimate). That's more than twice as many as die in automobile accidents.

You might say, """Well, my doctor is a nice person and he/she wouldn't give me anything that might harm or kill me. Would he?"

And the answer is, "Yes, he would!"

For two reasons: one, drugs are virtually all Western doctors have with which to control your symptoms and, secondly, they must follow the standard medical protocols (drugs and/or surgery) in order to stay in practice. An MD of my acquaintance didn't like to prescribe drugs but instead recommended that her patients try natural substances (like vitamin and mineral supplementation) and lifestyle changes to get well. When the Board of Medical Examiners in her state got wind of this, they stripped her of her license to practice medicine and drove her out of the state.

Surgery

Does the doctor say, "Come on down to the hospital and we'll remove some of those unnecessary parts for you." No!

But, 50% of all the surgeries performed in the U.S. could be avoided (some experts say it's 90%!) if doctors and patients learned to manage their problems in better, less invasive and expensive ways (a clue?). Surgery isn't always the quick-fix it is made out to be, and in my experience can sometimes lead to more problems than it solves, up to and including death. But it does accomplish one thing every time; it makes doctors and hospitals a lot of money.

Does this mean that every surgery is unnecessary? No, of course not; but a second, or even third opinion is valuable. I once had a patient whose leg was surgically removed above the knee. Some years after the surgery another doctor told her that she hadn't needed to have her leg cut off and that he could have saved it.

ORIENTAL MODALITIES

Herbs

One of the two pillars of Oriental Medicine is medicinal herbs and herbal formulas (the other is acupuncture). One of the great things about prescribing herbal formulas in constant use for over 1,000 years, besides the fact that they work, is the peace of mind it gives to the practitioner to use something long tested in the laboratory of Oriental culture. In that length of time (and some formulas are over 1800 years old) we not only find out what a formula will do *for* you, we find out what it won't do *to* you; like the dangerous side effects of drugs.

Drugs have been pulled off the market because of the scope of the damage of side effects; and believe me there have been many over the years. There are also drugs that should be removed from druggists' shelves, but the side effects take so long to develop, they can't be conclusively traced back to their origins in a specific medication.

In the Western culture, we have been raised with the idea that to solve medical problems you swallow a pill.

Even though Chinese herbs don't have unwanted side effects, it does not mean every herb is right for everybody and can therefore be used indiscriminately. This is simply not true.

Because herbs make a difference, we have to be sure that the difference an herb makes is what you need. Blood pressure, for example. If we thought your blood pressure was too low (yes, there is such a thing) and therefore gave you herbs to raise it, but we were wrong because it was really too high, then we would have given you a formula that was not right for you; not because of unwanted side-effects but because the principle known effect of that formula was not the one you needed! There was nothing inherently wrong with the herb, but there was something wrong with the diagnosis!

Because of the difficulty involved in making a proper diagnosis, we caution against the self-prescribing of herbs and formulas, and instead recommend that you consult with a medical expert. In the case of Oriental Medicine that person might be referred to as an Acupuncturist, or a Chinese/Oriental Herbalist, or a Doctor of Oriental Medicine (D.O.M., O.M.D., D.A.O.M.).

Even doctors of Oriental Medicine, who know the herbs and their actions, should not self-prescribe since it is impossible for a person to step far enough outside themselves for the proper perspective on their situation to make the right objective decisions. There is an old saying in Oriental Medicine: "The doctor who treats himself has a fool for a patient."

Acupuncture

You now know you want to have your organs and glands working as well as they can, so you might ask, "How does acupuncture effect changes in organ and gland function?"

The short answer is "by using the nerves of the meridian system to influence the actions of the **Autonomic Nervous System (ANS)**."

Autonomic Nervous System

It takes energy, in the form of electricity, running through nerves to cause anything to happen in the body. Let's say you wanted to move your arm, maybe so you could eat some food from the plate in front of you. First you would have to intend (a mental process) to move your arm, which would cause electricity to travel from your brain down through the nerves to the muscles in your arm causing them to contract, thereby raising the fork to your mouth. This action uses the voluntary nervous system; the one you have control over.

But what about all the things constantly happening in your body over which you have no control; your heart beating, lungs expanding and contracting, stomach producing acids, glands secreting the proper hormones at the appropriate time, and the myriad body functions you don't even know are taking place? These are run by the **Autonomic Nervous System (ANS)**—what we might call the involuntary nervous system. This system sets the functional levels of organs and glands and runs their actions on a moment to moment basis, and it is this system acupuncturists tap into to manipulate and correct the malfunctions of organs and glands.

The **ANS** has two branches: the sympathetic and the parasympathetic. The sympathetic branch increases function and the parasympathetic branch decreases function. Therefore, these two branches have to be in balance by providing approximately equal amounts of energy for an organ to operate in its normal range. Every organ and gland has a normal range of operation: your heart can beat too rapidly but it can also beat too slowly; your intestines can move too fast (diarrhea) but they can also move too slowly (constipation); your stomach can produce too much stomach acid and create an ulcer, or not enough acid leading to weak digestion; etc.

It is the balance of these two branches of the **ANS** that keeps things functioning properly, or improperly if the **ANS** is not sending a balanced signal.

Meridians

If you look at an acupuncture chart you will see lines indicated on the body and dots indicated on the lines. The dots show the location of the acupuncture points; the places that are stimulated by the tiny needles of acupuncture. If you follow the course of the lines down to the tips of the hands and feet (on most charts) you will find that each of these lines is identified by a name, like heart, lung, stomach, liver. These lines are the meridians (literally: energy channels) of acupuncture, and these dots are the points on those meridians acupuncturists use to stimulate the Autonomic Nervous System to alter and correct the malfunctions of the organs and glands.

Think of the meridians, which lie along the nerve pathways, as living electrical wires; they conduct measurable electrical current and it is electricity (energy) that makes things happen.

Localized Pains

Localized pains (hip, knee, etc.) can occur in someone with no major organic dysfunction, sometimes brought on by accidents or injuries, sometimes they just happen. The role of acupuncture here is to stimulate and direct the body to heal the area as quickly and thoroughly as possible by stimulating an increased circulation of blood and energy to the area. Your body knows how to heal anything but, for whatever reason, bodies sometimes need intervention. Acupuncture is a safe and effective means of intervention.

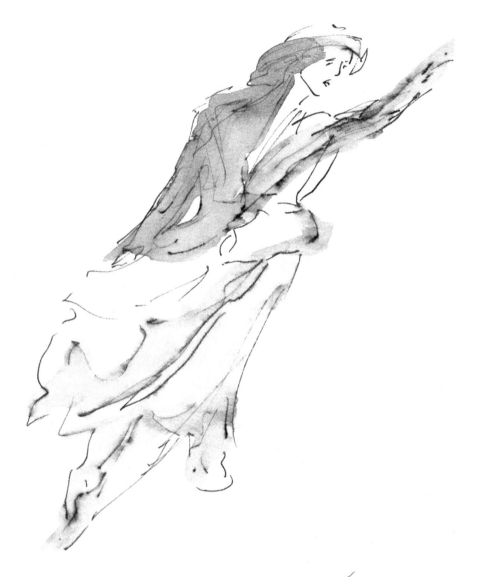

Chapter 12

It's Wrong—Period!

"Jennifer's" Troubles

Jennifer was the poster child for pathological periods! She not only had severe menstrual cramping for five days before her period began, but was severely depressed and very irritable during this time.

More importantly, her period itself lasted 8-9 days and 4-5 of those involved heavy bleeding (in other words, she was slowly but surely bleeding to death). Fortunately, she was only fifteen when her parents brought her in to see us so we could correct her difficulties before the occurrence of any long term damage. You'll see what I mean shortly.

Period Problems

In **Chapter 12 – It's Wrong, Period**, we discuss an issue of serious medical importance not clarified often enough, and that issue is *wrong* (medically pathological) menstrual cycles, or "periods."

I want to particularly discuss a problem not yet recognized as a problem, it seems, in Western Medicine and culture. In our modern civilized society, as we have increasingly lost our connection to the land and the cycles of nature, we have lost touch with many of our own cycles as well. Our principle methods of information dissemination increasingly concentrate in the hands of corporate controlled media, with its self-serving implications: all that matters is the accumulation and use of consumer goods.

We have lost our ability to accumulate and pass on culturally acquired knowledge and wisdom.

Correct Periods

To begin the discussion of a wrong period, let's define just what a correct period is. Not a "normal" period, mind you, as normalcy is a measure of the frequency of occurrence of a phenomenon, not its correctness. To be normal means to be like most people; so if most people were sick at any given time then it would be normal to be sick, but we wouldn't say that it was "good" or "correct" to be sick—it is never correct to be sick!

A correct period lasts 3-5 days, comes approximately every 28 days, involves no clotting, has no mental or physical discomfort and, most importantly, has one or two days of substantial (not heavy!) bleeding at most! That's it! End of story!

If this doesn't describe someone's cycle, there is something wrong... period! Here are some variations on a correct period; we'll look at what causes them, their meanings and long term consequences.

These would fall under three principal categories: pain, emotional disturbances, and incorrect amount of blood flow.

Pain

There should be no pain anywhere in the cycle; yet as we know, some pain somewhere is quite common—maybe even "normal." The most common pain I see clinically is uterine cramping, followed by breast tenderness and/or back pain, and lastly headaches (in extreme cases, migraines).

These pains can occur at various places throughout the cycle but mostly in the days (or weeks, if things are bad enough) just before the flow begins. They can, as in the case of migraines, be devastatingly painful and lead to the use of some serious drugs, or even visits to the emergency room.

Emotional Problems

Clinically, what we see most frequently falls under the category of premenstrual syndrome (PMS). This usually involves some combination of irritability (easily angered), depression, or just excess emotionality (crying easily, etc.).

These emotional problems, as well as pain occurring before the period itself begins, generally have as their cause a particular pathology of the liver so common that all of **Chapter 14 - Blocked Energy** is devoted to it.

Naturally, as in all these categories, a few of these problems may not be disruptive enough to require treatment, while on the other hand, whole families can suffer mightily if "Mom" or "Sis" suffer from these issues.

Incorrect Blood Flow

The most potentially serious of the period issues is the incorrect amount of blood flow. Problems may only seem inconvenient at the time but can truly have devastating long-term consequences. The most important issue is the absolute amount of blood discharged during the course of the period itself. Since we have already described correct flow, we could say that the two possible pathological variations would be either too little output of blood, or too great an output (by far the more serious).

Too Little Output is not itself a cause of difficulties but may be a sign of an underlying problem like blood deficiency (covered in **Chapter 13 – The Blood Speech**). Blood deficiency is a commonly seen and treated pathology in Oriental Medicine virtually always unrecognized and untreated in Western Medicine. It is an issue of the quantity of blood, not quality as with anemia, and is not detected through ordinary blood tests, but is detected by OM practitioners through our specialized diagnostic procedures of pulse and tongue analysis.

It is correct for women to have periods during a certain phase of their lives; if periods aren't coming around at the proper frequency and in the proper amounts, this is a sign of a problem.

Saved for last is the most significant menstrual problem I encounter, and the one with the most serious long-range medical consequences: **Excess Blood Flow**, meaning that the sum total of blood discharged per cycle exceeds the correct amount. Not only is this a sign of an underlying pathology but it can, and often does, have serious implications to a woman's future health.

Excess Period

Blood is a precious commodity (we'd all be dead without it) and the body cannot afford to waste it.

It takes two things to make something: raw materials and energy, to do the work necessary to convert those raw materials into the products or substances desired. If those products or substances are lost to us, for whatever reason, then this is a drain on our resources.

If General Motors took every fourth car they made and ran it off a cliff, it wouldn't be very long before they'd be bankrupt. Naturally, the Board of Directors wouldn't tolerate this, but we see essentially this same phenomenon tolerated in women's bodies in America all the time, only it isn't automobiles that are being lost. It's blood! If this is allowed to go on for years, as it often is, then we begin to see serious deficiencies of blood and energy and the myriad diseases and conditions that result.

Fresh Blood

Besides the output of blood exceeding the dimensions outlined in the first part of **Chapter 12 - It's Wrong, Period**, there is another circumstance that tells us if the amount of blood lost is in excess; and that is the presence of "fresh blood." If we cut ourselves and bleed, the blood we see is usually bright red—the brightness a result of a high oxygen content. When blood is in regular circulation it has been to the heart/lung complex in the chest recently and been re-oxygenated; hence it is fully oxygenated or "fresh" blood.

The flow of a woman's period represents the sloughing off of an accumulation of blood that lined the walls of the uterus for some time in anticipation of receiving a fertilized egg (getting pregnant).

This blood should be dark—the darkness shows that the blood has not been in regular circulation and re-oxygenated recently, but in fact has been in storage in the uterus. If a woman's period contains any significant quantity of fresh (bright red) blood, this is not the sloughing off of stored blood but is, in fact, simply bleeding through the uterus, and like all improper bleeding, this can pose serious health risks and should be stopped as soon as possible!

Replacing Blood

Both men and women must create a constant resupply of blood. Blood, like virtually all components of the body, is being lost, damaged, or worn out in the normal daily process of life, and therefore needs to be replaced. Women, however, have a special need (that men don't have) for blood replacement during a large part of their lives. To understand why a woman might have the problem of an excess period we must look at the working parts of the body most intimately involved with processing blood properly.

There is a saying in Oriental Medicine, "The heart rules the blood, the liver stores the blood, and the spleen governs the blood." In this saying are clues telling us where to look for the causes of excessive blood loss. In the case of an excess period, it isn't the issue of the heart malfunctioning in its ruling requirement, which has mostly to do with just pumping the blood around the body; rather it is a problem of either the liver storing the blood or the spleen governing the blood. In my clinical experience I rarely see an excess period brought on by the liver failing in its storage function, but much more commonly by the spleen failing in its governing function. In fact if anything, the liver is much more likely to be "victimized" by the blood deficiency brought on by the spleen's failings (more on this in **Chapter 13 – the Blood Speech**).

Governing the Blood

When we say, "The spleen governs the blood," what do we mean?

One of the spleen's functions is to keep the blood in its "proper course"—keeping the blood in the blood vessels. When it fails to do this and excessive bleeding occurs it is usually because of a weakness we call "spleen energy deficiency" meaning it is too weak to carry out this important function.

Another possible problem by the spleen weakening and blood not staying in its proper course is bruising easily. This does not usually have the potentially dangerous consequences of an excess menstrual flow because the blood, spilled out from the blood vessels into the surrounding tissues, is not lost to the body, but eventually reabsorbed and put back into circulation.

Compounding the Problem

Another very important spleen function is helping in the production of new (replacement) blood; but if it is too weak to perform its governing function properly and excess bleeding occurs, it is often also too weak to help produce the proper amount of replacement blood, and now we have the problem of a woman losing too much blood through her period and also unable to replace the lost blood adequately—a double whammy!

Even though the problem of an excessive menstrual flow can have serious ramifications (do I make myself clear?), it is often not that hard to fix.

The Solution

Even though it takes a qualified Oriental medical practitioner to differentiate between a liver storage problem and a spleen governing problem, it is worth discussing a Chinese herbal formula that strengthens spleen weakness thereby solving both the blood loss and replacement issues at the same time.

The formula I most often recommend is called Ren Shen Yang Rong. Ren Shen is the Chinese word for ginseng, and even though this formula usually substitutes Dong Shen (a cheaper substitute) for ginseng, the formula does share ginseng's spleen tonification (strengthening) properties. Ren Shen Yang Rong also provides blood building herbs like Dong Quai and others to help rebuild the blood supply.

I'll end **Chapter 12** by saying (once again!) that the problem of an excess period needs to be solved as quickly as possible. Mom and Dad, if you have a daughter in this phase of life, find out the facts of her periodic cycle, and if they don't closely conform to things outlined here, something needs to be done, and soon!

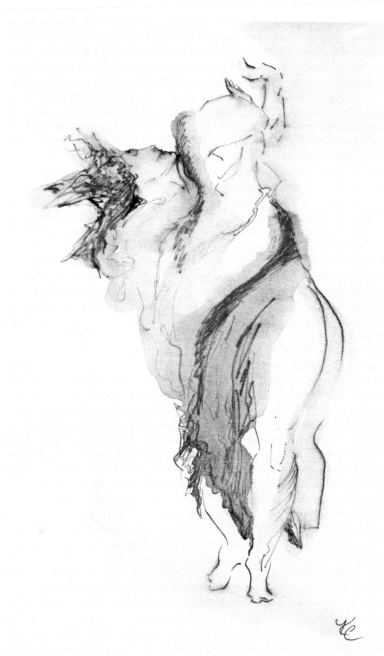

Chapter 13

The Blood Speech:
Blood, How Important Is It?

The case of "Awful Annette"

Symptoms don't have to be life threatening to be serious! Just disruptive enough to take the joy out of your life, or lead you to a significant program of drugs or surgery (both of which have the potential to cause serious harm).

Annette, aged 41, was in that kind of situation; she had so many different problems and was put on so many different drugs, which caused so many different side effects, that she felt "just awful." She was having trouble with insomnia, anxiety and panic attacks, palpitations, and PMS with irritability and depression.

All of Jane's symptoms were caused by an inadequate blood supply adversely affecting the performance of both her liver and her heart. Both of these organs demand a large blood supply in order to work properly, and as with Annette, it is common for them to malfunction at the same time if this requirement is not met.

Upon examination she was found to have significant "blood deficiency," caused by a period at least twice as big as it should have been. Unfortunately, this had gone on for many years.

Using acupuncture her menstrual flow was brought back into line, and with a combination of acupuncture and herbs her blood supply was replenished as well. Stopping the excess blood flow with acupuncture was the first step toward solving her problems, but just by itself it wasn't enough, which was why she continued taking blood building herbs for many months even after her excess period was staunched.

It's like, if every night after work you went home and hit your foot hard with a hammer, and you did that for a year, would you expect your foot to be fine as soon as you stopped? Or, might you expect to have to do something for some considerable time in order to correct the damage done over the year of your immoderate behavior? The same was true for Annette!

Even though she was not directly responsible for her excess period it had gone on for far too long, and as a result she had to do something for a considerable length of time to make up for the damage.

A general rule is, the longer you have a problem, or the longer it has built up as latent disease, the longer it takes to correct.

Blood Deficiency

Blood Deficiency is a common medical pathology known and treated in Oriental Medicine that remains unrecognized and untreated in Western Medicine. Blood deficiency means not enough blood in the body, or at a particular site in the body, to optimally carry out one or another of the blood's many functions. This is not an issue of quality, such as anemia or some other compositional irregularity that can be detectable by a blood test, but rather an issue of quantity. There are certain quantity problems detectable by blood test: for example, if a patient has suffered a recent considerable loss of blood, such as through a traumatic injury, this can be ascertained and the information used to determine how much blood to transfuse into the patient. But the blood deficiency we refer to here is a slow, gradual, long term development that remains undetected by current Western means. In **Chapter 13 - The Blood Speech**, we look at the consequences of this pathology as it impacts two particular organs.

First let me introduce you to a set of facts so fundamental to health which I have explained so many times over the years that I refer to it simply as ...

"The Blood Speech"

Every Living Cell in your body must have a blood supply in order to function properly and, for that matter, to stay alive.

Every Tissue in your body is made up of cells and, by extension, must have a blood supply as well.

Every Organ and Gland, made up of tissues which are made up of cells, must also have a blood supply; but two particular organs have a special relationship with, and a special requirement for, blood. These are the heart and the liver.

The Heart

The heart is a muscular organ sitting in the center of your chest pumping blood around your body. It is a set of four hollow chambers rightfully full of blood at all times. These chambers contract and pump blood via the arterial system to your every cell. The chambers of the heart should be full of blood; for them, that is the correct state. What about the stomach—it's hollow, too, should it be full of blood?

No, No! Certainly not!

The lungs? Nope!

The intestines, they're hollow, maybe they should be full, too?

Au Contraire!

So you see, it is only the heart that has this unique relationship with blood, and also a requirement for blood such that if, because of a generalized blood deficiency, it does not have a full complement of blood in its chambers it will begin to malfunction. In Oriental Medicine this condition is referred to as "heart blood deficiency" and can bring myriad heart symptoms including but not limited to: palpitations, tachycardia, insomnia, anxiety, panic attacks, menopausal symptoms, arrhythmias, and problems of mentation—like forgetfulness and difficulty concentrating.

The Liver

The Liver also has a special relationship with and requirement for blood. The liver is not hollow like the heart, but is rather a large spongy fibrous mass absolutely engorged with blood. The liver holds a tremendous amount of blood at all times. When you are in bed at night fully one third of your total blood supply is in your liver at any one time; up to three pints! Naturally, it's not the same blood all night long because the blood is constantly being worked on and circulated.

This does not mean that all the other cells in your body can be denied their ration of blood: if your toes don't get all the blood they need, they will die and you will lose them. Clearly your body can't allow this to happen, so if any one body part is going to get shorted because of a generalized blood deficiency it is likely to be the liver. We call this condition "liver blood deficiency" and it can lead to a wide range of liver symptoms including but not limited to: fibromyalgia, insomnia, clinical depression, migraine headaches, **PMS**, menstrual cramping, and even an increased risk of cancer.

Solving Blood Deficiency

One of the most common causes of blood deficiency, tolerated repeatedly in the U.S., is an excess blood loss during a woman's menstrual cycle. This is by no means the only cause of deficient blood as men can suffer the consequences of this as well. Oriental practitioners recognize this as a common problem and likely deal with its consequences multiple times a day.

The pathology of blood deficiency is readily detectable through the specialized Oriental diagnostic tecÛiques of pulse and tongue analysis and can often be inferred by the presenting symptoms of a patient. If you suspect you may be suffering from blood deficiency, I recommend an Oriental practitioner, as I am not aware of any other healing discipline that recognizes and treats this condition. If it is not practical to consult with someone at this time then you could try any of the blood building formulas that contain Dong Quai; one of the best but by no means only blood replenishers.

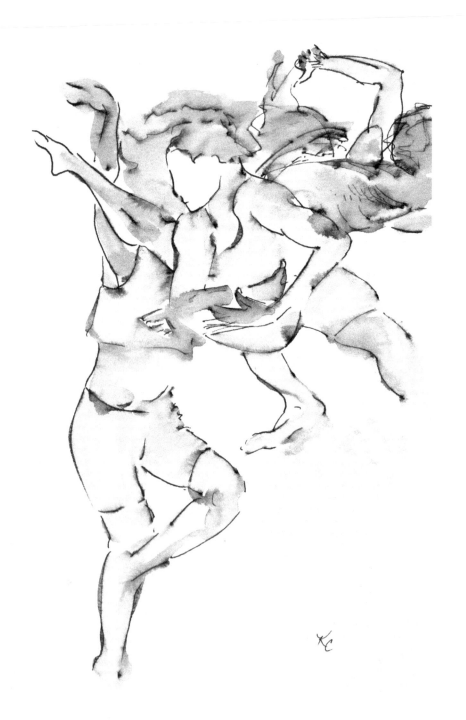

Chapter 14

Blocked Energy (Chi)

There are two principle things circulating in the body: blood and energy. As a general rule, anything that can circulate should circulate, and it should flow freely and without impediment.

We recognize this to be true of blood circulation and, in fact, there are certain disease conditions that are strictly a matter of impeded blood flow. Probably the most important of these is a blockage (impeded flow) in one or another of the arteries of the heart. This condition leads to many hundreds of thousands of heart bypass surgeries and, if left untreated, to many heart attacks and deaths. (Incidentally, surgery is not always the only way to deal with this condition.)

Other blood circulation problems include phlebitis and intermittent claudication, numbness or tingling in hands or feet, memory loss, muscle cramps, constipation and even fatigue. The circulation of blood is under the control of the heart, as can be easily demonstrated by dissecting a cadaver and tracing the blood vessels back to their source in the heart. Energy circulation, however, is another matter!

Energy Circulation

Energy (in the form of measurable electricity) circulates in the nervous system; nerves are living electrical wires. **The Central Nervous System (CNS)**, which includes the spinal cord running down through the vertebral column, has its origins in the brain and can be physically traced back to there in a cadaver. Energy also circulates in the meridian system of Oriental Medicine which utilizes some components of the nervous system. Meridians do not, however, originate in the brain, and yet like all things that move, there must be some component part providing the motive force for that movement.

The circulation of energy in the meridians (and certain other tissues) is motivated by the liver. I have said many times in my classes, "The liver is to the circulation of energy as the heart is to the circulation of blood." As we shall see, this is of tremendous importance.

Liver Stagnation

Since unimpeded circulation is the medically correct state of affairs, then it follows that blocked, retarded, or impeded flow represents a pathology.

The problems that develop from energy flow retardation can be as consequential as those of impeded blood flow—even if not quite as dramatic as dropping dead from a heart attack.

In order for a free flow of energy throughout the body there must be a free flow through the liver itself; if this is not the case we refer to this pathology as **"Liver Chi Stagnation."** A partial list of conditions that develop from this includes: allergies, fibromyalgia, menstrual cramps and PMS, migraine headaches, the formation of cysts, fibroids or tumors (either benign or cancerous), and clinical depression; depression that is not motivated or sustained by negative external circumstances but rather by an imbalance in the system.

There are three principle causes of Liver Energy Stagnation; two of these are physical, and one is mental/emotional. Let's discuss these in a particular order, but recognize that this order is arbitrary and does not indicate a ranking of importance or frequency of occurrence.

Physical Causes

Blood Deficiency: The liver needs a tremendous amount of blood in order to function properly, and if that blood supply is lacking for any reason this can lead to a retardation of the circulation of energy through the liver and, consequently, throughout the system. As you saw in the **Chapter 13 – The Blood Speech,** blood deficiency is a common occurrence—especially among women. The Chinese herb Dong Quay, or Dong Quay based formulas, are good for correcting blood deficiency.

Storage of Toxins: The liver is the largest and most functionally complex organ in the body. It is literally a miniature chemical factory performing many thousands of sophisticated chemical processes every second; among other things it must deal with the myriad toxins getting into our blood streams every day. Ideally the liver breaks these contaminants into harmless component parts or neutralizes them in some other way; but barring that, it may for various reasons remove them from circulation and simply store them. It is good for the rest of the body to not have to be subjected to these harmful substances floating around in the bloodstream; but ultimately harmful to the liver.

It's like on the Oregon/Washington border there is a nuclear waste storage facility called Hanford Nuclear Reservation (the largest nuclear waste dump in the Western Hemisphere). It's good for those around the country who generate this deadly waste material to have it hauled away and stored at Hanford, but bad for the immediate Hanford area to be the repository for these dangerous materials. Something like this goes on with the liver.

If enough toxins get stored in the liver this can, among other things, cause a stagnation of energy through the liver. The strategy for solving this pathology is to cause these toxins to be dumped by the liver into the bloodstream for eventual removal from the body. During this dumping process one might experience any number of unusual or unpleasant feelings or conditions, as whatever is in your bloodstream at any moment is what you're "on," and you will experience the consequences.

Acupuncture, as well as herbal formulas, are effective at facilitating the elimination of toxins from the liver. I particularly like the Oriental herbal formulas Hsiao Yao Wan or "Relaxed Wanderer" for this.

Mental/Emotional Causes

The liver, along with the heart, is a very emotional organ, meaning that certain emotional circumstances impact it profoundly and can have a significant impact on your own emotional state. Let's look at two emotional issues that can lead to liver energy blockage.

Abuse: To be on the receiving end of what I call an "abusive unequal power relationship," is a particular life circumstance easily leading to a blockage of energy circulation in the liver. Some examples of unequal power relationships are: employer/employee, teacher/student, parent (or other adult)/child, government/citizen, and certainly some husbands and wives. The problem develops when one person is dominant over the other and if the dominant person or agent is abusing (mentally or physically) the subordinate person; stagnation of the liver accrues to the person on the receiving end of the abuse.

Put another way, if the person on the bottom has to "take it" then that creates the problem. For instance, if your boss is a total jerk (or worse), and you'd love to tell him/her where to go, but you really need this job so you keep your mouth shut and stuff those feelings somewhere deep inside, that "somewhere" is the liver and this will lead to stagnation.

Another tragic example is a child sexually abused by a parent or other adult. Typically, but not always, this happens to girls. If this goes on for any length of time it always causes serious blockage. I believe that people who've had this circumstance in their childhood have a seriously increased incidence of cancer (as liver blockage is a contributor to this deadly disease).

Frustration: Webster's dictionary defines "to frustrate" as "to prevent (someone) from achieving an object...foiling...being thwarted...having some fundamental need unsatisfied." In other words, to block someone from realizing some need or goal.

Now, we all have had some aspects of this in our lives. The romantic dreams of adventure and excitement we had when younger have turned out to be unrealistic and we are living fairly ordinary lives (working, looking after a family, a periodic vacation or two, etc.). In most cases, we have slowly but surely modified our goals to conform with our daily responsibilities and obligations; we are therefore living the lives we have chosen, so we don't feel frustrated. It is only when someone's goals and desires have been actively blocked that frustration ensues and the liver's circulation is stagnated.

The way to address blockages brought on by mental/emotional causes is some combination of the following: eliminate the circumstance as quickly as possible; get emotional counseling; use acupuncture and/or herbs to unblock the liver. I would also recommend treatment for the heart, as all strong emotional circumstances will have an impact on the heart as well.

The Last You'll Hear of "Poor Jane"

We now know that Jane's formidable list of symptoms came from a functional pathology of her liver, and it can be revealed just what that pathology was and why she had it.

Jane was troubled for many years with a period much too large, which led to blood deficiency, but to top it off, she was in a psychologically abusive marriage for fourteen years; so having two of the three causes of liver stagnation, her liver was really stuck! Fortunately, she was now in a supportive relationship, so we just had to control the size of her period, rebuild her blood supply and get her liver circulating again with acupuncture and herbs. Once these things were accomplished she felt "…good as new!"

So now "Poor Jane" has become "Happy Healthy Jane."

The moral of Jane's (and others') stories?

If you have a problem, find someone who can help you fix it!

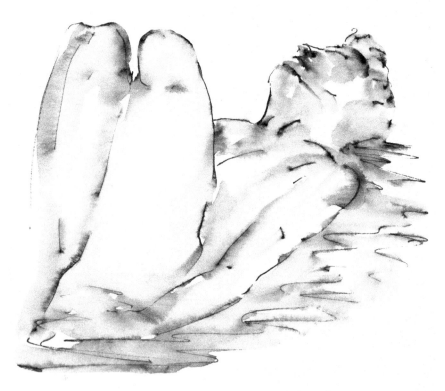

Chapter 15

The Big C:
Reducing Your Risk of Cancer

By the "Big C" I don't mean the vitamin. I mean the C that can take you, or your family and friends, to the cemetery. Not only can it, but it will and I'll tell you why. The incidence of cancer has reached epidemic proportions in America today.

The Special Case of Sally

Sally had developed breast cancer as a result of taking hormone replacement therapy (HRT) and had a mastectomy and chemotherapy. Even though both of these procedures are radically invasive, and in the case of chemotherapy quite harmful to the whole body, in Sally's case they were necessary; and that is because of the special and unique nature of cancer as a disease.

In virtually every other serious degenerative disease (arthritis, asthma, colitis, MS, etc.) the treatment strategy is the same as the preventative strategy. In other words, what you do to treat the disease is exactly the same as what you do to prevent it. You just have to do a lot more of it once the problem develops. An ounce of prevention *is* worth a pound of cure!

Cancer is a special case, however. With cancer, just the preventive strategy is not good enough to correct the disease once it has developed. With cancer a new entity has formed and is growing inside your body. It's almost as if your body has been invaded by an alien parasitic being, feeding on it with the ultimate goal of destroying it. Now you have to do something extraordinary; something more than just the effective recommendations for reducing the risk of cancer outlined later here.

Now you have to do something to conquer or destroy this invader; if you can. Cancer is so deadly, and the Western treatments (chemotherapy, surgery, and radiation) so potentially harmful, it is foolish not to adopt a preventative strategy. In our new more "cancerfied" world it is just too dangerous to do otherwise!

The Cancer Epidemic

In the year 1900 three percent of people in the U.S. developed cancer; the figure today is closer to forty percent and climbing. That's something like a thirteen hundred percent increase. Look around you, count your family and friends, do the math and you will see how many of the people you care about are going to end up with this disease; and realize that a percentage of them will die from it.

One might say, "Of course there is more cancer now than there was in the old days because people live a lot longer today and have more time to develop it. In the early 1900s the average life span was only about fifty years and today it's 78.9 (81.3 for females and 76.3 for males)." This sounds convincing but it is only part of the story. In these misleading numbers, statisticians have factored in the deaths at childbirth and deaths from childhood diseases; this serves to artificially skew the data.

For instance, in 1900 one third of children born didn't live to see their fifth birthday; today that figure is one percent. Naturally, this fact, when averaged in, will alter the data to make it look like people died, on average, so much younger in the old days than they do today. The fact is if you lived to adulthood then, your life expectancy was not terribly different than it is today.

Causes of Cancer

Let's look at some of the causes of the cancer epidemic (which will kill a larger percentage of the population than the Bubonic plague in Europe in the Middle Ages). If you understand the causes, it is easier to adopt a preventive strategy to protect yourself and your loved ones from this deadly menace. The causes of the increased incidence of cancer can be summed up in two words—*increased toxicity!!*

More poisonous agents are introduced into our water, air, domestic environment, and natural environment than ever before, and all this is done with compounds we ourselves have created! In the past one hundred years there have been more than one hundred thousand (100,000) new chemical compounds introduced into our lives; substances that do not generally exist in nature or certainly haven't existed in their present concentrations. These human-generated compounds, which we used to call "man-made," are unnatural to our bodies and, in a number of instances, harmful. On average there are thousands of new chemicals invented every year.

Toxins enter our bodies in one of three ways: ingested in what we eat and drink; absorbed through the skin; or breathed into our lungs. Either way they ultimately find their way into our blood streams. What can you do to protect yourself from this chemical onslaught? For a start you can avoid them, so let's analyze some of the places where you are likely to encounter potentially harmful chemicals.

Water

In the early 1970s, when I lived for a time in New Orleans, there were dozens of known carcinogens (cancer-causing substances) identified in the city's drinking water, and that was many years (and thousands of new chemicals) ago. Of course, New Orleans is at the tail end of the Mississippi River which picks up tons of agricultural and industrial run-off every day. The water supply in your city may be better than that, but your municipal water supply is undoubtedly introducing toxins into your body, as many of these harmful substances are not monitored or even identified yet.

To protect ourselves we can drink water that we "improve" at home. There are many home filter units and home distillation units available at moderate prices. The advantage of distillation is that it also removes heavy metals like lead and aluminum. While these metals may not be in your city's water supply, they may be in your home water if older lead pipes are present. I have my doubts about bottled "designer water"— among my reasons is that it is usually bottled in plastic, which creates its own set of problems. A 2018 study conducted by the State University of New York found that 90% of water bottled in plastic contained microplastic particles.

Personal Environment

We pick up toxins in our homes, cars, stores, work sites, places of worship, etc. Most of the chemicals that enter your body in these places are in the air you breathe. In part, these chemicals get into the air from "off-gassing" newly made products.

Some of the worst offenders are materials introduced during new construction or remodeling; including new carpeting, furniture, vinyl flooring, particle board, plywood, sheet rock, plastics, preserved woods, paints, stains, sealers, glues and insulation. As a general rule the older things are, and the longer they've been in place, the safer they are, as emissions decrease over time.

The solution is to exchange the contaminated air in these places for fresh air as much as possible, which may mean leaving doors and windows open, fans and heat pumps operating and exhaust fans in kitchens and bathrooms going as much as practical. Air-treatment devices are available, like filters, ion generators, etc.

An interesting fact relating to this issue was cited in a study showing pesticide contamination in household carpeting can be up to fifty times the outdoor level because these substances get carried in on shoes and don't get watered in or broken down by sunlight, as they would outside. To solve this problem there are three possibilities: remove all shoes at the door; vacuum daily with a good vacuum cleaner with a beater that agitates the substances up to the surface so they can be sucked in; or (my favorite) use only organic yard and gardening products.

Body Care Products

We encounter toxins in two ways; through the air (if you can smell it, it is entering your body), and through the skin in the case of topical applications. Products that may pose a risk include lotions, shampoos, conditioners, soaps, make-up, perfume, deodorant, after shave and hair spray. Incidentally, make sure your deodorant doesn't contain aluminum (a heavy metal); many do.

The safest way to resolve this is to use increasingly available "natural" body care products. Look in your local health food or natural foods store, nutritional product outlet or co-op for safe products. Be aware that the word "natural" has no legal definition and can be applied, as a marketing ploy, to anything. Always read the list of ingredients and if there are words you can't pronounce, or lots of numbers, be suspicious. Also, the more ingredients listed as organic the better.

Household Cleaning Agents

Soaps, bleach, fabric softeners, ammonia, cleansers, drain openers, furniture polish, carpet cleaners, spot removers, toilet bowl cleaners, etc. Another endless list. What are these things made of and do we know they are safe for us and our children? Not a chance!

The Solution: Use "natural" products from brands you trust. Since the word natural has no legally binding definition it behooves us to check out the manufacturer's commitment to real chemical safety (and probably their concern for the environment as well). This might eliminate many of the major producers and brand names, as most of them have shown a consistent disdain for the health of their customers and the environment.

There are safe products that could probably replace at least half of your old chemically questionable cleaning products.

Lastly in this section, I'd like to share with you the story of a chemical mishap of extreme medical significance brought on by the mixing of two common household cleaning products that may be sitting side by side in your home right now!

A young man in his mid-twenties came to me suffering from kidney failure. How deadly is that? Real deadly!

It was brought on by applying ammonia and chlorine bleach at the same time in an enclosed space.

Did you know that this is a deadly combination?

Well, neither did I!

But I know it now, and now so do you.

Why don't they don't teach us this stuff in school?

Food

Whole books have been written on the subject of the many questionable practices in food production, so even though what I have to say may not add any startlingly new information to the field, some of this will be new to you, and will be useful information you can adopt into your strategy of self and family protection.

In this category we include all beverages other than water.

There are *two broad areas* where toxins are introduced into the food chain: during the growing or raising of food products and during their processing for eventual distribution and sale.

Growing and Raising Phase: Toxins introduced into foods at this stage include chemical fertilizers, pesticides (including herbicides, fungicides, and insecticides), antibiotics and, in the case of cattle at least, the **Genetically Engineered (GE)** substance called "bovine growth hormone." All of **Chapter 23 – Sneak Attack** is devoted to potential dangers inherent in tampering with the genetic codes of our food supply.

Processing Phase: The list of added substances is long, but many of them fall into the categories of: stabilizers, preservatives, emulsifiers, artificial flavors, flavor enhancers (even including some "natural flavors") and more. The bottom line is, the less tampered with the better. I am reminded of an old adage with more than a little truth in it: "Don't eat anything advertised on TV!" Ever seen a carrot or broccoli advertised on TV?

There are literally thousands of chemicals that enter our bodies through the foods we eat, and yet the long range consequences to our health from this chemical feast are unknown. I am not convinced that the manufacturers of these substances, or the producers/processors who use them, place as much value on our health as they do on the health of their own bottom line.

The solution to the introduction of toxins through your food can be summed up in just three words: Organic, Organic, Organic!

Food Preparation and Storage

Cookware—Don't Use!

Aluminum: Aluminum is a heavy metal (like mercury and lead) harmful to (at the very least) the nervous system. Many researchers conclude it is a clear contributor to Alzheimer's disease as well as Parkinson's, multiple sclerosis, and even Lou Gehrig's disease. To be fair, there are other means by which extra aluminum can enter the body but it is prudent to minimize our exposure in any way we can, so get rid of your aluminum pots and pans.

Cookware with Non-Stick Coatings: These products are known to emit carcinogenic (cancer causing) agents and poisonous substances (including PF1B, a chemical warfare agent!) when heated to temperatures easily reachable on your stovetop. Many pet birds die as a result of inhaling fumes from heated non-stick cookware. Birds have extra sensitive lungs which is why they used to bring canaries into coal mines; when poisonous gas levels got so high the canary died, they knew it was time to get the humans out of there.

So, the bad news is, these coatings give off breathable toxins; the good news is they only do this when heated. So as long as you don't heat them they are safe! Do you (like me) have a problem with the logic here?

DR. GERALD SENOGLES

Cookware—Do Use!

Stainless steel, cast iron, glass or Pyrex, porcelain, enamel, or ceramic pots and pans.

Food Storage—Don't Use!

Plastic Containers: These create various problems, not the least of which is a significant reduction in sperm count in men and an increase in abnormal sperm cells; two of the reasons for a serious decline in birth rates in developed countries where we have the luxury of these modern conveniences. If your restaurant leftovers happen to come home with you in a styrofoam container, transfer them to something from the list below.

Minimize: Aluminum foil and plastic wraps.

Food Storage—Do Use!

Glass, Pyrex, ceramic or stainless steel containers.

Drugs

And then there are drugs! Whether legal or illegal, recreational or medicinal, prescription or over the counter, drugs are, by their very design, unnatural and harmful to one or another parts of your system. One thing for certain is, at the very least, your liver is going to be adversely impacted by every drug you take.

An example of a legal recreational drug directly linkable to cancer is tobacco, which clearly leads to an increased risk of lung cancer. Also, did you know that excess coffee intake is directly linked to pancreatic cancer—another real deadly one?

An example of a medicinal prescription drug linkable to cancer is hormone replacement therapy **(HRT)**. **HRT** increases the risk of both breast and uterine cancer, as well as other medical problems (for more on this see **Chapter 21 - Men... a Pause**). Anecdotally, in a conversation with a Registered Nurse friend of mine who often works in the oncology (cancer) ward in a local hospital, she commented on the many cancer patients in their 30s and 40s. She also noticed that the majority of these relatively young cancer victims had spent significant time on antidepressant drugs. Interesting, yes? Not hard scientific data, but surely food for thought.

So, when we look at what we are doing differently now than in 1900 that might account for the increase in this dreaded disease, we might also look at our radical increase in drug use, and our belief (promulgated by the pharmaceutical industry) that every little problem requires a drug for its solution.

Nuclear and Chemical Waste

Chernobyl, Three Mile Island, Love Canal, Bhopal (India)—all are sites of nuclear or chemical disasters; sometimes responsible for considerable loss of life, or an increase in the incidence of serious disease. How much of this are we subjected to and don't even know it?

Take Charge of Your Cancer Probabilities

Besides the recommendation to reduce or avoid various sources of toxicity, other, more proactive measures can be employed to reduce our likelihood of getting cancer. To understand these measures, below is a general picture of the mechanisms of cancer's beginnings and growth.

Our bodies are made up of trillions of living entities called cells; like all living beings they share certain characteristics like growth and reproduction. Each cell contains strands of DNA called chromosomes, and on these are units called genes that carry our hereditary characteristics.

Cells periodically split and replicate themselves to provide for growth and the necessary replacement of cells injured or dead. For myriad reasons, this process of replication can go awry and create "rogue cells" that reproduce incorrectly or at accelerated rates, causing neoplasms (new growths of excess tissue), some of which can be malignant. As we look at the cellular level, there are several things to consider: the way cells replicate and how this can go wrong and the methods the body has of protecting itself and correcting potential problems.

Fortunately, one of the best ways to assist both of these mechanisms is through a diet rich in fruits and vegetables. The Wall Street Journal informs us that even the staid American Cancer Society promotes this as one of the best ways to avoid cancer. Their recommendation is to eat a minimum of five to seven servings of fruits and vegetables per day.

The ways fruits and vegetables provide this protection are twofold: the positive effects on cellular reproduction and their support of immune system function.

DR. GERALD SENOGLES

In each fruit or vegetable there are thousands of different phytochemicals & nutrients, most of which are yet unknown and un-catalogued. Alone or in combination, they provide our bodies with a wealth of usable substances (like antioxidants) that reduce the "oxidative stress" each and every cell is subjected to thousands of times each day. Oxidative stress is a result of free radicals generated by normal biological processes, as well as the chemical stresses introduced by our increasingly chemicalized world. Many believe these oxidative "hits" to our chromosomes are a definite factor in the aberrant replication and proliferation of rogue cells.

The second way phytonutrients help us is by strengthening the immune system. We are aware that these nutritional elements increase T-cell activity, as well as the activity of "natural killer" (NK) cells; the cells that seek out and destroy cancer cells.

Whatever the mechanisms at work, one thing is very clear: over two hundred epidemiological studies from around the world demonstrate that the richer your diet is in plant foods, the lower your risk of developing cancer and many other serious diseases, including those that can bring on life threatening events, like stroke and heart attack.

For many of us with busy lives, and limited appetites, it may be impossible to eat five to ten servings in a day, so I recommend a "whole food" supplement (not to be confused with a vitamin/mineral supplement). There are several whole food supplements on the market; some are available at stores but some are only available through distributors. Check the internet!

Prevention

Prevention is the smartest strategy when dealing with disease; we only need treatment if prevention fails.

In Western (allopathic) Medicine, with its principle modalities of drugs and surgery, there really is no preventive strategy, as drugs and surgery are not good for your health in general, unless you get in so much medical trouble that you need them, and you hope you don't!

Western Medicine's concentration is on attacking disease already developed, so it is to the world of "natural" medicine we must look for prevention. We define a natural medical system as one that doesn't focus on attacking a particular disease, but rather on assisting the body in protecting and healing itself.

Natural practitioners believe the body has the inherent wisdom and capacity to take care of itself—it just may need a little help and guidance from time to time. Oriental Medicine is firmly in this camp, as are many other "alternative" therapies like homeopathy, herbology, chiropractic, Ayurvedic Medicine, iridology, therapeutic massage, and even vitamin and mineral supplementation.

To help understand how Oriental Medicine aids in the prevention of cancer let us first examine the scientific concept of "necessary but not sufficient" as it applies to cause and effect.

If something is necessary to a cause and effect relationship it means the relationship cannot occur without it. End of story!

If an element is not sufficient in a cause and effect relationship it means that it will not bring about the effect without other contributory factors. For example, it may be necessary to step onto a street to get hit by a car, but alone it is not sufficient; there must also be a car driving down the street that we can step in front of.

In Oriental Medicine we recognize two necessary (but not sufficient) preconditions that must exist in your body for cancer to develop: an energy deficiency and an energy circulation problem. Since both of these are necessary for cancer to establish itself, if we can ensure at least one of these is not present, then you cannot develop cancer!

Energy Deficiency can be in specific sites within the organism, or in the whole organism. One can feel energetic and still suffer with this pathology. To remove this precondition we must build energy. Besides all of the obvious methods to maintain good energy, like proper diet, exercise, rest, mental and emotional balance, etc., it is useful to build our energy supplies with natural substances and procedures.

In Oriental Medicine we use acupuncture and herbal tonics to build energy. An excellent herbal formula called Bu zhong Yi Qi Wan (literal translation: Tonify Center [digestion] to Invigorate Energy Pills) contains the powerful energy building/cancer fighting herb, Astragalus.

As always, every herbal formula isn't right for everybody so best be analyzed by an expert to make sure it is appropriate for you.

Circulation Problems: As it applies to cancer it is an energy (as distinct from blood) circulation retardation issue. The circulation of energy in your body is under the control of the liver, so it is to liver circulating formulas and acupuncture we look for prevention and correction.

There are some very powerful acupuncture points for improving circulation through the liver, and some valuable and effective herbal formulas. Because energy circulation problems are so common and so disruptive, all of **Chapter 14 - Blocked Energy** is devoted to this subject.

Cancer and Heredity

A common misconception goes something like this: "I don't have to worry because cancer doesn't run in my family." The problem with this statement is it implies genetics as the principle determinant of your risk of getting cancer, and this simply is not true!

The huge increase in the incidence of cancer in the last one hundred years is not a result of genetic change (genes don't change that much in only 4-5 generations), but rather a result of our increasingly toxic environment. The fact that "Grandma" didn't develop cancer does not afford you much protection, if any, but rather reflects the fact that she was born and lived most of her life in a less toxic and therefore less cancer prone world! Whatever way one chooses, it behooves us to do something to actively reduce the probabilities of developing cancer—it is just too dangerous to do nothing, given the risks involved!

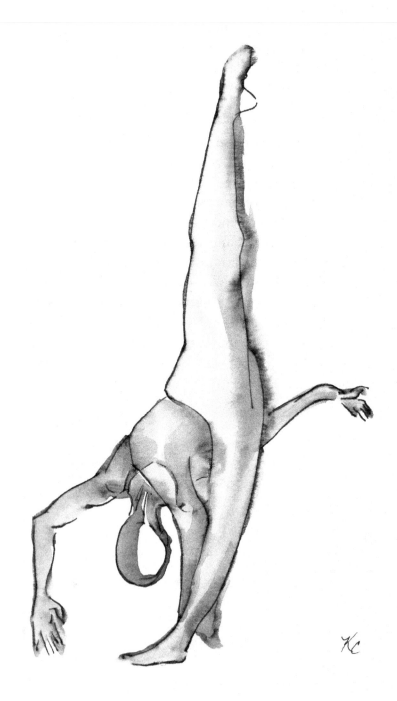

Chapter 16

Getting Well: What Does It Take to Really Solve Health Problems and What Do You Have to Go Through?

The Path to Wellness

What might you need to do to get well? Or, what program would work for you to achieve the maximum state of health of which your body is capable?

Because I work in a particular field, I will principally speak of a realistic program in that field, which does not imply it is the only discipline, but that it is one of the best and should, I believe, be consulted by anyone before launching into a program of drugs or surgery.

Naturally I cannot tell you, the reader, what would be the correct program for you at this time, but we can begin by discussing some of the considerations in determining how much correction a particular body needs:

1. The Nature of The Problem

Fibromyalgia, or even asthma, certainly requires more of a corrective program (read: more treatments) than an "arthritic" knee or a tennis elbow; the latter two, more confined to a localized area of the body, would likely not involve such serious systemic malfunctions. As a general rule, the more serious a problem, the more serious (and therefore lengthy) the solution.

2. How Long Has The Problem Existed?

Generally speaking, the longer a problem has existed, the more work it will take to correct it. Problems can build up for years (referred to as "latent disease") before a symptom shows up, so many conditions have been around much longer than just the presence of their symptoms indicate. The exception, of course, is a problem brought on by an accident or injury. Even though these may have been with someone for only a short time, they often require considerably more time and treatments to correct than exactly the same problem (a sore neck or back for instance) that just started spontaneously.

3. The General Health and Energy of the Patient

Any medical system trying to facilitate real healing (and Oriental Medicine is certainly one of these!) must take into account, and work within the limitations of, just how much healing capacity exists in the body of a particular patient at a particular time.

For example, if a patient is very sick, perhaps frail or feeble, then their energy level is severely diminished and only so much energy can be directed toward the healing process at that time. We must, therefore, work to increase that diminished amount of energy so the patient gets a little better.

With some patients, it is a slow, gradual building process, just to get enough energy available to facilitate healing. If one tries to push a body to heal faster than its capacity at a given time, the patient will probably feel slightly worse (extra tired) after a treatment.

In fact, not properly assessing a body's healing limitations (and therefore over-treating) is one of the most common mistakes young/new practitioners in the healing arts make. In the beginning years of my medical practice I was certainly guilty of this myself.

The Length of a Treatment Program

I've heard guidelines proposed in other natural healing professions where they say, "Expect one month of a treatment program for every year you have had your problem." This doesn't seem unreasonable to me, but I don't make such hard and fast statements.

I know Chiropractors who propose three adjustments/week for 6-8 weeks, then two adjustments/week for 6-8 weeks, then one adjustment/week for 6-8 weeks and then recommend monthly maintenance. I rarely propose such an extensive program, but I certainly have seen patients who require that much work to truly get well.

The point is, it can take real effort and dedication, and yes, even money (but I don't consider money worth much if you don't have your health), to achieve the real state of health and wellness that makes life the really fun and exciting adventure it can be.

DR. GERALD SENOGLES

The Right Questions

We are all healthcare consumers. Most people wouldn't buy a car without having a few basic questions answered first, like: how long will it last, how much will I have to spend on maintenance, and how much will it cost me in the first place? These are not bad questions to ask of a healthcare provider, either.

And one more: "When should I be able to experience some improvement so I know your program is making the difference my body needs?"

Remember, patience is a virtue when it comes to real healing, so don't expect things to improve greatly right away. After all, it took you your whole life to get in the condition you're in.

To my impatient patients, I sometimes say, "What I'm doing here is medicine and that takes time and work; if you're looking for a miracle (instant healing) go to church and pray for it, but don't be surprised if you don't get it."

My advice is, find a knowledgeable and honest practitioner and commit to following the proposed program and give them a real chance to make the corrections you need. When things don't work out it is more often because the patient has failed to commit and follow through with the program recommended by a practitioner.

Don't Quit!

Be a Winner!

Good Luck and Good Health!

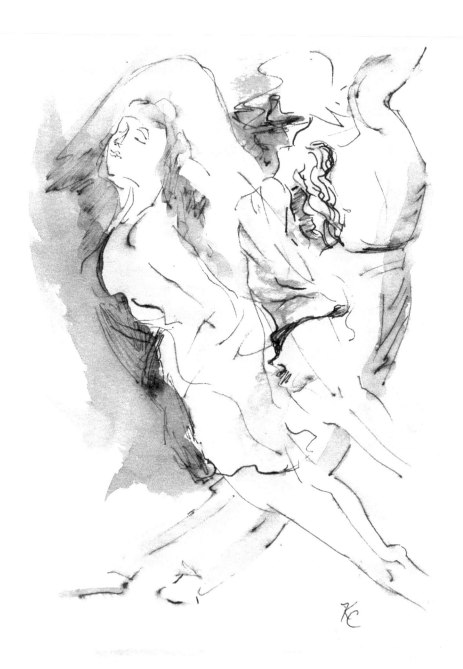

Chapter 17

Hot and Cold Colds

The Case of "Sorry Steve"

Steve was a truly sorry looking sight, and he felt miserable to boot! It seemed that every cold and flu season Steve got one or two colds, and each one lasted 3-4 weeks.

Even though many people think winter is the principle season for colds and flus, they are actually more prevalent in the spring and fall, and usually die down with the really cold weather of winter or really hot weather of summer. So each spring and fall Steve was sick multiple times and getting sick and tired of being sick and tired.

Because his colds always wound up in his lungs with the symptom of coughing, we determined his lungs and defensive energy ("wei chi," discussed in **Chapter 5 - The Digestive System**) were weak. We also discovered that he had a weak digestive system.

The digestive system is a very important source of our basic energy; since Steve's digestion was not working well he wasn't getting enough energy out of the foods he ate and, consequently, his storehouse of defensive energy was not being replenished. Strengthening his digestion and lungs helped Steve get back on track.

In Oriental Medicine we will tolerate one or two 7-10 day colds a year. If people don't get too sick we feel this is acceptable and not worth undertaking a large program of systemic strengthening to correct.

I don't mean to imply that it's good to have a cold or two a year, but that it's within an acceptable range. Steve's circumstance illustrates how symptoms that show up in one organ can be caused, or exacerbated by, malfunctions in another part of the body altogether, as his digestive weakness was part of the reason he got sick so often.

Outside vs. Inside Conditions

Every medical system has various ways to categorize and organize symptoms or diseases, so a proper strategy of treatment can be applied. Oriental Medicine is no exception.

While there are many different categorizations in Oriental Medicine I want to introduce one particular one here in **Chapter 17**, and that is: **Outside vs. Inside Conditions**. This refers to the difference between diseases we "catch" from the outside as opposed to ones we develop on the inside.

Outside Conditions include colds and flus; pneumonia and other bacterial or viral respiratory infections; stomach or intestinal flus (which include the symptoms of nausea, vomiting and/or diarrhea); food poisoning; allergic responses to external allergens (hay fever, etc.); and problems brought on by accidents or injuries.

Outside Conditions share certain characteristics even when the symptoms are quite different: diarrhea vs. a cough for instance. Outside conditions often come on suddenly; one day (or hour) you are fine and the next thing you know you are sick as a dog. Also, they are often self-limiting; which means, even if left untreated they will likely clear up on their own in a relatively short period of time (if they don't kill you first). Because of the suddenness of their onset, as well as their possible severity, these are also referred to as "acute" conditions.

Inside Conditions are problems we develop rather than catch. They include all degenerative conditions like: diabetes, insomnia, PMS, cancer, heart disease, MS, arthritis, asthma, constipation, Parkinson's disease, headaches, acid reflux, etc. This large category of conditions usually take a longer period of time to develop and often come on more gradually. They are usually not self-limiting (they don't go away on their own) and if left untreated can be very disruptive or even deadly. These are also referred to as "chronic" conditions. Inside Conditions usually involve structural or functional problems with the organs and glands.

Colds

One small class of outside (acute) conditions is the common Cold. I refer to colds as a "class of conditions" because in Oriental Medicine we categorize colds into more than one type and treat them differently according to their symptoms; one person's cold is not necessarily the same as another person's cold.

Also true is that one person's cold may not necessarily manifest the same symptoms as another person's cold as it runs its course. A cold may begin as a tickle in the throat or a funny feeling in the sinuses, but end up a few days later as a serious cough producing lots of thick yellow sputum. Because there is a fairly predictable sequence we refer to these changes as the "stages" of a cold. And because colds have different symptoms at different stages, they require different strategies of treatment as they progress.

Here are some characteristics of different types of colds and the different stages.

The Surface Stage

One differentiation we make with outside conditions is the level of penetration of the disease process. For our purposes, there are two: the surface level, and the deeper (interior) level (this is the level of the organs and glands). By the surface level we mean the musculo-skeletal system. The organ level speaks for itself.

Colds tend to start at the surface level. Symptoms here include a sore throat, sinus issues, sneezing, headache or body aches, slight chills or fever, etc. At this level, if the proper strategy is applied, the penetration of the disease process can often be stopped and the cold driven out completely. If this occurs, of course, the cold never reaches the level of the organs and glands (with colds, that's the lungs). Some of you may have driven colds out at this stage with the use of Vitamin C, zinc, or another substances that work for you, but I'd like to introduce some other Surface Relievers.

Surface Relievers

When a cold is at the surface level you can use **Surface Relievers** to drive it out. Part of the strategy of surface relief is diaphoresis: to cause a sweat. Some Chinese herbal formulas accomplish this, as does aspirin — the problem with aspirin, however, is that you bleed a teaspoon of blood into your intestines with every one you take. This is one of the reasons that aspirin kills thousands of Americans every year.

A better way is to take either western herbs with a diaphoretic action, or the venerable Chinese herbal formula Yin Chiao Chieh Tu Pien. If taken in substantial doses this formula will often end a cold before it barely begins. It is necessary to take it immediately at the first sign of a cold, so keep it on hand. If the cold does continue its penetration, this will at least make it milder.

Hot and Cold Colds

We also categorize colds as either **Hot Colds** or **Cold Colds**. At the surface level they often don't manifest strong tendencies either way, so a good surface reliever like Yin Chiao is always appropriate. If a cold is not driven out at the surface but continues to penetrate towards the interior level, it often begins to show clear signs of either heat or coolness and indeed, can change from one to the other; most likely from cold to hot.

Cold Colds

Forget about them! 1) They are usually not that serious, and 2) I almost never see them (at least in America) and I'll tell you why. Even though it is true that many colds arrive at the surface with a cold nature, they usually transform into hot colds as they penetrate deeper toward the lungs. The reason is that as they penetrate, our bodies begin to "imprint" their own natures onto the cold, and that means in America (and I suspect much of the Western World), they begin to get hot. American culture is generally overheated, over-stimulated and excessive, and this influences our body's physical nature.

Some of the excesses contributing to this over-stimulating (heating) process are caffeine, sugar, alcohol, tobacco, meat, deep fried foods, and television. Television is not just over-stimulating because of the program content, but also from "fast cut" editing that never allows any one image to remain on screen for more than a few seconds. This continual abrupt change in visuals is a stimulating "hit" to your nervous system, the intended consequence is to continually draw you back to the program, which it usually does, with the unintended consequence of over stimulating (heating) your nervous system, and by extension, your whole body.

Some signs of a *cold* cold are: body aches, mild sore throat, headache, thin watery nasal discharge and substantial chills.

Hot Colds

If colds are not driven out at the surface but continue to penetrate into your body, they are liable to show signs of heat, and also may penetrate to the level of the lungs. Some indications that a cold is *hot* include: a severe sore throat, thick colored phlegm, burning pain in the bronchial tubes when you cough, and/or a substantial fever accompanied by the desire to avoid heat.

As always, it isn't necessary that you manifest all of the signs of heat to establish this diagnosis; in this case just the severity of the throat pain or the colored sputum would be enough.

Many of the signs of heat are considered signs of an "infection" in the West, but if you follow the heat reducing strategies outlined here your "infection" will likely clear up without resorting to the use of drugs. In fact, one of the reasons antibiotics work with these conditions is because they are very cold in nature. You may also know that antibiotics are vastly over prescribed, have no effect on viral diseases (like colds), and destroy the "good" bacteria, which you must have in your body.

A general principle in Oriental Medicine is to treat a disease with its opposite. If a disease is hot (or excess) treat it with cold (or reductive) procedures or substances, and if a disease is cold (or deficient) treat it with warming (or toning) substances or procedures.

Treating Hot Colds

If you are sure your cold has reached a hot stage you can treat it with heat reducing strategies, like avoiding caffeine, meat, spices, sugar, alcohol, and deep fried foods, and to emphasize cooling foods like fruits and vegetables (except phlegm producing bananas and oranges).

One of the fastest ways to reduce heat is through acupuncture. Acupuncture also helps relieve cold symptoms, including headaches, sinus pressure and congestion, body aches, sore throat, cough and just that general sick feeling.

Heat reducing (cold) herbs or herbal formulas are also effective. A good Western herb is goldenseal while Huang Lien Shang Ching Pien is an excellent Chinese herbal formula.

In Oriental Medicine we know the important connection between the colon (large intestine) and the lungs, and this factors in especially with a

Hot Cold. It is important to keep the colon emptying well with a **Hot Cold**, so a small amount of mild laxative can be useful. Also, Huang Lien Shang Ching Pien includes the gentle but effective laxative herb Rhubarb Root.

If you don't have access to a mild laxative, emphasize laxative foods in your diet, like prunes, figs, pears or peaches, and avoid constipating foods like milk and milk products, white flour products and bananas. I tell my patients to determine the proper level of laxatives or laxative foods by the actions of their intestines (we are not trying to create diarrhea here, just a good emptying out). I tell them that it is okay to have one more (possibly looser than usual) bowel movement per day than they normally do while treating a **Hot Cold**. It is also wise to drink plenty of liquids to stay well hydrated when dealing with this or any hot condition.

A note of caution: one must be very careful when giving laxatives to children, as too many loose stools can quickly lead to dehydration, especially in little ones. Give only small doses of mild laxatives to children and only if the child is missing bowel movements altogether. Huang Lien Shang Ching Pien should never be given to children under ten years of age.

DR. GERALD SENOGLES

THE DANGERS OF ANTI-INFLAMMATORY PAIN RELIEVING DRUGS.

NSAIDs (nonsteroidal anti-inflammatory drugs), like Aleve, Advil, ibuprofen, aspirin, naproxen, etc. cause gastrointestinal bleeding leading to the deaths of tens of thousands of Americans every year.

While I am on the subject of the potential dangers of over-the-counter (OTC) pain relievers I want to share some recent information on Tylenol (acetaminophen).

This information is from a newsletter published by Dr. Joe Mercola on March 26, 2014: "Each year acetaminophen overdose is the leading cause of calls to poison control... it is responsible for more than 56,000 emergency room visits... is responsible for nearly half of all acute liver failure cases in the US. It can be toxic to your liver even at recommended doses when taken daily for just a couple of weeks."

I think the message here is that all pain relieving drugs, and all drugs for that matter, are to some degree harmful to your body and need to be taken as sparingly as possible. Plus, keep an eye out for any unusual or unpleasant changes in your health and consult a medical professional to see if they may be from something you're taking.

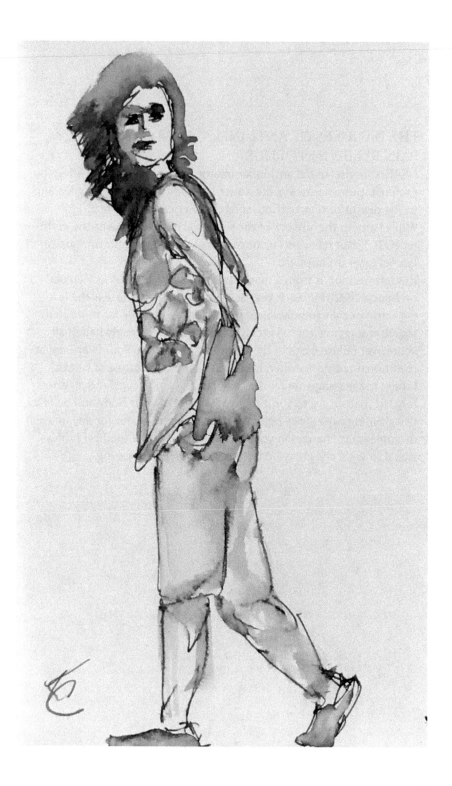

Chapter 18

Phlegm Fatale:
Phlegm Diseases and Their Cures

Phlegm—It's More Troublesome than You Think.

Is phlegm potentially fatal? Really? The answer is, "Yes, it is!" Even though most of us who encounter phlegm in a disease process, like a cold or a sinus infection, aren't likely to die from that disease, there are other diseases, potentially fatal, where phlegm is a major or causative factor.

The Case of "Goopy Glenda"

Glenda came in because she was tired of having multiple "sinus infections" every year, and being repeatedly put on antibiotics. About every 6-8 weeks she had another "infection" and ended up on drugs. After three or four years it became clear to her that her current method of addressing this problem wasn't working, and she was taking many more drugs than were good for her. Her doctor was also at a loss as to how to break this cycle of disease.

Upon examination we determined her "sinus infections" were really the result of her system creating much too much phlegm. We could tell this because she blew out copious quantities when she was sick, and also had lots in her sinuses and throat between her acute episodes.

There is an old adage, "Flies don't create garbage, they just show up where it collects." In this same way the bacteria/viruses of her infections were just proliferating where they had a nice nutritious medium in which to propagate. Phlegm is not, after all, a massive accumulation of germs but, in fact is a massive accumulation of undigested food that can play host to a large number of harmful microorganisms.

After a combination of acupuncture, herbal formulas (particularly Ehr Chen Wan), and dietary modifications over the course of several months, she didn't need any more drugs, and eventually controlled her problem (which would want to recur periodically) with the herbal formulas used on an "as needed" basis, plus a little maintenance acupuncture.

Chinese herbs can be used over a long period of time—years if necessary. Every herb is certainly not right for every body but if you find something that makes your disease condition *behave better*, you can be pretty sure that it just helping your body *work better*. As always, it is best to consult with an expert while undergoing any long term medical regimen.

The Mucusless Diet

When I first began medical studies in the early 1970s, I was introduced to an alternative medical classic called *The Mucusless Diet Healing System* by Professor Arnold Ehret. In the Mucusless Diet, the good professor proposed that mucus (we shall use the terms mucus and phlegm interchangeably) was a significant factor in many degenerative disease processes, and a cause of much suffering and even early death. He determined that certain foods were more likely to form phlegm in ones system than others, and advised people to eliminate those foods from their diets.

A table in his book shows the mucus forming tendency of individual foods and assigns numerical values (based on scientific tests) to show the likelihood of their becoming phlegm in your body.

Professor Ehret advises us to remove highly mucus forming foods from our diets. Unfortunately his list of taboo foods includes meats, eggs, milk and cheese, fats and oils, cereals (by which he means all grain and flour products), legumes (all beans and peas), potatoes, rice, and nuts. Perhaps if we removed all these foods from our diets we would live longer, *or perhaps it would just feel that way!*

You will be glad to know there is another way to solve problems of excess mucus or phlegm production other than removing more than half the foods you eat and that a certain amount of mucus in the system is the correct state of affairs.

Mucus Membranes

Certain cavities (hollow spaces) in our bodies are lined with a tissue called a "mucus membrane." This type of tissue exudes a thin moisture coating called "mucus" that keeps the lining of these cavities moist and this is as it should be. For instance, there is supposed to be a thin moisture coating inside your sinuses and when the amount is correct you are not even aware it is there. You would, however, be aware if it were not there: your sinuses would feel unpleasantly dry, or perhaps even burny or achy, and you would know something was wrong.

In other words, when the amount of mucus coating is correct you just feel "normal." But what about the opposite circumstance? What about when there is too much moisture?

Phlegm

There can be copious quantities of thick gooey stuff issuing forth from our sinuses that we can clearly recognize as pathological. This gelatinous goo is not the desired thin moisture coating but is instead a pathological byproduct of incompletely digested food.

The purpose of digestion is to take large substances (food) and break them down into small enough particles to be absorbed into the blood stream through the walls of the small intestine. If this function is not performed properly, and the food is only partially broken down, it can become a thick gooey gunk that can circulate out of the stomach and go to other parts of the body and create problems.

So we see what Professor Ehret called "mucus forming foods" are just foods that can be, in some systems, particularly hard to digest and therefore likely to become phlegm. The Oriental strategy to resolve this problem is not to eliminate most foods from the diet, but instead to strengthen the digestive process so even these hard to digest foods will be broken down into usable component parts. Anything that aids the body in this breaking down process (like supplementing with digestive enzymes) could serve to help eliminate phlegm disorders.

Acupuncture is an especially powerful tool for strengthening the digestive system, plus there are certain points that particularly target phlegm reduction. Ehr Chen Wan is specially formulated for this purpose.

Phlegm production issues can be especially resistant to solution, so it is recommended that one try this formula for up to three months to determine if it is helping, and for whatever amount of time thereafter that is required to solve the problem.

As always though, it is best to consult with an expert while undergoing any long term medical/herbal regimen.

Phlegm Diseases

There are certain places we tend to encounter phlegm and therefore know that we have a phlegm-based problem. Typically these are the sinuses, throat, lungs, or possibly the stool. It is easy to see the contribution phlegm makes to asthma, emphysema, respiratory infections (colds, bronchitis, pneumonia), sinusitis, mucus colitis, post nasal drip, etc. But phlegm can circulate to other parts of the body, where we do not overtly encounter it, and contribute to a number of other disease states including dizziness or vertigo, Parkinson's disease, epilepsy or other seizure disorders, leucorrhea, some schizophrenias, arteriosclerosis, pain or stiffness in the joints, lymphoma, and even breast cancer.

Until the digestion can be strengthened enough to eliminate excess phlegm/mucus production, it is best to minimize phlegm forming (difficult to digest) foods in one's diet. This includes sugar, milk products, corn syrup, white flour products, fatty meats, cheap or hydrogenated oils (including margarine), and bananas and oranges.

DR. GERALD SENOGLES

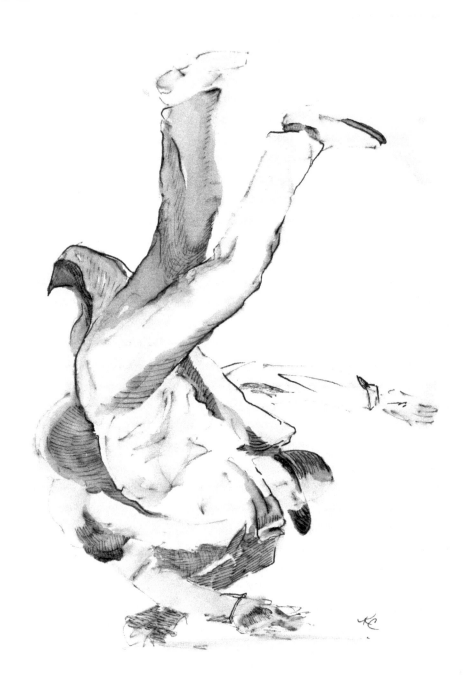

Chapter 19

Don't Need a Break:
Bone Health and Strength

Broken bones—Who needs 'em?

B roken bones can be anything from pretty disruptive to deadly and are at least going to interfere with life for some considerable time. Besides just being careful to avoid them, is there anything one can do to minimize risk in this area? The answer fortunately, is yes!

One of the keys to bone health and strength is mineral density: the denser our bones are, the stronger they are and the less likely to break. The easiest way to discuss bone density is with the problem of loss of density, such a common problem it has been given its own name, **Osteoporosis**.

Osteoporosis

The U.S. Surgeon General warns of a serious decline in bone health in the United States. His report states 10 million Americans over the age of 50 have osteoporosis while another 34 million are at risk. Risk factors for developing osteoporosis include age, diet, lifestyle, menopause, drugs, alcohol, and tobacco. Even though both men and women sustain a half a percent bone loss per year after the age of 50, women are 6 times more likely to develop osteoporosis than men.

Why is that?

The answer in a word is "menopause."

Menopause

The changes in a woman's body at the time of permanent cessation of the menses (menopause) include an accelerated bone loss. Women lose 1-3% of their bone mass density every year for 5-7 years after menopause. Believe me when I say that this is a very meaningful statistic; it is also why women need to do something proactive at this time (and beyond) to counter the deleterious effects of this event.

So, while it's true that both men and women experience bone loss as they get older, women are "ahead" of men by virtue of the accelerated bone loss following menopause.

Maintaining/Increasing Bone Density

Some other factors in determining bone density (and therefore improving it when needed) are: the amount of dietary calcium (plus certain other factors like phosphorous, magnesium, boron, and vitamins A, C, and D), the body's ability to absorb and assimilate minerals and the amount of weight-bearing exercise in someone's lifestyle, which causes the minerals to be deposited on the bones.

A particular contribution from Oriental Medicine is that the status and strength of the kidney/adrenal complex also helps determine bone strength and density. More on this connection later.

Dietary Calcium

The main issues here are how much calcium is in your diet and how much is actually absorbed by and made available to your body. Minerals are "cold" by nature and cold substances are hard to digest. Ever try taking a bite out of an oyster shell? The point is, it isn't just the amount of calcium in some particular food you eat but whether your body can absorb and utilize it. This is the problem with pasteurized cow's milk; it has a high calcium content but is virtually indigestible in many bodies so very little, if any, of the calcium is made available to increase bone density.

While it may be useful for some people to take calcium supplements, the most usable source is from our foods. To help you get started, here is a partial list of foods with good calcium content—the numbers represent milligrams (mg) of calcium per serving:

30-80 mg: soy, cheese, greens, lobster, oranges, spinach, apricots, broccoli, beans, sunflower seeds.

150-300 mg: oat flakes, clams, ocean fish, sesame seeds, peanuts, garbanzo beans.

More than 300 mg: tofu, almonds, collard greens, shrimp, brazil nuts, broiled skinless chicken, bone meal.

1000-25000 mg: kelp, salmon, and beef liver.

Because of serious problems with food production in the modern world, I strongly recommend buying organically grown food when possible.

Bone Density and Drugs

There are some medications that adversely affect bone density. Some examples include steroids (including inhalers for asthma), blood thinners, anti-seizure medications, thyroid drugs, chemotherapy, and anti-depressants.

Go online to find out if any of the drugs you take have this side effect, or ask your doctor, the less desirable of the two options as doctors are not always up on the latest research or may not want to admit that something they recommend may prove harmful to you.

There are also drugs prescribed to increase bone density but, as always, you must weigh the supposed benefits against the potentially damaging side effects to see if the risk is worth it.

The most common class of anti-osteoporosis drugs are called bisphosphonates (Fosamax, etc.). These do seem to increase bone density at various sites around the body but it isn't clear how long the effects last if someone stops taking it, as the increase goes away after a time.

A recent discovery is that a small percentage of people taking these drugs develop osteonecrosis (literally: "bone death") of the jaw; a condition where whole sections of the jaw and teeth can die and need to be surgically removed. A not very common but very serious complication. When it comes to drugs there is no free ride!

Studies have also found that people who took proton pump inhibitors (Nexium, Prilosec, Previcid, etc.) for acid reflux had a moderately greater incidence of hip fractures. Apparently, the longer it is taken and the higher the dose, the more problematic it is.

Kidney/Adrenal Complex and Bones

As you already learned in **Chapter 7 - The Kidneys,** the kidneys are very important to your health. For our purposes, what matters here is that they "rule" the teeth and bones. By rule we mean that the status of your bones (their strength and proper functioning) is partially dependent upon the strength and functioning of your kidneys.

Besides acupuncture to strengthen kidneys and bones I also recommend the use of herbal supplements especially designed for this purpose. One of my favorite Chinese herbal formulas is *Osteo 8* by Evergreen Herbs, as of this writing, only available through Oriental medical practitioners. This, or a similar formula, can be used to speed the healing of bone fractures.

Oriental Medicine is the primary system (so far) that understands the kidney/bone connection, so look under acupuncture or herbs (Oriental) in the yellow pages for a practitioner. In whatever manner you choose, proactively addressing bone density and supporting kidney strength is a valuable strategy.

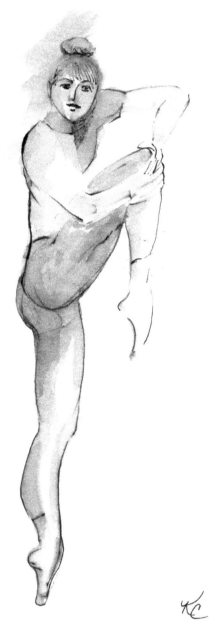

Chapter 20

Shelf Defense: The Basics of Nutrition and Protecting Yourself from Fake Food and Other Dietary Abominations

Our bodies require things that must be provided by what we ingest (eat and drink). One requirement is fuel in the form of glucose, for energy; another is the raw materials necessary for the replacement of weak, injured, or dead cells and for growth.

Therefore, it should come as no surprise that the quality of the foods you eat and drink is an important factor in your overall health profile. Unfortunately, many of the products on your grocer's shelves represented as food are not really food and do not help meet your daily requirements for fuel and nutrients. Some may even be doing more harm than good.

Basics of Nutrition

The bulk of the nutrients you need are provided by foods that fall into three categories: carbohydrates, fats and oils, and proteins.

Carbohydrates

All sugars and starches, and most fiber, consist of carbohydrates. There are two types of "carbs"—simple and complex.

Simple carbohydrates are known as sugars. There are many forms of sugar besides just the white stuff (sucrose) sprinkled on cereal in the morning. (In fact, this is one of the worst kinds. Any ingredient listed in packaged, canned or processed food that ends in …ose, is a sugar.)

Digested sugars enter the bloodstream through the walls of the small intestine and travel to the cells and the liver. The cells, with the aid of insulin, absorb the glucose and convert it into energy. Some glucose is stored in the liver and muscles in the form of glycogen, which can be readily converted to glucose when needed. Any excess glucose is converted to (and stored as) fat.

Because of the speed of absorption and conversion to energy (glucose or "blood sugar") in the body, we must be thoughtful in the use of all sugars including sucrose, honey, maple syrup, high fructose corn sweetener, dextrose, maltose, lactose, etc.

The "quick hit" of glucose the body receives from simple carbohydrates can cause the pancreas to oversupply insulin, thereby bringing blood sugar down too low, too rapidly, leading to the roller coaster effect of a sugar rush followed by a real energy low, tempting us to go for the quick hit of energy from sugar again; and on and on it goes. This recurrent over-stimulation of the pancreatic function can eventually lead to pancreatic exhaustion and disorders like hypoglycemia, or even diabetes, in the future.

Complex Carbohydrates are known as starches, actually long chains of sugar molecules strung together. Starches are digested and absorbed more slowly than sugars and provide us with a more steady, balanced source of energy over a longer period of time. Also, this doesn't overtax the pancreas and lead to the high/low roller coaster ride that simple carbohydrates do, making this the preferred way to get our energy. Starches also tend to come in more nutritionally rich foods like bread, pasta, beans, rice, potatoes and vegetables, while sugars tend to be in nutritionally empty foods like cookies, cakes, and candy.

Fats and Oils

For simplicity's sake let's refer to these somewhat separate but clearly related foods as "fats," even though in our culture, this word has negative connotations. This anti-dietary fats crusade might stem from the fact that fats are a large category of foods; some are good for us and some aren't. We absolutely need fats in our diets, so the question becomes, "How do we tell the good fats from the bad?"

As a rule of thumb, the more liquid a fat at room temperature the better it is for you, and vice versa. This also brings up the issue of saturation.

Saturated Fats (the not very good for you ones) are loaded with hydrogen atoms that make them hard to digest and utilize. They are much more likely to be solid at room temperature and come mostly from animal sources; although some tropical oils like coconut and palm kernel oil fit in this category as well.

Unsaturated Fats are from vegetable sources and are liquid at room temperature; these are the good fats (usually referred to as "oils"). We still must be thoughtful in our use of even the good fats, however, because of their high caloric content: nine calories per gram versus four calories per gram for proteins and carbohydrates. That said, the judicious use of some extra virgin olive oil is a marvelous thing, and good for you as well!

Hydrogenation is a process by which we can turn an unsaturated fat (which is good for you), into a saturated one (which isn't). Adding hydrogen atoms to a liquid oil might make it solid at room temperature, but it also renders it virtually indigestible. This may suit the purposes of some food manufacturers but does not promote good health, so watch for this and avoid it.

Hydrogenated oils are also referred to as trans fats and are linked, along with saturated fats, to an increased risk of coronary heart disease, which is one of the leading causes of death in the U.S. Another reason to always read the labels on the products you buy! Hydrogenation is what makes margarine (fake butter) solid at room temperature, and responsible for that dead (and dead-looking) white stuff called vegetable shortening used in much deep fried food.

Proteins

Proteins come in many forms and are needed to build, repair, and maintain muscle tissue. There are many thousands of different proteins made up of different combinations of twenty-two amino acids. The human body produces only thirteen amino acids; the remaining nine (the "essential" amino acids) must be supplied from the foods we eat.

Proteins from animal sources often contain all nine essential amino acids, and when this is the case, they are called "complete" proteins. Individual plant foods often don't have all nine, but it is easy enough to combine them to get the complete package. Grains and legumes (beans and peas) are a common combination that serves this purpose; which is why it is a standard diet in many cultures. Beans and rice; tofu and noodles or rice; lentils and rice; and even the classic peanut butter sandwich meet this criteria.

In spite of our need for essential amino acids it is possible to consume too much protein in our diets. Only about 15% of our total daily calories should come from protein or we can over stress our kidneys and liver.

THE RIGHT WAY TO EAT

Fad Diets vs. Traditional Diets

Fad Diets are restrictive dietary recommendations that quickly become popular and often just as quickly recede from view; often touted for weight loss, but also for solving various (or virtually all) medical problems. The common thread is the recommendation of the consumption of one type of food at the expense of others , or the elimination of one or more essential food groups altogether. Examples include the *Low Carbohydrate Diet, Blood Type Diet, Zone Diet, Prolo Diet, Low Fat Diet, Pritikin Diet, Scarsdale Diet*, etc.

I suggest you approach these with a healthy skepticism and research them thoroughly before adopting one or the other.

Traditional Diets are combinations of food items proven to provide the nutrients necessary to maintain the body in reasonable health. These are diets evolved in the laboratory of traditional cultures over millennia. Some examples include the *Mediterranean Diet, East Asian Diet*, etc.

The "Latest and Greatest" may be the latest but it isn't necessarily the greatest (or even life sustaining). In general, Fad Diets should be avoided altogether, or only used for a short period of time.

Shelf Defense

Shelf Defense means defending yourself against the deleterious effects of many of the items on your grocer's shelves; items sold as food but containing none of the nutritional components real foods provide. Food quality is of increasing concern to many in the health field, as well as to others who pay attention to recent trends in food production.

To some extent, problematic developments in food production are occurring throughout the world, but the U.S. seems to be leading everybody in really bad ideas. We cover some of these dangerous developments in other chapters: the introduction of toxic materials into the food chain in **Chapter 15 - The Big C,** and we discuss the growth of the BiotecÚology industry and the truly frightening proliferation of **Genetically Modified Organisms (GMOs)** in **Chapter 23 - Sneak Attack.**

One more category of problematic food inventions (can you really invent food?) to discuss:

Fake Food

By **Fake Food** I mean a set of substances combined to approximate an existing real food item, or simply to appear to be food when it is not. It's almost as if there is some chemist sitting in Akron, Ohio (motto: "Rubber Capital of the World") thinking to himself, "What combination of rubber byproducts and coal-tar derivatives can I mix with sugar and sell to the American public as food?"

In the category of resembling existing real food, a classic example is margarine: fake butter.

Margarine begins with a food item—namely vegetable oil, such as corn, soybean or canola oil. It is hydrogenated so that the oil, usually liquid at room temperature, becomes a solid (like butter! Get it?).

Then different chemicals are added to make it look, act and taste like real butter. And there you have it: a Fake Food (just one of many, I'm afraid).

It is well established that hydrogenating oils renders them indigestible, thereby negating any potential food value while also causing harm.

There are many problems with Fake Food. After more than 40 years in the medical field, I posit that the human body has evolved (or was created, if you prefer) needing certain foods existing in nature. By manipulating elements, in an effort to trick the body into thinking it is getting real food, we may be risking our health, since the consequences to the body of these "manipulants" is unknown.

THE MEANING OF "NATURAL"

You have likely seen the word natural applied to many food, health and beauty products, but what exactly does this mean?

According to Wikipedia, "A natural product is a chemical compound or substance produced by a living organism... found in nature...produced by life." But it also states that these compounds "...can also be prepared by chemical synthesis..."

Since natural products can be synthesized I would submit that they aren't natural at all! In the 1990s a genetically modified tomato was invented with a gene from a flower and a bacteria spliced in. Does that sound natural to you? This, however, meets the above definition!

There are also many natural poisons—search the internet to see the wide range. To me, natural labels refer to something that exists, or was extracted or synthesized here on earth. In other words, it's not from outer space!!!

I suggest that you approach any products labeled "natural" with a healthy dose of skepticism.

Beware—"food" may be hazardous to your health!

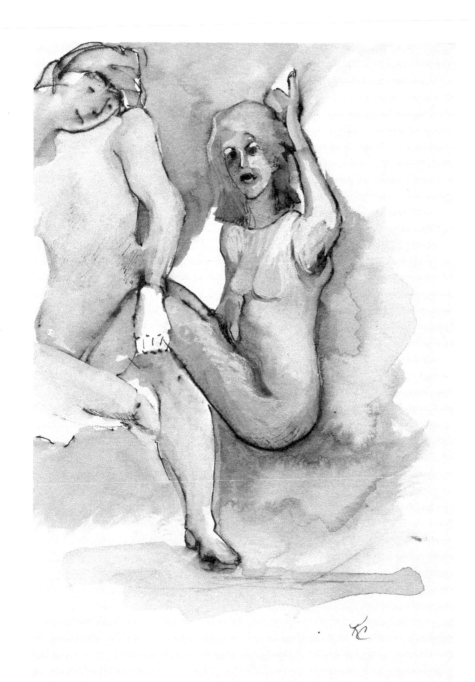

Chapter 21

Men... a Pause! Why Some Women Get Symptoms and Others Don't

Yes, men, let us pause and consider the plight of our female friends (wives, mothers, daughters, etc.) who may suffer the slings and arrows of outrageous menopausal symptoms: a partial list includes: daytime hot flashes, night sweats, insomnia, mood swings, depression, irritability, pain with intercourse, decrease in libido, vaginal dryness, and decreased bone density (osteoporosis). Not a pleasant thought, indeed!

Miserable Mary

Mary, age 49, complained of night sweats pursuant to her menopause. For almost 18 months she was awakened four to five times a night ringing wet with perspiration. In fact it was so bad, at least once a night she had to change her nightgown and sometimes even the sheets on her bed. Because of their dangerous side effects, Mary didn't want to go on hormone replacement therapy even though her symptoms were severely impacting her quality of life.

She was also troubled by irritability, insomnia and low energy in the daytime. Though these three extra symptoms could have been about menopause as well, I judged they were just a result of being awakened so many times at night, and losing so much sleep. I was proven correct when all of her secondary symptoms subsided as we got her night sweats under control using a combination of acupuncture and herbs!

Hormone Replacement Therapy (HRT)

The standard Western medical interpretation of this menopausal syndrome is that it is caused by a reduction in the production of female sex hormones—particularly estrogen and progesterone. Therefore, the standard Western treatment is to supplement these reduced amounts with similar substances (drugs) that mirror the actions of these naturally occurring hormones—thus **Hormone Replacement Therapy (HRT)**.

However, it has become increasingly obvious that this is a dangerous strategy possibly leading to more serious problems than it solves. At the very least, **HRT** has been shown to increase the risk of breast cancer, uterine cancer, ovarian cancer, endometrial cancer, gallbladder disease, and serious circulatory disorders. Is there a better way to reduce menopausal symptoms than by giving something that increases the risk of developing life-threatening diseases? The answer is ... Yes!

First, let us examine the assumption that menopausal symptoms are "caused" by the reduction in hormone production (which is, after all, a natural occurrence in a woman's body at a certain stage of her life), and therefore can only be treated by replacement with similar (but unnatural and dangerous) substances.

Cause and Effect

The dictionary says a cause is "that which brings about a result" and an effect is "the result produced by a cause." A cause/effect relationship has a certain inevitability built in: the same causes cause the same effects, and the same effects are caused by the same causes!

Here's an example from nature:

Gravity causes apples that fall off trees to fall down—this happens every time! It's not like sometimes, on a whim, gravity may decide to cause the apple to fall up or sideways. This doesn't happen because the cause/effect relationship is a constant.

Another example: Given enough strycÚine, a person will die. We can give enough of this deadly poison to *anyone* to kill them. Cause and effect! Inevitable!

Given the inevitable character of cause and effect relationships, how do we account for the fact that some women get only one or another menopausal symptom when their hormone levels decrease, while others get them all! Many of my women patients don't get any at all! If this were truly a cause/effect relationship, every woman would get every symptom every time going through menopause with their hormone levels dropping. Inevitably!

Could there be a flaw in the Western interpretation? Might there be something else at work here, and therefore a safer way to correct these symptoms? Fortunately the answer is, YES!

DR. GERALD SENOGLES

Like Pulling Teeth

It was extremely difficult for me to finally sit down and write this chapter. I put it off for a long time. I knew something was wrong with the standard medical model and treatment, and I knew what was really going on, because Oriental Medicine understands the body's processes at a truly profound level, but I didn't know how to explain the fact that **HRT** does make the symptoms of menopause go away, even though I knew that it was not truly correcting the underlying causes of those symptoms. I am indebted to my friend, Bob Burch, a chemist at Kodak, for providing me with the answer; and that answer is masking.

Masking

To *mask* something is to hide, cover up, or conceal it. We will discuss the underlying pathologies responsible for menopausal symptoms in a moment, but first let's look at how the naturally occurring female hormones (and the unnatural substitutes prescribed in their place) can mask these conditions. The female sex hormones have powerful, positive roles to play in a woman's body. They not only help develop secondary sex characteristics and produce an environment suitable for the fertilization, implantation and nutrition of an embryo; but they also help a woman's body bear the extra burdens that menses, childbearing, and nursing can bring. In other words they support and aid women's bodies during the years when considerable extra burdens can cause the need for help.

The loss of this hormonal support at menopause can lead to the emergence of various difficulties. For an explanation of how this change can allow the development of menopausal symptoms I am again indebted to Bob for an elegant analogy clarifying the circumstances.

A Rising Tide Lifts All Boats

It's like if you had a boat on a lake and the bottom of the lake was covered with rocks and debris that could damage the boat, but the water level is high enough to support it above these obstacles so it doesn't come in contact with them. Should the water level drop low enough for your boat to contact them however, then it would get damaged (develop symptoms). In our analogy the boat is, of course, a woman's body; the supporting water level represents the female sex hormones; and the rocks and obstacles are the underlying conditions that cause the menopausal symptoms, which just aren't being encountered while the body enjoys the extra support—whether naturally occurring or artificial hormones (**HRT**)—provide. Please note that the underlying conditions to create symptoms are already there, but are being masked (covered up) by the powerful supportive effects of the hormones!

The Western strategy is to pump in artificial hormones to metaphorically "increase the water level" (with **HRT**) to raise the boat above these obstacles, thereby avoiding the symptoms of menopause without really resolving their underlying causes, at the same time increasing the risk of life-threatening diseases! The Oriental medical strategy is to fix the underlying causes of whichever menopausal symptoms occur so they go away naturally and safely.

The Causes of Menopausal Symptoms

Let's consider the symptoms one by one and discuss their individual causes. The fact that each has its own separate cause explains why one woman will get one or another of the symptoms while another woman doesn't get any and someone else gets them all. The determining factor is which underlying pathology built up over the years has been masked by the hormone support, so the symptom hasn't shown up until that support is withdrawn at menopause.

Here is a list of symptoms, including their ultimate causes and some ways to help correct them:

Night Sweats: caused by an imbalance in the Autonomic Nervous System, we address and correct through the kidney/adrenal complex. Acupuncture can help with this, and two good herbal formulas are Liu Wei Di Huang Wan or its stronger cousin Chi Pai Di Huang Wan.

Daytime Hot Flashes: from a pathology in the heart's blood supply. We recommend acupuncture and possibly Tien Wang Bu Xln Wan.

Depression/Irritability/Mood Swings: brought on by problems in the heart and/or liver. Acupuncture, and perhaps Tien Wang Bu Xln Wan for the heart and Xaio Yao Wan or Relaxed Wanderer for the liver.

Osteoporosis/Bone Loss: covered in depth in **Chapter 19 - Don't Need a Break.**

Vaginal Dryness: Acupuncture, Aloe Gel, Wild Yam Cream, Agecom or similar herbal formulas can usually bring relief.

Menopausal symptoms can be complex and resistant to change in some women. Seek help from an Oriental Medicine practitioner or another non-drug oriented health professional, but be prepared to be patient as they work to resolve your problems. It can be a real trial and error process because what works beautifully for one person may do nothing at all for the next.

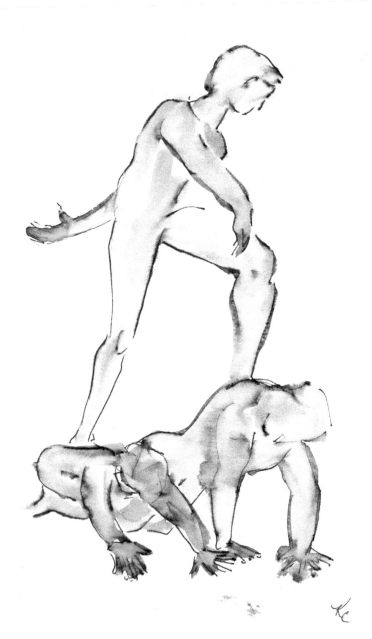

Chapter 22

Your Back! Managing Back Problems

"You're Back!"

"**Y**eah Doc, you did such a great job solving my shoulder problem I thought I'd give you a shot at solving my back pain—it's killing me!" I can't count the times I've heard something like this. Low back pain (with possible hip and leg involvement) is the number two reason people seek medical help.

Let's get down some statistics to show how common it is:

- Eighty percent of Americans will get this problem at one time or another in their lives.
- In America alone it is responsible for *100 billion dollars* in medical bills, disability payments, and lost productivity.
- Low back pain is the second most common reason for doctor visits; right behind colds and respiratory infections.
- 480,000 fusion surgeries (a type of back operation) were performed in 2017 alone, at an average cost, including testing, re-hab and meds, of $100-160,000.
- There was a seventy percent increase in these surgeries in the U.S. between 2001 and 2011. In other words, this little money maker is getting more popular all the time.

Is surgery the only (or for that matter even the best) way to solve this problem? The answer in my experience is, "No, not in most cases." Why is this so, and what might we do other than surgery to manage back problems? Most of what is said in this chapter is based on four sources: a study published in the New England Journal of Medicine, an article in Newsweek Magazine, an interview conducted (while working on her low back pain) with a high-powered Ph.D. Nursing Professor, and the author's more than forty years of clinical experience working with low back pain.

The Journal Study: Ninety eight (98) people of various ages and lifestyles who had no back pain were given an MRI (Magnetic Resonance Imaging) test to determine if they had disc (the fibrous material between the vertebrae) irregularities. These tests are commonly given to patients with pain in the region of the spine; if certain irregularities are found surgery is commonly recommended. Much to the surprise of the researchers they found that twenty-seven percent of the ninety-eight subjects had herniated discs, and another fifty-two percent had bulging discs! Remember, these subjects had no pain at all, but if they had pain for any reason (and there are lots of other reasons not detectable by an MRI) many of them would have had surgery recommended.

Dr. Scott Bode, an orthopedic surgeon at Emory University states that, "The MRI should never be used as a screening test, which is unfortunately the way it is very commonly used today."

From the Horse's Mouth: Several years ago I worked on the low back pain of a woman with fifteen years experience as a head surgical nurse, and another fifteen years as a Ph.D. Nursing Professor. In the course of our interaction, I made the comment that I thought that fifty percent of back surgeries performed in the U.S. were unnecessary; after all I had fixed many patients who were told they needed surgery to be out of pain.

I was surprised at the vehemence with which she shot back that, "Ninety percent of back surgeries are unnecessary!" She said that after all she had seen, no one was going to operate on her back and that, furthermore, most of the surgeons she knew wouldn't get back surgery either! Interesting, don't you think?

The back is a very complex interaction between muscles, bones, tendons, discs, capsules, ligaments, nerves, and blood vessels. A problem in any one of these components can lead to pain. In fact, disc issues are the real cause of back pain in only an estimated ten percent of low back cases; including the ones that get surgery for disc irregularities shown on MRIs.

Now What?

So what are we to conclude here? That back surgeries are never justified? No!

Should we conclude that there are many more surgeries performed than are really necessary? Unquestionably!

Might we conclude that Orthopedic Surgeons and Neurosurgeons with their MRIs and scalpels perhaps should be the last people you consult if you develop back pain? That's what I think!

Do you remember the old saying that to someone whose only tool is a hammer every problem looks like a nail? Should you exhaust every other possible method to resolve your difficulties before even considering surgery? I think so!

Might it behoove you to get a second, or perhaps even a third opinion before you go under the knife? Undoubtedly a very good idea!

Alternatives to Surgery: According to the Newsweek article most back problems can be resolved with less invasive tecÚiques than surgery: acupuncture, massage, chiropractic, physical therapy, reflexology, stretching, yoga, and just plain time are other methods that just might give someone the relief they need.

The Case of Painful Patty

"Patty" was in town from Alaska visiting a relative. She had received 5 low back surgeries and was in extreme pain. Surgeries #1 and #2 were for her original problem, surgery #3 was for the scar tissue generated by the first two, #4 was for scar tissue from 1, 2 and 3, and #5 was for... I think you get the picture.

There was no relief from surgery #5 performed 3 months before I saw Patty. Her doctors proposed a sixth when she realized that this strategy was a dead end and she came to me. With a modest series of 10 treatments I was able to relieve at least 75% of her pain.

ACUPUNCTURE AND BACK PAIN

In more than 40 years in Oriental Medicine study and practice, the number one problem I have treated has been what I call back-hip-leg pain—some combination of those three.

On an ordinary day, I treated 2 to 5 of these cases and gave significant relief to 80-90% of the patients who allowed me a realistic opportunity to help them.

Some people think they only have to come in one time to solve their 20 year old back problem—in other words they want a "miracle cure." What I say is, "If you're looking for a miracle, go to church and ask for one, but don't be too surprised if you don't get one! What I do here is medicine, and like many other things we do medically, this requires dedication and repetition."

How many acupuncture treatments might it require? 5 to 15 sounds reasonable, except for the most difficult cases, but when you compare that to the months or years one has suffered with this problem that seems like a modest number to me.

Incidentally, whether or not someone has had prior surgery doesn't seem to impact my percentage of success. I have seen plenty of those scars on patients' backs.

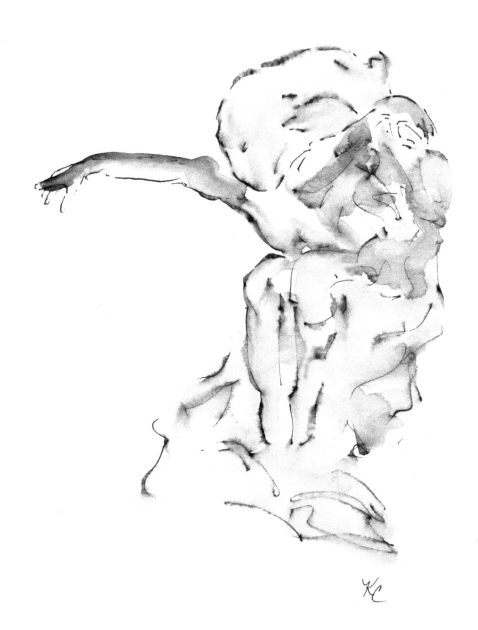

Chapter 23

Sneak Attack!
Assaulted by the BiotecÚology Industry

Ladies and Gentlemen, you are under attack and your very life is in danger, but many of you probably don't even realize it. You are an unwitting participant in the largest medical experiment of all time and, as with all experiments, the outcome is unknown, but will likely prove to be significantly detrimental to your health.

The Experiment: Take foods that have evolved over millions of years of natural interaction with animals and humans and arbitrarily splice in genetic materials from other species (and even other Kingdoms—as in the Animal, Vegetable, and Mineral Kingdoms), and create some new "Frankenfood" you can fool people into buying so your corporation can make more money. And then stand back and see what happens. An appropriate name for this experiment would be "Genetic Roulette."

The Participants: You and everyone else in the world alive today, and all future generations of plants, animals, and people. In a good scientific experiment we might call these "variables," but of course this is not a good scientific experiment but more of a diabolically stupid gamble.

The Stakes: cancer, heart disease, stroke, neurological diseases like multiple sclerosis and Parkinson's disease, asthma, diabetes, birth defects, genetic mutations, and a host of others (known and unknown) too numerous to mention. Also the possible loss of your life and those of your children and your children's children.

The Experimenters (or Should I Say Perpetrators): include chemical and biotecÚology companies with names you know; aided and abetted by the Food and Drug Administration (FDA) and numerous politicians (We do have the best politicians money can buy!).

The Results: aren't in yet, but you can bet that there will be many, and they will be varied, and some of them will be really serious.

Here is a partial list:

1. Increased Use of Pesticides and Herbicides and therefore more pollution and poisoning of our environment. An example: the dreaded genetically modified soybean, an organism invented and patented by a well known chemical company. To a variety of soybeans they spliced in genes from a bacteria, a virus, and a petunia and made a soybean plant that doesn't die (like real soybean plants) when it is lavished with their famous toxic herbicide. This accomplishes two things—more poisons into and on to the part we eat and more poisons into the ground, the water, and the air we breathe. It also makes a lot more money for these well-known chemical companies (but I'm sure this is just an accident—they must be running this experiment just to be part of the "final solution" to issues with food production).

Maybe it's time to modify my old rule from, "Don't eat anything advertised on television," to "Don't eat anything advertised on TV or patented by a chemical or biotech company." When the stuff you're eating is patented by any of the usual suspects, you can bet you are in trouble!

2. Increased Pesticide Consumption: Not only can more poisons be sprinkled on the growing plants (and into the environment), but some poisons are built right into the "food" itself. For instance, the "New Leaf Superior Potato." In this instance the insecticide Bt (bacillus thuringiensis) is built into each one of its cells so that it kills every Colorado potato beetle that tries to eat it, and incidentally, also gives the chemical company a nice insecticide enriched potato to sell to you. Does the fact that this potato is registered with the U.S. Environmental Protection Agency (EPA) as a pesticide tell you anything?

Bt is built into one of their varieties of corn as well. It's hard to keep up!

3. Risks to Other Species: In a 1999 study at Cornell University, scientists found if they dusted milkweed leaves with GMO corn pollen nearly one half of all the Monarch butterfly caterpillars that ate the leaves died within four days, and the ones that survived were undersized and underweight. One can only imagine the myriad other disasters waiting in the wings.

4. Risks of Allergies: Someone may know they are allergic to a particular food, like peanuts, and therefore avoid that food. But what if the specific

Dr. Gerald Senogles

allergic "trigger" from peanuts were spliced into another seemingly un-related, "Food." The person with the allergy could suffer years of reaction until the connection was found, if found at all.

5. Ethical Issues: As plant and animal genes are interchanged willy-nilly, what happens to people who don't eat meat, or certain types of meat? How would they know that the tomato sauce on that slice of pizza is made from tomatoes with a pig gene spliced in? There is such a tomato!

What does this do to vegetarians who don't want to eat meat? What about Muslims or Jews who have a specific religious injunction against eating pork? This partial list of problems is just the tip of the iceberg and there is even scarier stuff.

Metaphorically speaking, your house is on fire and your children are trapped inside, as all future generations will likely pay even more dearly than we for this monumentally foolhardy experiment.

The Magnitude of the Experiment: Big and getting bigger fast! Even though the first large scale harvest of **Genetically Engineered (GE)** "foods" wasn't until 1996, by 1999 more than 25% of all American grown crops were **GE**. Here are some percentages from that period: 35% of all corn, 55% of soybeans, 50% of all cotton. As of 2018, these percentages were : 93% corn and soy; 95% sugar beets; 94% cotton; plus others. If you think cotton is not a food (and you're right) that doesn't mean you are not eating it. Look for the infamous "cottonseed oil" in the list of ingredients of your foods on the grocer's shelves.

The **U.S. Department of Agriculture (USDA)** has already approved many **GMO** foods for production, including beets, canola, corn, cotton, flax, rice, soy, potato, tomato, papaya, squash, watermelon and zucchini, and these are grown and eaten in America today, with a host of others on the way!

If you think these foods are easy to avoid, think again. Soy alone finds its way into about 60% of all processed foods. It is estimated that as of 2018 at least 75% of all processed items on supermarket shelves contained **GMO** ingredients. Here is a partial list of substances commonly used in processed foods made from soy or corn: lecithin, soy oil, soy flour, textur-ized vegetable protein, corn oil, corn starch, fructose, and the ubiquitous "high fructose corn syrup."

The Solution (If There Is Any): Buy (or grow) and eat exclusively organically grown foods or, at the very least, foods identified as containing no **GMOs**. These biotech profiteers will stop at nothing in their pursuit of the almighty buck: the industry pushed to have its unnaturally produced products included in the USDA's "organic" designation, and it was only after the largest public outcry in that agency's history (over 200,000 letters) that they were excluded.

Pesticides (designed to kill living organisms) do not belong in our diets. Become knowledgeable and more active in the fight to stop this travesty. At the very least, products containing GMOs should be labeled as such so you would have the choice of whether or not to buy them. A Time Magazine poll in 1999 showed 81% of Americans favored labeling; it also showed that around 60% of the poll's participants would avoid these foods if they were identified. It's no wonder producers have fought (so far successfully) against labeling and your right to choose what you eat.

According to Wikipedia, "**The Precautionary Principle** states that if an action or policy might cause severe or irreversible harm to the public, in the absence of a scientific consensus that the harm would not ensue, the burden of proof falls on those who would advocate taking the action."

Furthermore, this is "… most often applied in the context of the impact of new tecÚology on the environment and human health, where the consequences of actions may be unpredictable." It also points out that new tecÚologies can be dangerous because of "the fallibility of human understanding."

Let's put this principle into plain English: "If you don't know the probable outcome of an action, and it might be harmful—Don't Do It!" How well do you think the **GMO** experiment meets this criteria?

The importance of this leads to the suggestion of regular research on the internet to learn about **GMO** foods recently added to this list.

THE MEANING OF ORGANIC

There are several definitions of organic, only one of which is used in *Body Wisdom* when referring to diet.

Some definitions:

1) "...containing carbon...of biological origin..." (This is an older definition, used in chemistry);

2) "relating to a bodily organ or organs;"

3) "food... produced without the use of chemical fertilizers (defined as "any inorganic material of wholly or partially synthetic origin"), pesticides (defined as any chemical preparation for destroying plant, fungal or animal pests—this includes insecticides, herbicides, fungicides etc.), or other artificial agents."

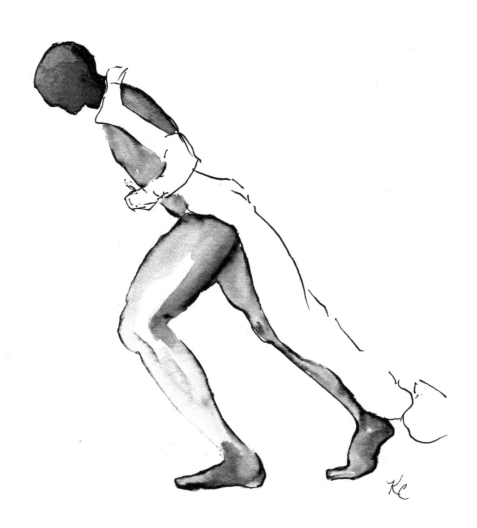

Chapter 24

Getting Up Again:
The Use and Abuse of Stimulants

The "getting up" referred to here is "uppers" to boost your energy level. Unfortunately, we do this increasingly in modern society by abusing various kinds of stimulants.

Stimulation, as defined in the dictionary, means "to quicken or promote an increase in activity of a physiological process as by a drug." In other words, as far as it applies to your body, to increase the functional level of some part of your body, or your system in general, in order to gain access to more energy. The problem with this strategy is that even though stimulation appears to give you more energy, it is really depleting your energy in the long haul. Some of the most commonly used (and abused) stimulants are caffeine, alcohol, tobacco, sugar, and some legal and illegal drugs.

Energy Storage

We constantly use energy as we go about our daily lives, so we need a constant resupply. Even while we sleep, our bodies are using energy to digest food, breathe, circulate blood, and perform trillions of metabolic functions every second. Not unlike the energy storage function of a battery, our bodies store energy; specifically in the kidney/adrenal complex in the back. Also, just like in our cars, we take energy out of our kidney/adrenal "battery" at some times and put it back in at others. Unfortunately, as with all batteries, we can never put back in quite as much as we remove, therefore every battery (and every body) eventually runs out of energy and dies.

Draining Our Batteries: The problem with stimulants is, they don't really give us energy; they just drag energy out of storage and make it accessible to us when we can't really afford to spend it. Let's say it's the end of a long and tiring day and your body tells you it really wants to just go home and rest, but you have this big party to go to, so you take another cup of coffee (or a few drinks when you get there) and lo and behold you're the last one to leave. This strategy works, but there is a hidden cost.

It's like in the old days, if you had a mule to plow your field and at the end of a long and tiring day that mule needed to rest to rebuild her energy supply for the next day, but you got out a whip and whipped that mule to get more work out of her tonight. Well, you'll get more work out of her now, but you are going to shorten the life of that mule. In the same way we can "whip" our kidney/adrenal battery with stimulants to make more energy available to us right now, but we surely are going to shorten its (and our) life.

Use versus Abuse

I'm a fun guy and I don't want to wreck the party, so I'll note the difference between using (not so bad), and abusing (bad) stimulant drugs like caffeine, alcohol, sugar, chocolate, etc. Most of us are in good enough health and have generally healthy habits so we can periodically take that drug to have a little more fun, or get a little more work done, and still be just fine. It only becomes a problem when some of us (you know who you are!) overdo it. If you need one more cup of coffee to get over the letdown because that last cup wore off, you are probably abusing caffeine.

One way to find out for sure if you are abusing a substance is to see if you have become addicted to it; a simple test for that is to see if you suffer withdrawal symptoms when you try to go without it. The most common withdrawal symptom from caffeine is headaches; if you try going without coffee (or tea, chocolate, cola beverages, etc.) for a couple of days and get a headache, you can be sure you are using an abusive (harmful) level of that substance. You can also use the method of testing to lower your use to a non-abusive level by stepping down your intake until you no longer experience withdrawal symptoms when you go without.

Prescription Drugs: Another whole group of stimulating (and therefore weakening) substances is doctor prescribed drugs, not necessarily to give a person more usable energy but instead to stimulate some particular organ or gland to function at a level it no longer capable of on its own.

A classic example is diuretics (commonly called "water pills"). Diuretics force the kidneys to put out more fluid in the urine when they are too weak to perform this function adequately on their own (otherwise they would have set the proper fluid balance in the system already, as this is one of their primary functions).

There are also oral medications for diabetes that cause the pancreas to produce/secrete more insulin; this is used sometimes in lieu of the other Western treatment strategy of injecting synthetic/animal insulin to make up for the pancreatic shortfall (this creates its own set of problems).

To understand the danger of applying these strategies to your kidneys and pancreas, just think of that poor mule; when you force something to work beyond its current capacity you weaken it in the long haul.

Fortunately, there are other more natural and health-promoting substances and procedures to help you achieve these same ends without shortening the functional lives of important (as in, you can't live without 'em!) components of your system.

Tonics

To tonify something means to strengthen it. To some extent anything you do that is good for you, like proper rest, diet, and exercise, is tonifiying to your body. In natural medicine we also have a large array of tonifiying substances and procedures to strengthen a particular part, or function, in your system, or just build energy in general. Tonics (and tonification) have gotten a bad rap in our culture and we have become suspicious of them. Beware of "Dr. Smith's Snake Oil Tonic!" I believe this putdown of tonics is part of a deliberate effort by the medical industry (doctors and drug companies) to discredit something they are incapable of doing (strengthen), in favor of something they can do (stimulate /weaken).

Along with acupuncture, which can increase function and energy, there are many tonic herbs in natural medicine. The best known (but by no means only one) of these is ginseng. There are many effective formulas that utilize ginseng (or similar tonics) to build energy in general or to strengthen the functional ability of some particular part. Bu Zhong Yi Chi Wan is a good, safe general tonic.

*A **word of caution***: any considerable medical problem can cause someone to experience a diminution in available energy. Get checked out by a competent medical practitioner if you feel you do not have enough energy. For some medical problems, energy tonics would be contraindicated. Sometimes what is needed for increased energy is to solve an underlying medical problem tying up or blocking access to energy. This is also discussed in **Chapter 1 – The Ways of Energy**.

In our modern societies with electricity-driven 24 hour entertainments, some people may seek an unrealistic, or unnatural activity level. After all, proper rest is one of the requirements of a healthy body.

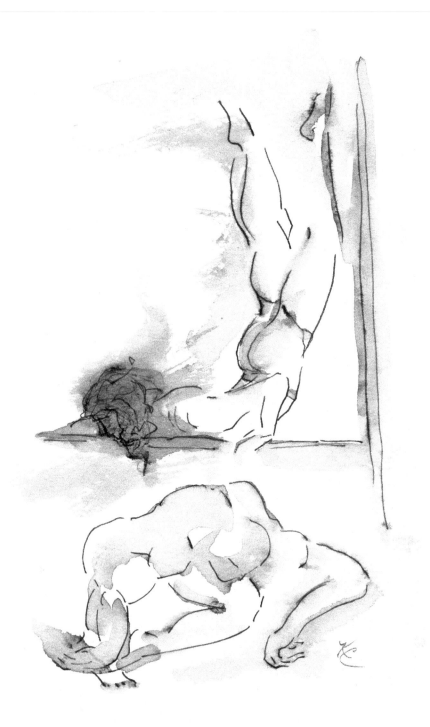

Chapter 25

Bleeding Injuries: The Treatment of Bleeding, Bruising, and Swelling

Not all injuries involve bleeding, but some of the more troublesome (and dangerous) ones do, including anything from sprains, cuts, breaks and dislocations to any blow strong enough to cause a blood vessel to rupture and spill blood into the surrounding tissues or out of the body entirely.

In **Chapter 25 - Bleeding Injuries** we will look at things we can do for ourselves to address these problems, but please be aware these are meant to be used along with normal common sense first aid procedures, as well as the appropriate medical intervention; whether that involves an immediate trip to the emergency room or a scheduled visit with your regular medical provider.

Bleeding can be internal or external. In common parlance, if bleeding is external (blood leaves the body) we call it bleeding, but if it is internal (blood spills out of the vessels into the surrounding tissues) we call it bruising.

Either way it represents the blood leaving its proper channels (blood vessels) and is a problem. This can be serious or even life threatening and require immediate medical intervention, but even in that circumstance there is something you can do for yourself to minimize the danger.

Repeat after me: "Yunnan Pai Yao."

This is the name of a famous Chinese herbal formula that can help slow down or stem emergency traumatic bleeding. It can truly make the difference between life and death under certain circumstances. I first learned about this formula in 1983 while doing advanced study in Oriental Medicine in Hong Kong; and therein lies a tale!

During the Viet Nam War, American GIs found that many of the Viet Cong forces and North Vietnamese Regulars carried containers of a bitter tasting powder they used immediately if they were wounded to stop the bleeding and hopefully save their lives. I say, "hopefully" because there are some bleeds that nothing will stop. The Americans wanted this potentially lifesaving powder too, and began to stock up on it in Hong Kong, a city on the southern tip of China, where they took their "R&R" (rest and relaxation). As it turned out, the Communist Chinese government was supporting the North Vietnamese communist government and therefore began restricting the shipping of Yunnan Pai Yao to Hong Kong, thereby drying up the supply not only for the GIs but also for the etÚic Chinese population. A bad circumstance indeed as the Chinese do not want to be without the lifesaving advantage of this formula.

This story is to impress upon you the value of this miraculous substance and the need to keep it handy. No household should be without it. We even keep it in the glove compartments of each of our cars along with a bottle of water to wash it down should the need arise.

Yunnan Pai Yao

This near-miraculous herb comes in two formats: a package with 16 capsules; and in bottles with the same amount of powder uncapped. In each case is a tiny red pill to be taken if there is a danger of going into shock. I recommend having both formats; with the capsules it takes just a few for a moderate bleed, but for a more serious bleed I would take the whole bottle of powder (and it's not for the taste!). With a serious bleed one should take the red pill as well.

Recovery

With injuries, once all the bleeding has stopped (which can take days), we enter into the recovery phase, where we want to return to normal as quickly as possible. Where there has been a lot of bleeding there will be a lot of bruising, and swelling from the accumulation of other fluids in the area of the injury. Soon enough these extra substances in the injured area become an impediment to healing, as they retard the circulation of fresh blood to the area, and good blood circulation is always a key factor in determining how quickly we recover.

Fortunately we can do things for ourselves to speed along the recovery process.

The Uses of Heat and Cold

A good way to relate the therapeutic uses of heat and cold is to choose a particular injury and discuss how we might proceed; a sprained ankle is our example.

The Use of Cold: Immediately following and for several days after the sprain, the ankle will swell larger and larger. During this "expansion phase" we recommend the use of cold; cold retards expansion and growth; we don't want the swelling to get any bigger than it absolutely has to. The injury won't be fully healed until all the swelling dissipates and the ankle returns to normal size. In most instances the expansion phase lasts a few days to a week, after which we switch to...

The Use of Heat: Once the swelling and bruising reaches its full size and begins to recede we use heat to speed the process, as heat stimulates circulation and causes the extravasated (out of the vessels) blood and fluids to be picked up and returned to their proper places. Acupuncture is also very useful at this stage.

An important exception to the rule of using heat at this time is if there is a presence of heat at the site of the injury; we don't add heat to an already hot inflammation. It is easy to determine if heat is present by simply feeling the area with the palm of your hand and the underside of your fingers and comparing it to the temperature of the uninjured side. if significant heat is present then continue to use cold until such time as the use of heat becomes appropriate.

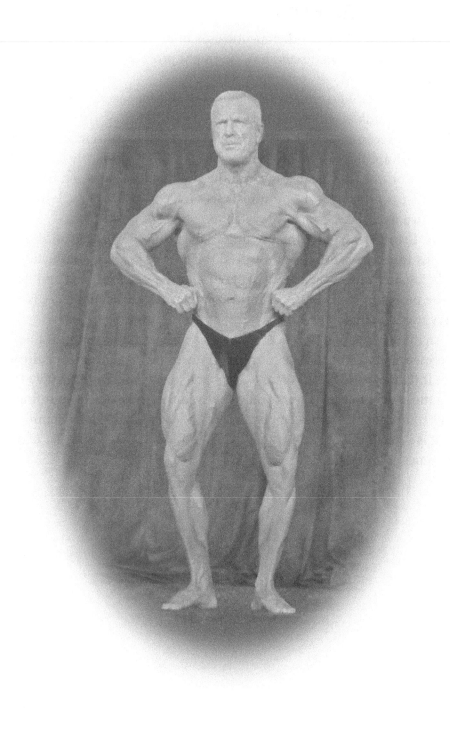

Chapter 26

My Friend, Friend: An Interview with World Class Bodybuilder, Jack Friend

In **Chapter 26 - My Friend, Friend**, we receive ideas about health from a multi-award winning athlete I have had the pleasure to know and interview, Jack Friend.

A Total Lifestyle

Body Building is a sport. The goal is the development of a strong, balanced, powerful physique with each muscle defined and in proper proportion vis a vis the others. Although most of us don't have the goal of developing our musculature to the same degree as Jack's, I believe most of us would like to maintain good health and strength as long as possible. As Jack pointed out to me, this requires a total lifestyle commitment.

Commitment is a word he uses a lot. If you don't adopt a healthy lifestyle, you don't get to the upper echelons where Jack competes. For Jack a healthy lifestyle means a balanced diet, regular sleep habits, no drugs (including alcohol and performance enhancing substances), lots of water, cardiovascular exercise and, of course, strength training.

Let's examine his regimen to see what he does to develop such a powerful body.

Balanced Diet

For Jack, this means a protein source, vegetables, and a complex carbohydrate with every meal. Jack says to maintain current muscle mass you need about one gram of protein a day per pound of body weight; more if you want to build muscle, as protein builds muscle.

For protein he usually eats a lean chicken breast (or sometimes beans or tofu). He also eats a wide variety of fresh vegetables for their nutrient content; and then a source of carbohydrates, which is mostly sweet potatoes

Photo by Dan Ray, courtesy of Jack Friend and RxMuscle.com. Used by permission.

or brown rice.

Each meal consists of equal portions, with the portion size about what would fit in the palm of your hand. He eats this every two hours for a grand total of seven medium sized meals a day! Jack says that if you wait six hours between meals your body goes in to "starvation mode" and holds on to fat because it's afraid you will never feed it again. This is also true for water so he drinks 2-3 gallons a day!

Exercise: Jack's day starts with one hour of cardiovascular exercise before breakfast, because, as he says, "That way you burn fat rather than the food you just put in your stomach for breakfast." He does "cardio" three days on and one day off.

And now for the amazing part! Jack does strength training six days a week for no more than one hour a day! He says if you over-train, you can't grow. He devotes each of those days to a different body part: one day for abdominal muscles, calves and chest; one for back and trapezius muscles; one for shoulders, triceps and biceps; and two for legs.

Building Muscle

There are two phases to Jack's program: one is what he does in the ten weeks leading up to a competition and the other is for all the rest of the time.

Before a show he gets his metabolism up high and his body fat low (3-5%). At this level you cannot build muscle mass but only maintain what you already have. At all other times (when he wants to build muscle) he lets his metabolism slow down and his body fat get to 6-8%, which is not a problem for most of us.

The American Council on Exercise states that "for each decade after age twenty-five, 3-5% of muscle mass is lost." That is for the average person though, and Jack is anything but average, so he has opted to contradict that tendency. Even though he is over fifty he is still adding substantial muscle yearly. He currently competes in the Heavyweight Division at five feet eleven inches tall and 225 pounds.

No Shortcuts

Jack tells about young men (and women, too, he and his wife both compete and have won numerous trophies as a couple) who come up to him and want "the secret" (read: shortcut) to attaining his level of achievement. When he starts talking to them about a healthy lifestyle: good diet, regular habits, hard work, commitment, and consistency, they don't want to hear it. It's like they're attached to the idea of having what Jack has but not to the idea of working to get it. But Jack knows that work and commitment are what it takes.

The founder of the martial art of Aikido used to tell his students, who professed the desire to know "the secret" of mastering the art, to show up and train the next day, at which time he would reveal the secret. He came in the next day and just started training, saying again he would "reveal the secret tomorrow." Maybe the secret is to just show up and train every day. Jack says, "Habits and consistency are everything."

Giving Back

To quote Jack, "At a point in your journey you ask yourself, 'How do I give back?'" Part of his commitment to his sport is to help others progress. As he says, "There are a lot of young people out there with dreams." Jack makes it a point to "lend a hand."

Competing

Another quote showing the quality of the man, Jack Friend, is in regard to competition in the sport of bodybuilding. He says, "If you absolutely have to win that First Place Trophy, then you'll probably give up and not compete at all. There's always going to be somebody better than you out there. You only compete against yourself; if you're a little better than you were last year then you're a winner!" Spoken like the true winner he is—my friend, Jack Friend.

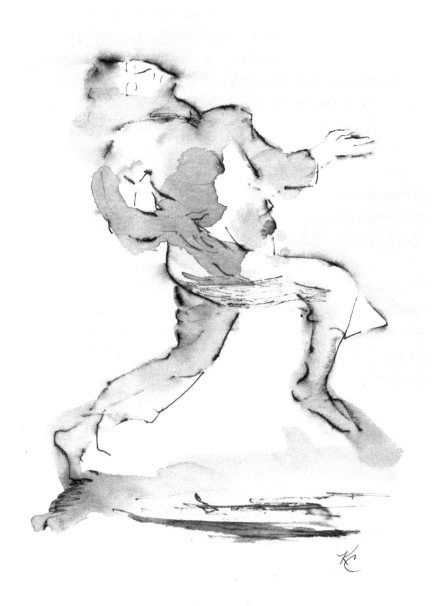

Chapter 27

Knee/Joint Pain:
Investigating Some of the "Modern"
Supplements Used for this Problem

Much of the information on the substances we discuss in **Chapter 27 – Knee/Joint Pain** is anecdotal, not based upon a large body of rigorous scientific research and, consequently, should be viewed as preliminary. If you choose to investigate the use of these substances for yourself, results may vary, and may or may not meet your expectations.

New Products

A medical professional is fairly inundated by "information" promoting the sale and use of literally dozens of new products or substances touted to solve a wide variety of human ills. Some are promoted as solving a narrow range of problems (joint pain, depression, etc.), and some presented as fixing virtually every problem to which the human body/mind is heir. The people who send me this "information" want to sell me these products and recommend them to my patients to further increase sales.

Being involved in a medical system tested in the laboratory of Oriental culture for more than 4,000 years (a certain peace of mind goes along with recommending an herbal formula used effectively and safely for at least 1,500 years), I consider these new products with a "wait and see" attitude. If this "stuff" is really effective (whatever it is), in a few years I'll hear more about it from real people not just sales personnel. I value one patient telling me something worked for her more than all the glossy brochures and audios put together.

That said, here are some thoughts on some new supplements aimed at promoting joint health: specifically Glucosamine Sulfate, Chondroitin Sulfate, MSM, and SAMe.

For certain of the following information I thank Mark Abell, an Oriental Medicine practitioner from Ashland, Oregon, specializing in Sports Medicine. Mark kindly consented to be interviewed for this chapter. Thanks, Mark!

Knee Pain

One of the common sources of knee pain is what is called "degenerative joint disease" characterized by a loss of cartilage and the possible formation of bone spurs. Cartilage is a tough, fibrous connective tissue covering the ends of bones at the joints; it acts as a protector and shock absorber to keep the bones from rubbing against one another and causing pain. The loss of this covering is one of the causes of knee pain; so the basic strategy of all four of these supplements is to provide your body with the building blocks needed to create more cartilage. The key ingredient in each is sulfur, as the supplementation of usable sulfur is a major component to regenerating cartilage. Incidentally, all of these substances are generated naturally in the body.

Sulfur is the fourth most abundant mineral in the body, right behind calcium, phosphorous, and magnesium. Emphasizing sulfur rich foods is another good way to provide this necessary ingredient; garlic, onions, broccoli, cabbage, Brussels sprouts, and asparagus in your diet are recommended.

It is important to note that none of these substances under discussion are pain relieving drugs; rather they are supplements aimed at joint regeneration; so they naturally take time to work. It is recommended that you take them for up to three months before judging whether or not they are helpful and then you will likely need to take them for months longer to get their full benefit.

Dosages

There is no "exactly right amount" of anything that is correct for everybody (as every body is unique), but we can suggest some guideline dosages. Thanks again to Mark for these. These dosages are predicated on a body weight of about 150 pounds, so if you are significantly lighter or heavier you can adjust the dosage accordingly.

We also include the disclaimer that if you feel you are not getting along with any of these after you begin taking them (nausea, vomiting, headaches, etc.), you should stop them immediately.

Glucosamine Sulfate: 1500 mg a day, and if you are over fifty you could add 500-1,000 mg of **Chondroitin Sulfate**.

MSM: a metabolite of DMSO, can be started in the 1-2 gram range. Start slow and build up until your body is accustomed to this substance, as some people can experience gastrointestinal problems or even headaches.

Warning: MSM can also amplify the blood thinning effects of drugs like coumadin (warfarin), or even aspirin. If you take any of these be alert for signs of excess bleeding or bruising and reduce the dosage of MSM, or stop it entirely, if this occurs.

SAMe: According to an extensive article in the July 5, 1999 issue of Newsweek Magazine, a dose as low as 400 mg daily may help joint problems. SAMe is also touted as helping depression and correcting liver problems. but the dosage required is considerably higher; up to 1600 mg a day may be needed for depression.

NSAIDs

If you have been relying on **Nonsteroidal Anti-Inflammatory Drugs** (aspirin, ibuprofen, naproxen, etc.) the bad news is twofold: they have lots of side effects, and they inhibit cartilage repair and accelerate cartilage destruction. Also, at least 107,000 Americans are hospitalized each year for NSAID induced gastrointestinal problems, and over 16,000 people die as a result. This doesn't seem like the best way to go.

Another Way

Now that we have discussed some of the *new* ways to treat knee/joint pain, I will say that by using acupuncture I have been able to help the majority of my patients, including a number who were told they needed surgery and, in some cases, even knee replacement. In fact, I have relieved knee pain in people still suffering after knee surgery.

This again demonstrates the multiple ways to solve virtually every problem and that surgery should almost always be your last resort.

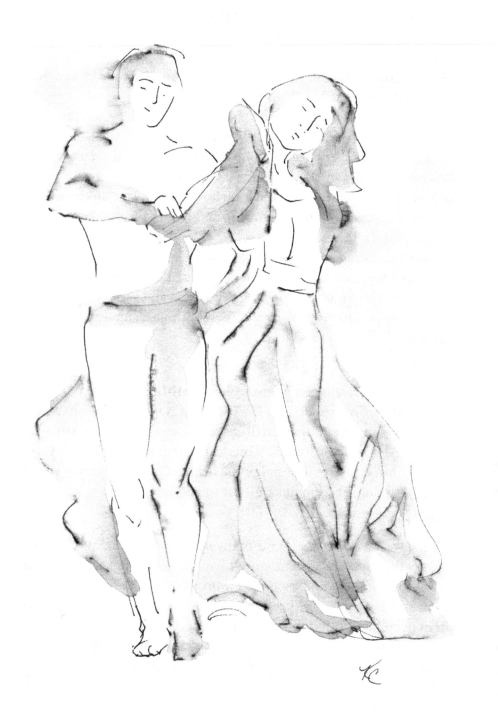

Chapter 28

Yin and Yang: The Elemental Dance

O ne of the most fundamental philosophical concepts in Oriental thought is the complementary opposites of yin and yang.

Let's analyze the familiar symbol used to represent these two ends of a polarity. The symbol you see below is usually printed in black and white but it's actually meant to be red and blue.

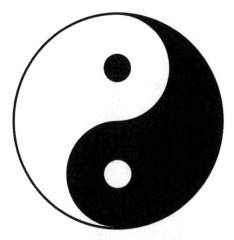

The One

The circle enclosing the duality of yin and yang is symbolic of The One, unending, formless, undifferentiated principle/mind/being/spirit behind all manifest reality. In Western thought we call this "God," or "The Creator." In Chinese thought it is "The Tao."

In Taoism they say, "The Tao that can be spoken of is not the true Tao," while in Buddhism they say, "Those who talk don't know, and those who know don't talk." I'll leave the rest of this part of our exposition up to you to understand and interpret according to the particular cosmology to which you subscribe.

The Two

If God, the Tao, is the one single reality behind manifestation, its first breakdown into form is its division into The Two: the complements of yin and yang. This differentiation continues until we reach the level of what the ancient Chinese called, "The Ten Thousand Things," by which they meant everything there is.

Nowadays, in our complex cultures, we recognize there are more than ten thousand things. A magazine article about a ship transporting military hardware to Europe in World War II stated it was carrying over 200,000 different items. Still, it is not too hard to imagine someone living in a peasant culture thousands of years ago thinking ten thousand things covered just about all there was.

Yin and Yang

Listing some characteristics of yin and yang is the best way to begin to understand this duality in action:

Yin	Yang
water	fire
cool	warm
dark	light
female	male
night	day
receive	give
defend	attack
matter	energy
inside	outside
passive	active
below	above
blue	red
right	left
front	back

Opposites Required!

As you can see, these opposites imply one another, require one another, complement one another and cannot exist without one another. To see this better let's look at the example of right vs. left. Let's draw a line and mark the left (L) side, the midpoint (M), and the right (R) side.

Thus: L   M   R

Now, if we wanted a line without a right side we would erase that part of the line that is to the right of the midpoint and we would have a line with only a left side.

Wouldn't we?

Wait a minute! This didn't turn out as we had hoped, because the former midpoint is now the right side of the line. Looks like we'll have to chop it in half again to get our line with only a left side. Well, we can chop away at that line all day until we end up with just a point (.) but that point will have a right side, too!

You can't have a left without a right, just like you can't have a top without a bottom or a front without a back. That is just the way it is in the phenomenal world—polarity is universal!

The terms yin and yang can be used to describe absolutes, but they can also be used to describe relativities. As absolutes, fire is yang and water is yin; but if we stack three identical objects on top of one another the one in the middle is yang (above) relative to the one on the bottom, but yin (below) relative to the one on the top.

Yin and Yang in Medicine

When it comes to the human body the two most important yin/yang complementarities are: blood and/vs. energy; and the sympathetic and/vs. the parasympathetic branches of **the Autonomic Nervous System (ANS)**. Since blood and energy are covered in depth throughout this work it just remains to examine the two branches of the ANS as they relate to one another.

The Autonomic Nervous System is the part of the nervous system that runs the myriad organ and gland functions beyond our conscious control. You don't tell your pancreas how much insulin to secrete to properly balance the amount of blood sugar in your bloodstream; nor do you consciously decide how much stomach acid you will require to digest a particular meal. Your **ANS**, however, is involved in these decisions and many more of the day to day and moment to moment decisions your body parts make in order for your body to function properly. Interestingly, the **ANS** has two distinct branches: the sympathetic and the parasympathetic.

The sympathetic branch (**yang**) increases functional levels while the parasympathetic branch (**yin**) decreases functional levels. It is the balance in the strength of the electrical signals in each of these branches (nerves are living electrical wires) that sets the proper levels of function of the components of the body. To demonstrate this, let's use the example of the heart.

The Heart: The correct rate of the heartbeat is 72 beats per minute (**BPM**), even though we accept anywhere from 60-80 **BPM** as being within the normal range. One of the reasons the rate of the heartbeat gets out of the normal range is if one of the branches of the **ANS** sends a stronger (or weaker) signal than the other. If the sympathetic/yang signal is too strong (or the parasympathetic/yin signal is too weak) to balance it, the heart will beat too rapidly; on the other hand if the parasympathetic/yin signal is too strong (or the sympathetic/yang signal is too weak) to achieve balance, then the heart will beat too slowly.

Just as elsewhere in the universe, the balance of yin and yang in the body must be maintained for there to be order, harmony, and correct action. Oriental Medical practitioners analyze for this balance in the two branches of the ANS and work to reestablish it at its proper level, if necessary. We call it "balancing yin and yang."

Since **the Kidney/Adrenal Complex (Chapter 7 - Kidneys)** is ultimately the repository for the basic yin and the basic yang of the body, it is by adjusting the functional level of this pair that we correct any **ANS** imbalance in a person's body; a more common circumstance than you might imagine, as I estimate fully half of the patients I see have this problem. Like most conditions this tends to develop more often as we get older.

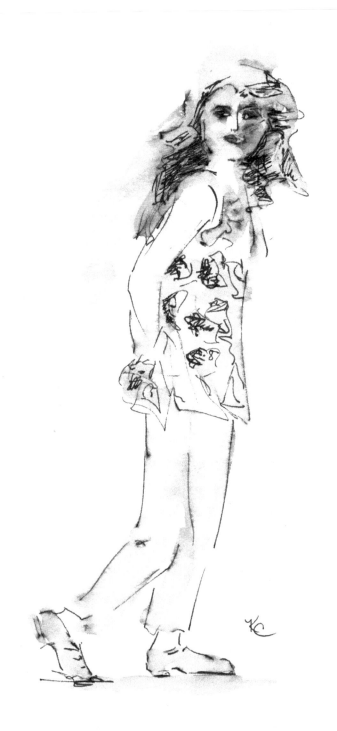

Chapter 29

Why Me? Why Do Bodies Develop Medical Problems in the First Place?

Someone said to me the other day, "I now know which organ malfunctions I have, but why do I have them?" I had given her a lot of information (*Body Wisdom* wasn't in print yet) so I was surprised by her statement; I thought I had explained things thoroughly enough. Perhaps for her (and your) benefit I need to spell out one more thing, namely: why do bodies develop the problems they do?

Two Principle Factors that Determine Your Health

1. Your Genetic Inheritance. We all inherit bodies with certain strengths and weaknesses, by which I don't mean muscular strength but rather the functional strength of the organs and glands. Some people inherit bodies so weak they don't live to see their first birthday (tragic but true), while others live to be a hundred or more with little effort. Even inheritance, however, doesn't usually mean you must develop a particular disease (like diabetes, cancer, or MS) just because various members of your family have. Think of it more as a proclivity for or a tendency toward a certain problem; hopefully it will just stimulate you to take proactive steps to avoid or prevent that particular illness from developing in your future.

Also, inherited conditions can respond to treatment just as well as any other. Your inheritance is not a death sentence!

2. What's Happened to Your Body Since You Got It. Some things you have done to yourself and some are rather beyond your control.

Within Your Control are diet (amount, quality, and type), exercise (or lack thereof), smoking, drinking alcohol, and the mental and emotional content of things you regularly subject yourself to, including the movies or TV shows you watch, books and other materials you read, and the people with whom you regularly spend your time.

There are very negative (or worse) images and ideas passed off as news or entertainment in our culture which can adversely impact your health. It is especially important to control the content of programming for young children, as children up to the age of seven can't really differentiate between make believe events and reality.

As an example of the possible medical consequences of "entertainment," frightening or very emotionally charged programming can and will adversely affect the heart and kidney/adrenal complex in small children. A child suffers functional damage as a result of this exposure—and that's a fact!

Beyond Your Control are things like pollution and environmental toxicity, gravity, radiation, injuries, emotional traumas, and even the way you were treated growing up in a particular family or household. The emotional content of your environment in your early formative years can influence your subsequent health picture for good or bad.

There are forces at work on earth that constantly pressure your body to break down, which is why everybody eventually dies. Every machine, as it gets older, doesn't work like it used to—and it never changes for the better! if you bought a new car, would you expect it to improve year after year, and work better when at 20 years old than the day you bought it? Hardly!

Think about it! Even though your great, great grandparents lived in a relatively toxin free world with pure air and water, ate only organic food (that's all there was), and got lots of good exercise, they still died!

One last point often misrepresented and misunderstood is that there is no problem you have to have because you are a certain age. ("After all Gladys, you are 76 so you are bound to have some arthritis.") Doctors regularly say things like this, but it just isn't true. In fact, if you hear this from a medical practitioner I suggest you look further, because you are talking to someone who doesn't know how to fix your problems.

What is true however, is that problems tend to develop over time; therefore the older you are the more time you have had to develop trouble (we usually do have more health issues at 66 than at 16).

This does not mean these problems aren't correctable, because they almost always are if the right means are employed.

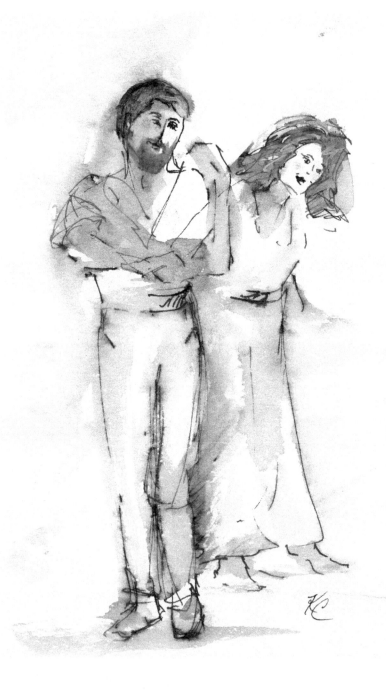

Chapter 30

Conclusion

Well, there you have it!

M y goal is to make your body understandable to you and I know if you have read this far, you are a lot more knowledgeable than when you first picked up *Body Wisdom*.

I hope I have helped you realize that vibrant energetic health and enthusiasm are available to you and the majority of your friends and loved ones.

I hope you have also figured out that almost all the myriad diseases catalogued in Western Medicine (fibromyalgia, Parkinson's disease, myofascitis, multiple sclerosis, polycystic ovary disease, coronary artery disease, etc.) have as their causes the breakdown in function of the basic component parts discussed throughout *Body Wisdom* and that, by correcting (or preventing) these organic malfunctions, we can go a long way toward solving these and many other medical problems.

Perhaps you also realize the road to true wellness is not paved with the mountains of drugs lavished on the sick and unhappy by the medical establishment, but that real health comes from understanding how your body works and what it needs to function correctly, and knowing how to make better lifestyle and health decisions (which may include consulting with alternative healing practitioners).

Am I telling you to throw away all your prescription and over the counter drugs? Certainly not! Drugs are like crutches, they just artificially prop you up without really fixing anything; on the other hand you can't pull a crutch out from under someone until they are well enough to walk on their own, otherwise, they just fall down!

But, do I think that you can likely find a way (or a practitioner) to help you achieve better health with fewer (or no) drugs?

Yes, I do!

Might there be some people who are so sick and weak, or whose disease processes are so advanced, that they may need to stay on drugs? Unfortunately, yes!

There is an old saying in natural medicine: "There are no incurable diseases, only incurable patients." To me, this means one of two things.

ONE: Some problems have advanced so far before they are discovered, or before the patient seeks treatment, that it is just too late to reverse the disease process. Some cancers are certainly like this.

TWO: There are some people who aren't willing to do whatever it takes to get well. Maybe they won't make the lifestyle changes necessary to improve their health, or they are too closed minded to seek out and consult with an alternative medical practitioner who may be able to provide a real solution to their problems. Some people are their own worst enemy!

I like to think that you are the kind of person who, after reading *Body Wisdom*, will do whatever it takes to get well.

I certainly hope so!

Good Luck and Best of Health To You!

Dr. Gerald J. Senogles, D.O.M.

Index

body care products, 90

bones, 117–120, 131, 134
    deterioration, 35–36
    knees, 164

bovine growth hormone, 91

bruising. *See* injuries: bleeding, bruising, swelling

butter, 50, 125, 127

Bu Zhong Yi Chi Wan, 151

C

calcium, 118, 164
    dietary, 118

cancer, xii, 28, 45, 50, 77, 84, 87–97, 173, 178
    causes, 88–95

carbohydrates, 123–124. *See also* sugars
    complex carbohydrates, 124
    simple carbohydrates, 123–124

carcinogen, 89, 92

cartilage, 164, 165

cells, 94, 95

central nervous system (CNS), 81

chemicals, 24, 47, 48, 82, 88–89, 91–92, 94–95, 127, 128, 143–146

chi, 81–82

chiropractic, 96, 139

chronic obstructive pulmonary disease (COPD), 27, 56

circulation, 4–6, 10, 19, 48

circulatory system, 3, 4, 14, 15, 19–20

clinical depression. *See* depression, clinical

colds, 28, 103–108
    hot colds and cold colds, 106–107

colitis, xi, 16, 21, 25, 87, 114

complex carbohydrates. *See* carbohydrates

concentration problems, 20

congestive heart failure, 33

cookware, 92–93

corn, 52, 114, 124, 127, 144, 145

coronary artery disease, 177

counseling, 21, 84

CT scan, 16, 49

D

death, 11, 15, 28, 31, 32, 35, 36, 41, 81, 88, 109, 112, 119, 125

depression, clinical, ix, 16, 47, 48, 57, 68, 75, 77, 82, 131, 134, 165

development, 32, 35, 51, 76, 159

diabetes, 16

diagnosis, 16, 23, 31, 63, 64, 107

diaphoresis (sweat), 105

diarrhea, 21

diets, 112, 124–126

digestion
    and liver disorders, 48
    colds and, 103
    herbs and tonics for, 96
    imbalance of, 65

phlegm and, 113
process of, 25
purpose of, 24

digestive system, 4, 5, 15, 23–25
phlegm and the, 113

disease, x, xi, xii, 14, 15, 16, 21, 27, 28, 43, 111–114, 132, 134, 143, 164, 173, 177, 178

diuretic drugs, 33, 151

Dong Quai, 72

Dong Shen, 72

drugs, ix, x, xii, 10, 36, 44, 49, 56, 61, 62, 63, 68, 75, 95, 99, 107, 111, 117, 119, 149, 150, 159, 164, 165, 177, 178
and bone density, 119
dangers of, 93–94
side effects of, 165

dying, 41

E

edema, 33

Ehr Chen Wan, 111, 113

emotion, 21, 44, 48

emotional, 19, 20, 44, 68, 96, 173, 174
causes of illness, 82–84

energy, 3–6, 9, 10, 24
and stimulants, 149
assessment of, in healing, 100
Basic Energy, definition of, 41
blocked (chi), 81–85
carbohydrates and, 123–124
circulation of, 5–6, 96–97

deficiency, 96
definition of, 3
digestion and, 103
distribution of, 6
pathologies of, 5
source of, 4
stimulants and, 149–152
storage of, 149

exercise, 19, 36, 96, 118, 151, 159–160, 173

F

fad, 126

fad diets, 126

fake food, 123, 127

fats, 48, 112, 124–125

fats and oils, 48, 112, 124–125

fibromyalgia, 13, 16, 49, 57, 61, 77, 82, 99, 177. *See also* arthritis

food additives, 92

food preparation and storage, 92

free radicals, 95

Friend, Jack, 159–161
photo, 159

frigidity, 34

frustration, 21, 84

function, 3, 4, 6, 9, 14, 19, 21, 23, 25, 27, 28, 33, 47, 76, 82, 94, 124, 150, 169, 170, 177
definition of, 15

functional, 5, 10, 15, 16, 20, 24, 31, 32, 34, 36, 48, 49, 51, 64, 82, 84, 104, 149, 151, 173, 174

G

gall bladder, 15, 24, 25, 47, 48

Ganoderma, 45

gastroesophageal reflux (GERD), ix, 16, 25, 47, 48, 53, 104, 119

gastrointestinal bleeding, 109

gastrointestinal tract, 4, 48

genetically modified organism (GMO), 59, 127, 128, 144, 145–146

genetics, 91, 127, 128, 143, 144, 145, 173

GERD. *See* gastroesophageal reflux (GERD)

ginseng, 72

glands, 3, 4, 14, 16, 20, 23, 24, 55, 57, 64, 104, 105, 173

glucose, 27, 123–124

God, 167–168

Gomez, Selena, 34

Goopy Glenda, 111

H

headaches, ix, 6, 16, 21, 47, 49, 150
  causes and origins, 49

health, ix, x, xii, 109, 177–178

hearing loss in aging, 35

heart, 16, 21, 27, 28, 50, 64, 65, 70, 83, 84, 170
  and blood, 75–78
  angina pectoris, 10
  blocked arteries, 81
  blood deficiency, 77

function of, 19–20
  myocardial infarction, 15
  pathologies, 10–11, 20
  The Blood Speech, 76

heart attack, 11, 81, 82, 95

heart blood deficiency, 77

heartburn, 25, 48

herbal, 96

herbal formulas, 20, 21, 37, 63, 83, 97, 105, 107, 111–112, 119

Herbicides, 144

herbs, 37, 45, 63–64, 72, 75, 84, 106, 120, 131, 151

heredity and cancer, 97

He Shu Wu, 45

high fructose corn syrup, 145

hormone replacement therapy (HRT), 87, 93, 131–135

Hot Colds. *See* Colds

hot flashes, 131, 134

household cleaning agents, 90

hydrochloric acid, 25

hydrogenation, 125

hypertension, 16

I

ibuprofen, 109

immune system, 27–28
  defensive energy, 27

impatience, 48

incontinence, 33, 36

infections, hospital acquired, 28

injuries: bleeding, bruising,

swelling, 155–157

insomnia, ix, 16, 104, 131

ion generators, 90

iridology, 96

irritability, 68, 75, 131, 134

J

jing (essence), 32, 45

joint pain, 163–165

K

kidneys, 9, 31–38, 170
    function, 32
    pathologies, 33–35
    strengthening of, 37

knee & joint pain, 163–165
    NSAIDs, 165
    supplements for, 164

L

latent disease, 76, 99

laxatives, 108

life expectancy, 88

liver, 15, 21, 24, 25, 34, 47–51, 123, 125, 134, 165
    anti-inflammatory drugs, dangers of, 109
    function and physiology, 47–48
    pathologies, 48–49
    structure, 47

liver and gall bladder, 24

liver stagnation, 82

longevity, herbs for, 45

Lou Gehrig's disease, 92

lungs, 4, 9, 15, 20, 27–28, 89, 103, 105, 114
    cold colds, 106
    defensive energy, 27
    function, 27
    hot colds, 107
    pathologies, 56

lupus, 34

M

margarine, 114, 125, 127

menopausal symptoms, 134

menopause, xii, 59, 117, 131–135
    bone health and, 117–118
    symptoms, 134–135

metabolism, 4, 9, 24, 27, 32, 41, 160

migraine headaches, 21

Miserable Mary, 131

multiple sclerosis (MS), 87, 104, 173, 177

myocardial infarction, 15

myofascitis, 177

N

NAET, 53

naproxen, 109, 165

natural, xii, 13, 36, 62, 88, 95, 100, 128
    body care and household products, 90–91
    food, 91–92

nerves, 6, 11, 64, 81, 138, 170

nervous system, 5–6, 81, 92, 106, 134, 169

autonomic, 64–65

night sweats, 131, 134

nonsteroidal anti-inflammatory drugs (NSAIDs), 109, 165

O

off-gassing, 89

old age, 31, 35

Old Ed, 31

organic food and products, 90, 92, 146–147, 174
    definition of "organic", 147

organs, 3, 4, 14–16, 20, 23, 24, 64, 75, 105, 147, 173
    structure vs. function, 15
    vital organs, 15

Oriental Medicine, 16, 28

osteoporosis, 35, 117, 119, 131, 134

oxygen, 4, 9, 27, 41, 70

P

pain, ix, xi, xii, 5, 11, 109
    acupuncture for, 140
    angina pectoris, 10
    back, 137–139
    in knees and joints, 163–165
    menstrual, 68
    wandering, 13–14

Painful Patty, 139

pains, 49, 65

palpitations, 20, 53, 75, 77

pancreas, 24, 124, 151, 169

parasympathetic nervous system, 65, 169–170

Parkinson's disease, 16, 177

periodic cycle, 67–72
    and the liver, 48
    correct, 67
    excessive, 69
    headaches, 49

pesticides, 90, 91, 144–146

phlegm, 111–114

phytonutrients, 95

polarity, 167, 169

polycystic ovary disease, 177

Poor Jane, ix, 47, 84

precautionary principle, 146

pregnancy, 35

premenstrual syndrome (PMS), 16, 48, 68, 75, 77, 82, 104

prevention, 20, 51, 57, 87, 95–97

prostate gland, 31, 34

proteins, 123, 125

proton pump inhibitors, 119

R

reflux. *See* gastroesophageal reflux (GERD)

reishi mushroom, 45

Ren Shen Yang Rong, 72

respiratory system, 15. *See also* lungs
    function, 27–28
    pathologies, 28

W

wandering pain, 13
water, 144, 156, 159–160
    pills, 33, 151
    pollution, 88, 144
    quality, 89

Y

yin and yang, 167–170

The Author

D r. Gerald Senogles graduated from the New England School of Acupuncture in 1977 and is one of the first 50 graduates in Acupuncture and Oriental Medicine in the United States. He apprenticed with Dr. Cheung Wai Tak in 1977–78.

Dr. Senogles was a member of the acupuncture sub-committee of the Oregon Medical Board for six years. In 1988, he received his Doctor of Oriental Medicine Degree from the International Acupuncture and Chinese Medicine Research Institute in Hong Kong.

Dr. Senogles has been in private Oriental Medicine practice in the Rogue Valley of Southern Oregon since 1979. To learn more, visit his website at **www.medfordacupunctureclinic.com**

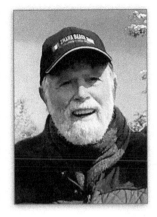

The Artist

K aty Cauker creates art developed around the ideas she finds relevant to her personal life and the world we live in. Her paintings often utilize natural forms as images symbolic of the concepts and emotions she is working with.

She has art in public places, and paintings in collections in the U.S., Canada, Europe, and Argentina.

Her work is widely shown and can be found on the world wide web at **www.katycauker.com**.

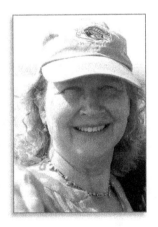

CPSIA information can be obtained
at www.ICGtesting.com
Printed in the USA
JSHW011134160220
4251JS00004B/34

9 780578 507774

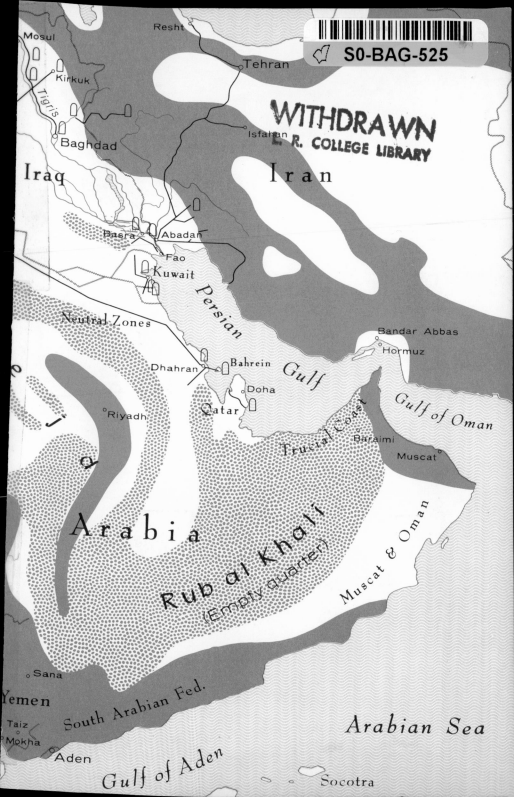

Mosul

Resht

Kirkuk

Tehran

Tigris

Baghdad

Isfahan

Iraq

Iran

Basra

Abadan

Fao

Kuwait

Neutral Zones

Persian

Dhahran

Bahrein

Gulf

Bandar Abbas

Hormuz

Doha

Qatar

Riyadh

Gulf of Oman

Trucial Coast

Baraimi

Muscat

Arabia

Rub al Khali
(Empty Quarter)

Muscat & Oman

Sana

Yemen

South Arabian Fed.

Arabian Sea

Taiz

Mokha

Aden

Gulf of Aden

Socotra

es and the Arab world ₍by₎ William R.
Harvard University Press, 1965.

929–

aps (1 col.) 22 cm. (The American foreign

p. ₍297₎–311.

₍neral₎ with Arab countries. 2. Arab coun-
with the U. S. 3. Arab countries—Politics.

956

₍65₎14₎

65—16688

The United States and the Arab World

THE AMERICAN FOREIGN POLICY LIBRARY

CRANE BRINTON, EDITOR

THE
UNITED STATES
AND THE
Arab World

William R. Polk

HARVARD UNIVERSITY PRESS

Cambridge, Massachusetts

1965

956
P 75 u
53215
mar. 1966

For Ann—

There lies Syria

FOREWORD

The American Foreign Policy Library was founded in 1945 by Sumner Welles, then undersecretary of state, and Donald McKay, professor of history at Harvard, then on leave with the Office of Strategic Services in its Research and Analysis branch. Both men had had direct experience of the relative unpreparedness of the United States for the grave responsibilities in international politics thrust on her by the war. They designed the Library primarily as a series of handbooks directed toward the formation and guidance of an enlightened public opinion on important and difficult problems of American relations with specific countries or areas. One of the first volumes issued was *The United States and the Near East* (1947) by E. A. Speiser of the University of Pennsylvania, then a colleague of Professor McKay's with Research and Analysis in the OSS. Professor Speiser, a distinguished historian of the ancient Near East, had excavated and traveled widely in the region. During the war he had concentrated on the study of the area's modern and contemporary aspects. His book, which very successfully achieved the compromise between the scholarly monograph and the broad popularization of journalism that the Library aims at, has long been out of print. Moreover, it dealt with an area in which fundamental changes in the last two decades have been at least as significant as those in any other part of the world. The essentially contemporary character of the Library required that our treatment of the Near East be brought up to date.

The present editor, with the kind consent of Professor Speiser, who has returned to his studies of ancient history, decided to divide the materials of the original study into two books, one on the United States and Israel and another on the United States and the rest of the old Arab World. The first, written by Nadav Safran of Harvard, appeared in 1963. The second, by William R. Polk of the Policy Planning Council of the State Department, is now before the reader.

Dr. Polk has lived in the region he writes about, and has gone successfully through a long apprenticeship in Arabic and Islamic studies. He has that intimate personal knowledge of what he writes about that the founders of the Library regarded as essential in their writers. He has also something even more important than technical mastery of language and history and personal experience of the lands and peoples he deals with; in discussing this very important region, divided by the moral dilemmas set by the establishment of Israel as an independent nation in the heart of the Arab World, Dr. Polk maintains the detachment of the scholar, the fairness of the judge. Such an attitude is not easy to achieve toward the basic problem of Israel and the Arabs, a problem in one sense like that of the Spanish Civil War in the 1930's, a *cas de conscience* for many Westerners of our time. Dr. Polk's is not an attitude of indifference, let alone one of "a plague o' both your houses." He likes and understands the people he writes about, but his sentiments do not stand in the way of his judgment. For the United States, involved directly ever since the war in the manifold problems of the Arab World, of which, as the reader will see, that of Israel is only one, the importance of the region has increased rather than diminished since Dr. Speiser's book appeared in 1947. It is a pleasure to welcome to the Library Dr. Polk's fine book.

Crane Brinton

PREFACE

When Professor Crane Brinton asked me to write this volume of the American Foreign Policy Library, I was teaching at Harvard University with a year's leave seemingly just ahead. In my mind's eye I saw myself ensconced on the lovely island of Rhodes, alternating a diving lung and a typewriter, as I leisurely prepared this book.

Now, four years later, I sit in my snow-bound study in Washington, D.C., never having been closer to Rhodes than a 35,000-foot-high seat in a jet. If less relaxed, I am nevertheless the richer by experience. For in January 1961 I was asked to join the Policy Planning Council to assist in planning American policy toward the Middle East.

Obviously, in many ways, some perhaps not clear even to me, my work in the council has altered my perspective, broadened my knowledge, and, perhaps for the better, chastened my thoughts. Additionally, of course, my appointment has imposed a degree of restraint on my pen. This will not, I believe, prevent me from accomplishing the task I set out to do in this volume, but it is fair to the reader to record the disability. Naturally the views expressed here are my own and do not necessarily reflect official opinion.

My work on the Policy Planning Council on all major aspects of American relations with the Middle East has posed the question to which this book is directed: what are the essential facts, ideas, emotions, and guesses which one needs to understand the relations between the United States and the Arab World?

A few words on the organization of the book may be of assistance to the reader. Part I sets out the basic human and natural factors of the Arab World. Part II is an episodic history of the

Arabs. No attempt is made, nor could it be made in this short space, to treat exhaustively the whole of Arab history. What I have done is to show the development of four pertinent factors of the modern scene, the social code, the religion, the heritage of a golden age, and the deep gulf between society and the state. Part III illustrates the impact of the West during which the traditional ways of life have been altered, thus moving the Arabs from a medieval into a modern period. Part IV documents, in more detail, the development of the Arab states as we know them. The mandate period was a school in statehood in Iraq, Transjordan, Syria, and Lebanon. The Arabian Peninsula stood apart in splendid isolation for which its people paid by relative lack of modernization. Egypt, the most modern of the Arab states, on the contrary, paid for its modernization by political subordination. Palestine, a special problem, has left deep imprints on several aspects of Arab thought. Formal independence has brought radical political changes. Part V gives the matrix of current social revolution in the Arab lands, the rise of new elements in society, changes in the economy, and the development of thought on the place of the Arabs in the world. Part VI discusses the new relationship between the Arabs and the United States and analyzes United States interests, offering some projections for the near future. It is followed by suggested reading. In each chapter I have made every effort to cut out all that I thought not essential to the reader in understanding the present.

My own work on the Middle East goes back to 1946 when I first visited the Arab World. It owes more than I can record to numbers of friends, colleagues, teachers, supporters, and students. Without sharing responsibility for my words I want to mention with gratitude John Badeau, Gabriel Baer, Leonard Binder, Charles Cremeans, Nabih Faris, Sir Hamilton Gibb, Manfred Halpern, Albert Hourani, J. C. Hurewitz, Adib al-Jader, John Marshall, Emrys Peters, Chaim Rabin, Walt Rostow, Herbert Salzman, and James Spain. I also wish to thank the John Simon Guggenheim Foundation, the Rockefeller Foundation, and the Ford Foundation.

The western or North African part of the Arab World is covered in a companion volume by Charles Gallagher, and Israel
is discussed in another by Nadav Safran. Therefore, except where
essential to the development of the discussion here, all issues relating to these topics are omitted from this volume.

William R. Polk

McLean, Virginia
December 1964

CONTENTS

MAPS

DIAGRAM

The United States and the Arab World

THE ARAB WORLD AT A GLANCE

UAR (Egypt) has a population of 28 million of whom 30 percent are literate, an area of 386,000 square miles of which 3 percent is arable, and a Gross National Product (GNP) of $3.5 billion or $125 per capita.

SAR (Syria) has a population of 5.4 million of whom 30–35 percent are literate, an area of 71,200 square miles of which 32 percent is arable, and a GNP of $920 million or $170 per capita.

Jordan has a population of 1.8 million of whom 30 percent are literate, an area of 37,300 square miles of which 10 percent is arable, and a GNP of $360 million or $200 per capita.

Lebanon has a population of 1.8 million of whom 80 percent are literate, an area of 4000 square miles of which 25 percent is cultivated, and a GNP of $756 million or $420 per capita.

Iraq has a population of 6.9 million of whom 20 percent are literate, an area of 172,000 square miles of which 13 percent is cultivated, and a GNP of $1.3 billion or $195 per capita.

Kuwait has a population of 340,000 of whom 30 percent are literate, an area of 6000 square miles of which 1 percent is cultivated, and a GNP of $1 billion or $2940 per capita.

Saudi Arabia has a population of 3–6 million of whom 10 percent are literate, an area of 620,000 square miles of which 0.1 percent is arable, and a GNP of $1 billion.

Yemen has a population of 4–5 million of whom 25 percent are literate, an area of 50–75,000 square miles of which about 4000 is cultivated, and a GNP of $360 million.

Qatar has a population of 60,000 of whom about 10 percent are literate, an area of 4000 square miles of which virtually none is arable, and a GNP of $80 million or $1335 per capita.

PART ONE INTRODUCTION

I. The People on the Land

The Middle Eastern Arab World—encompassing Egypt, the Arabian peninsula, Jordan, Lebanon, Syria, and Iraq—is a vast stretch of mostly barren land joining northeastern Africa to western Asia. Roughly half the size of the United States, the Arab World has a climate similar to that of the Great Plains. The summers are intensely hot and dry; the winters are often bitterly cold. From the point of view of the inhabitants, perhaps the most significant physical feature is the lack of sufficient rainfall to support agriculture in most of the area. This fact has had and today continues to have a profound impact on every aspect of life. From the perspective of outsiders even more significant is the fact that the Arab World is the junction between Africa and Asia and Europe. The linchpin is Egypt, through whose land, sea, and air routes pass much of the world's commerce. Taken together the area constitutes a great highway—or a roadblock.

These two factors, the internal poverty and the strategic importance of the area, have from the dawn of history brought invading armies to the Middle Eastern shores and today make the Arab World a scene of the Cold War. These same factors have also driven the people to occasional bursts of energy and inventive genius to which the world's civilization owes a vast debt. Indeed, civilization began in the valleys of the Nile and the Tigris and Euphrates. Occasionally, too, the people of the area, frustrated by their harsh environment, have lunged outward to conquer vast empires or create far-flung commercial links.

Every American school child is familiar with the Phoenicians, the Babylonians, and the ancient Egyptians, but the Arabs came upon the stage of history at a time when our historical focus had shifted westward. It is difficult, therefore, for Americans to speak with precision of the Arabs, their history, and their culture. But it is also difficult for the Arabs themselves to formulate a commonly accepted definition of Arab, Arabism, and Arabdom.

The Arabs, wrote one of their early poets, are "parasites of the camel." The true Arab was a nomad. Only in his veins coursed the pure Arab blood and only on his tongue the pure Arabic language. Corruption and weakness are the vices of settled life. When the plow crosses the threshold, said an Arab proverb, manhood departs. Thus, "nobility" could be measured by the distance of penetration into the great sand seas of western Asia.

Actually, however, the great majority of the people who speak Arabic are peasants and city dwellers. The bedouin nomads are today, as they probably always have been, a minority of the population. About as few Arabs today can trace their origins to the Arabian Peninsula as Americans can to England. Arabs, like Americans, are a mixed lot. The overwhelming proportion of those who are today called Arab are descendants of the native populations, once called Babylonians, Phoenicians, or Egyptians, who have adopted the Arabic language during the last fourteen centuries since the coming of Islam. Yet so deeply have the Arabs impressed their image upon those with whom they came in contact that the drawing of distinctions on ethnic or linguistic grounds is pointless. The Iraqi is, in a political and cultural sense, no less an Arab than is the Saudi Arabian. To understand the modern Arab world an appreciation of the impact of what has come to be called Arabism is essential.

It was not the desert which was the matrix of Islamic civilization. Islam was always an urban culture. To call a Muslim of the Islamic middle ages an Arab would have been an insult. His was a different order of culture, a different mode of life, and he held the nomad in a contempt tempered by fear. Some of his values he derived from the nomad, whose marvelous poetry, that thread on which Arabic civilization has been strung and in which are embodied the values of Arabic society, he relished. But the city man found in the Islamic order of society, in brotherhoods and guilds, and in fixity of dwelling new norms of life alien to those of the nomad.

Between these two, as wheat between grindstones, was the peasant. Taxed and exploited by the one, he was bled or evicted by the other. Lacking the organization and resources of the one, he was weaker and less warlike than the other. Never was he able fully to participate in the culture of either. Both despised him. Yet he literally furnished the wheat of Middle Eastern life. Upon his labor was built urban civilization and upon his resources the bedouin drew in the frequent lean years of drought.

These three, the bedouin, the peasant, and the city man, are the Arabs. Between them are wide and deep cultural, economic, and political schisms. Yet between them are also important bridges of mutual dependence. And across these bridges, throughout history, a steady stream of men have moved.

Impelled as they were by the harsh and unpredictable conditions of their environment and aided by the fierce qualities they possessed as warriors, the bedouin constantly encroached upon their settled cousins. The clash of the desert and the sown, the parable of Abel and Cain, is a persistent theme in Arabic history. Usually the bedouin were content to levy a tribute and retire when the coming of the rains and the absence of more powerful foes made the desert again safe, but periodically groups spilled into the settled lands and remained. Throughout recorded history there has been a tendency toward what has been called sedentarization. In the last century, sedentarization has increased, but only the scale not the fact of sedentarization is new.

Indeed, the gradations from a purely nomadic to a purely settled way of life are imprecise. Practically all bedouin plow some land. Even in the midst of the vast deserts, one encounters plots where water seepage, flash floods, or occasional rainfall periodically make agriculture possible. There men sow seed, move on with their herds, and return to harvest a crop. On the belt of steppe lands between the desert and the true agricultural lands the villages are semi-nomadic. Their populations fluctuate with the seasons. During the winter rains part of the village will move off to pasture the flocks, returning in the late spring to work the land and harvest the crops. Even in the "black lands," the irrigated plains, the villagers are in part herdsmen.

Yet in general terms the "frontier" between the desert and the sown land can be drawn with considerable precision on a map. In order to stay in one place to cultivate the land, a farmer must have the equivalent of at least eight inches of rainfall yearly. Where this much water is available from rain, oases, or rivers, men have settled. Where the water amounts to less than eight inches or is unreliable, men have had to move. In the Arab World the frontier between these two ways of life has been called the "Fertile Crescent" as it is a great arc running from Jerusalem northward to Aleppo, eastward to Mosul, and south to Basra. Inside the arc only by irrigation can men settle to farm.

Let us examine the area to see how the physical facts have shaped society and culture.

The vast majority of the Arab World is today, and has been throughout history, desert. In Egypt, for example, the total land area is the size of Texas and New Mexico but 97 percent of this is waterless sand and rock. More richly endowed are Iraq, about two-thirds the size of Texas, which is 70 percent steppe and desert, and Syria which is about half desert. Jordan is about 80 percent desert while Saudi Arabia and Kuwait, comprising about 630,000 square miles or an area one fifth the size of the United States, have an agricultural area only about twice the size of Long Island or one tenth of one percent of the total.

Scattered in the vast empty areas are "islands." Some are large oases where an outpouring of spring water makes settled agricultural life possible; others are merely cisterns where rain water is collected and stored for men and animals. Normally these cisterns and some of the oases are meeting places for nomads when the intense heat of the summer desiccates the desert's plant life. Then, as the winter rains come, the nomads and their flocks move out into the suddenly, and briefly, lush pasture.

The rainy season is short, normally about two months, and the summer is long, about six months, but the bedouin manage to

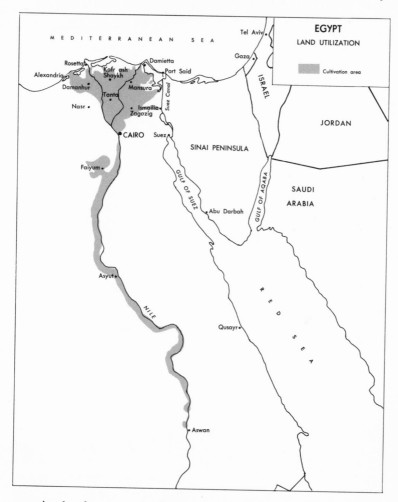

stay in the desert or the fringes of the desert upwards of eight months. Only by living in small groups and by moving about can men and animals live there.

Many, including settled Arabs, have thought of the bedouin as aimlessly wandering gypsies who, to avoid the hard physical labor of settled life, follow their animals around the deserts, stealing a bit now and then from their hard-working cousins, the peasants, and contributing nothing to the well-being of their fellow men.

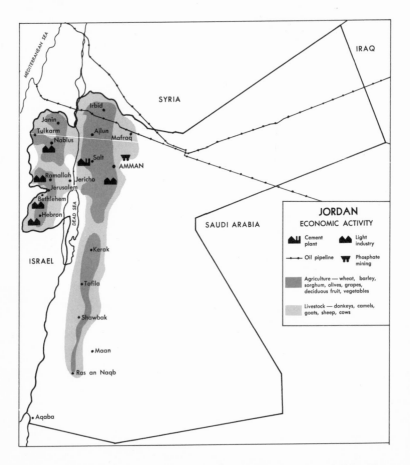

The reality is quite different. The bedouin way of life, like that of the Eskimo, is a highly sophisticated adaptation to an extraordinarily difficult environment. It takes great skill, daring, and perseverence to live in the desert. And unless one is constantly supplied from outside, as armies and explorers are, he must move

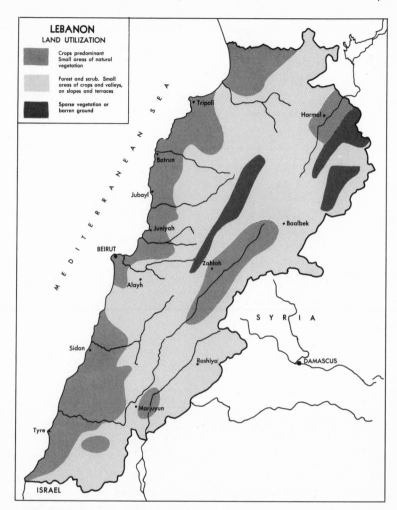

to live. The resources of the desert can be exploited only by the bedouin through his animals. The animals which can stand desert life are the camel, the sheep, and the goat. Others, even the horse, are, like man, ill-fitted for desert life. But, though the desert is harsh and poor in any particular area during most of the year, the resources of the desert taken in the large are immense. Winter rains create vast and lush pastures for short periods and fill water tanks and cisterns. Chance thunderstorms, with their telltale flickers of lightning, are watched as eagerly by the water-hungry bedouin as guides to green valleys as are thunderheads by the Polynesian sailors of the western Pacific as guides to unseen islands. When rain falls, the patches of desert

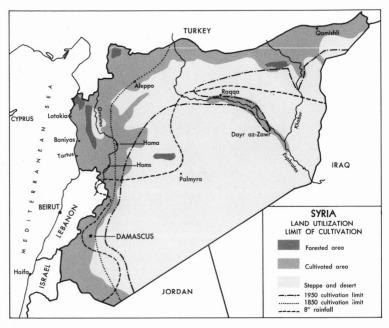

which receive it burst into meadow lands to which the bedouin and their herds must hurry before sun and wind destroy the grass and flowers. The Arabs, whose whole artistic powers have been channeled through their language, even have a particular verb, *shāma*, which means "to watch for flashes of lightning to see where the rain will fall." Few scenes in Arabic literature are treated with more care, sensitivity, and delight than the coming of a rain storm.

Apart from movement to take advantage of a chance rainfall, the bedouin must move for two other reasons. The animals quickly exhaust the pasture and both men and animals quickly drink up the water in wells and cisterns. If the season is cool and the vegetation wet, the animals drink little water and men live on their milk. But even camels need some water. The change of

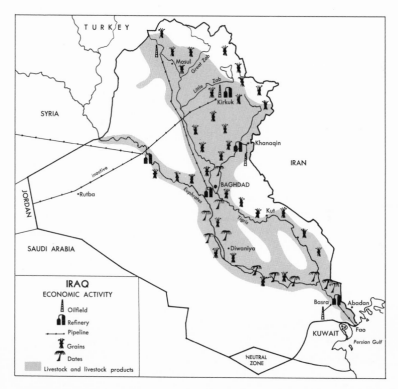

seasons provides another reason for migration. In the summer the desert is the literal hell described in the Koran. Scorching heat, suffocating sand storms, and raging winds bring unquenched and maddening thirst and are murderous to plants, animals, and men. The plants that grow in the desert survive underground but men and animals must move to the cooler areas of the hill

country where they can find water holes and some grazing. Even
there the water may be so brackish and undrinkable that men
must live on camel milk. (It is not without reason that the
bedouin has been called the parasite of the camel.) With the
coming of cold and rainy weather biting, icy winds drive them
back to the lowlands, for the camel needs warm areas to breed.
With rain the desert once again becomes the "Garden of Allah."

A true tribal map of the Arab nomadic areas would be unlike
any other land map. What it would show is the route of march
with an area of approximate winter pasture at one end and summer pasture at the other. Perhaps the best analogy would be a
map of the sea showing fishing areas: one could trace the route
of the boats and their general location but could not predict
exactly where they would be, for this would depend on where
the men found fish. So, for the Arabs, little or nothing is fixed
and their civilization traditionally has lacked the concepts, so
strong in our civilization, of home, homeland, and patriotism.
The sentiment which we find in place of birth, home, and death
exists for the nomad, of course, but it attaches to people not to
land. It is the family, the clan, and the tribe which capture
loyalty and devotion. In the classical literature, the pre-Islamic
poetry, the nomad is usually pictured as he happens upon an
abandoned campsite, but for him the place means nothing—on it
he lavishes no brilliant description—it only serves to remind him
of a loved one. It is to scenes of desert life as a prelude to the
glorification of his folk that the poet addresses himself. Land
per se has little meaning for him, and the Arabic word which
comes closest to meaning "homeland" has none of the emotional
overtones of *patria*.

In other ways, as well, the material conditions of bedouin life
are reflected in his social organization and thought. In the desert
no man can live alone. The bedouin is required by his harsh
environment to be a social animal. Resources are too scattered for
large numbers of people to live together, but efficient utilization
of those resources requires team effort. Under normal conditions
the "team" appropriate to the task is what the Arabs call the
qawm or the clan. The "tribe," of hundreds or thousands of men,

based on genealogy and on grazing areas and water rights, can have effective existence only when enough water and fodder is available—and that can only be sporadically. It is the clan that lives, herds animals, and fights as a corporate group. It normally is composed of several generations of children of a single man but often absorbs clients whom it agrees to protect and others who, in the Arabic expression, "put on its skin."

To the qawm the individual owes total loyalty and from his membership in it he derives social identity and legal standing. Since the primary function of the qawm is to enable the individual to live in a hostile environment, every cultural and social pressure is brought to bear on the individual to do his part in making the qawm cohesive, strong, and effective. Within the qawm property distinctions are minimal.

In a society without external institutions or means of coercion, a man's safety depends upon the ability and willingness of the clan to protect him. But, since the mode of life of the bedouin demands that he spend much of his time alone and far from his fellows, the notion of vengeance came to be substituted for protection. Failure to take vengeance, of course, would reduce the credibility of the threat and so undermine the safety of everyone. However, unlimited warfare and the taking of vengeance would destroy that minimum element of security which makes life in the desert possible. So, as we shall see in the next chapter, various other sorts of safeguards were created to give men a degree of tranquility.

Bedouin society has always been a pulsating organism, subject to rapid coagulation and to equally rapid disintegration. As one clan grows rich and numerous, other clans will ally themselves to it and it will absorb numbers of clients. When it outruns its resources or becomes politically unwieldy, the clan subdivides.

There never have been large numbers of bedouin and today their numbers are decreasing. Reliable statistics do not exist, but there are probably not more than a million bedouin in all of the Arab countries. Always, the lure of city comforts attracted and the unpredictability of the desert climate expelled some nomads. Now, with the tractor reaching out to plow the steppe lands and the pump bringing more areas under regular cultivation, with property rights of the settled peoples enforced by governments whose weapons are carried on airplanes, tanks, and trucks and who are guided by radios, the bedouin are held in check. As the market for camels has declined, with the coming of the airplane, railroad, and truck for transport and beef cattle for meat, the bedouin have ceased to command markets and perform services which once gave them an assured place in the economy. Moreover in the last century it has been the policy of governments to force the bedouin to settle so that they can be controlled, conscripted, and taxed. As a result the frontier of settlement has moved out into the desert areas further each generation, and by the 1930's a French sociologist could accurately say, "the contemporary Arab East is a vast peasant farm." About two thirds of the Egyptians, Syrians, Iraqis, and Jordanians today derive their living from agriculture.

Like the nomadic encampment the village is predicated upon the proximity of water; but unlike it the village is relatively fixed. There has been distinct and constant change in the location of villages. The frontier of settlement of Syria and Iraq as well as, but more dramatically than, Egypt has varied a great deal in the last century, and old tax registers of even such relatively stable areas as Lebanon show great changes over the centuries. Yet village life presents perhaps the most stable element in the area.

There is no "typical" village in the Middle East, but certain characteristics are sufficiently widespread to give an idea of peasant life. Most villages define themselves in terms of kinship, locality, livelihood, and religion.

Villages are small worlds unto themselves. Today, with the advance of the motor car and the radio, this is less the case than formerly, but it is still pronounced. Villagers tend to marry within their villages. Of the nearly 400 marriages contracted over the last century in one Lebanese village, for example, only 40 were with "foreigners" from neighboring towns. The vast majority were with cousins inside the large extended families or clans. Thus, the village and its component families achieve a high degree of homogeneity and control over people and resources which might otherwise have been alienated. Real or ascribed kinship becomes a conceptual scheme by which all contemporary relationships are explained and codified.

Subdivisions within a larger kindred among villagers, as among the nomads, re-enforce their kinship with neighborhood. In many mountain and hill villages in the Levant the neighborhood of a clan is a miniature fort whose houses present a windowless wall to the outside and front on a courtyard in which a well or cistern is shared by all. Within the court the women go about their daily chores unveiled and the children play as members of one family. Often the rules of inheritance will result in a graphic portrayal of the family tree on the ground. For example, one can observe in a Lebanese village the sort of "geography of kinship" illustrated in the accompanying diagram.

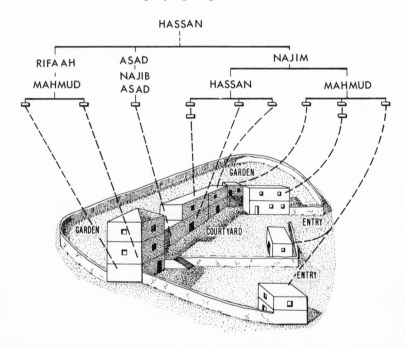

The geography of kinship in a Lebanese village

Other parts of the village may be held in common. In Jordan and parts of Syria and Iraq a sort of village commune has existed. In this system land is reapportioned among inhabitants from time to time. In other villages, where the custom of individual holdings is stronger, the village might hold grazing lands and a market place in common. Resources, such as access to a spring or cistern, would be carefully regulated by custom or even by a written "treaty" between the major clans of the village.

The fact of life most central to all is the community of the village: any threat to the stability or economic well-being of a part of the village is necessarily a threat to all. As in the nomadic life the rights of the individual are severely subordinated to those of the group; above all, the system is conservative. Major dislocations by migration, death, or impoverishment have to be righted by social means, so the village brings in or excludes outsiders as it sees fit, protects village rights to water or land, and endows shrines and religious organizations.

Whereas the bedouin can protect himself, his fellows, and his animals by moving, the villager, tied to his plot of land, his house, and his access to water, can not leave except in dire emergency and at high price. In times of unrest or anarchy villagers did become partly or wholly nomadic. The perceptive Swiss traveler John Lewis Burckhardt noted in 1810—a time of anarchy—that few Syrian peasants died in the same village in which they were born, so oppressed were they by the government tax collectors and the rapacious bedouin raiders. Even today and even on irrigated lands, the Iraqi peasant is at least semi-nomadic, partly out of the habits of insecurity and partly because for nearly a thousand years the central government has failed to regulate irrigation and drainage. But for most of the peasants in the Middle East, kinship has been replaced by geography and the central function of all organization is to protect one's little world from outside encroachment.

Among settled people, as among the nomads, those are most safe who are least easy to reach. And so the inhabitants of the remote mountain villages of Yemen, Hadhramaut, Oman, Iraq, Syria, and Lebanon have been able to preserve, through the changing times of many centuries, their culture and their independence, while the peasants of the open plains of Syria and the river deltas of Egypt and Iraq could not. It is not surprising, therefore, that the minority communities and religious sects are often to be found in the mountains while there is more homogeneity in the plains.

The large-scale, irrigated agriculture of the Middle East has, historically, given the area its wealth. Indeed, it is probable that the "birth" of civilization as we know it, in the sense of human organization on a large scale, is intimately associated with the need to control the mighty rivers of the Middle East. This problem, it has been suggested, is at the base of oriental despotism. It is certainly clear that the settled agricultural areas have always lived under highly centralized, autocratic governments which have closely regulated not only the commerce but also the details of agricultural production. In fact, so intimately have the governments, from ancient Egyptian and Babylonian times, intervened in the lives of the people that they represented the whole spectrum of organized life from economic, military, bureaucratic, and legal power to matters of personal status and religion. But the people fear and resent this interference and usually resist by withdrawal, having as little to do with government as possible while submitting to its outward power. As Father Ayrout observed in *The Peasant*, "They have changed their masters, their religion, their language and their crops, but not their way of life. From the beginnings of the Old Kingdom to the climax of the Ptolemaic period the Egyptian people preserved and maintained themselves. Possessed in turn by Persians, Greeks, Romans, Byzantines, Arabs, Turks, French and English, they remained unchanged . . . A receptive people, yet unyielding; patient, yet resistant." So accustomed are they to living apart from government and yet so pliant are they before government as to make both the development programs of today and the attempts at representative government of recent years extremely difficult.

The peasant is deeply suspicious of any move the government may make—even if, on the surface, it appears to be to his benefit.

When the governments tried to get him to register his lands, he often did so in someone else's name, fearing taxes and conscription. When modern governments have sought to get him to use better methods and seed, he has been reluctant, since the old ways, though perhaps not the best, were known, trusted, and reliable. The peasant can ill afford to gamble and is little disposed, in any case, to trust any government. And indeed governments of the last century, even when occasionally proclaimed in his name, nearly always were or became centers of power for the landlords to oppose all measures designed to help the peasant. It was, after all, the elected Iraqi parliament which in 1932, upon achieving independence, passed a law to convert free tribesmen into serfs, bound to the land and policed by machinery of the state. It was the elected Egyptian parliament which stoutly resisted to the bitter end any moves to enforce equitable taxation, introduce better and cheaper fertilizers, or to give the peasant a share in the land.

The city, as personified by the government, always has lived leechlike on the countryside and often gave little in return. Between the way of life in the cities and that in the countryside there has been always a vast gulf, unbridged even by a common culture, for the peasant actively partook little of the Islamic culture of the urban areas or the Arabic culture of the bedouin, although he was the passive recipient of both.

Like the bedouin, who was attracted to settled life, the peasant was constantly lured by the city. In times of rural anarchy and chaos men huddled in walled towns for protection. As economic opportunity or political considerations led them, they moved to cities or garrisons or palaces and, by encamping around them, created new urban areas. At several times in the Islamic period such movements have been particularly pronounced. During the Islamic conquests the early caliphate, to keep the hastily assembled tribal armies from fading into the countryside, encouraged them to settle around the garrison-administrative centers which gradually grew into such cities as Basra, Kufa, and old Cairo. When Baghdad was laid out in 762, its founder, the Abbasid Caliph Mansur, planned only a palace and an administrative center but founded, in fact, the core of a city. And, finally, in the period of rapidly expanding commerce that has extended over the last century the cities have grown considerably in size and, like magnets drawing together iron filings, have clustered around themselves concentric rings of shanty towns.

But, of course, rings of shanty towns are not cities. And the Middle East has had an unbroken urban tradition from the earliest historic times. This is particularly evident in Egypt and Mesopotamia but Damascus, Palmyra, Petra, Tripoli, Sidon, Tyre, Jerusalem, Medina, and Mecca have their roots deep in the past. Jerusalem and Damascus were well enough known, but Mecca, even before the birth of Muhammad in A.D. 570, was a great international entrepôt, controlling through diplomatic and military ties with the "nations" of Arabia, the bedouin tribes, and a caravan trade covering thousands of miles. This center had a sophisticated oligarchy dealing with intricate problems of commercial law, money, and banking, and an urban pride and sense of identity celebrated in the pantheon, the Kaaba, which long before Islam was a focal point of Arabian religion and commerce.

The coming of Islam provided a powerful stimulus to urban life. Muhammad was a city man who thought in urban terms. His "Constitution of Medina" was, among other things, an attempt to transcend the limits of kinship and neighborhood of the tribe and village by creating a sense of community which would embrace rival groups of kindred, men of different hamlets, and even men separated by the frontiers of religion. Inherent in the structure Muhammad created in Medina is the intricate social pattern of the medieval Islamic city, interlaced as it became with religious and craft guilds and neighborhoods centering on mosque schools, with its markets patrolled and organized by inspectors of weights and measures, police, and law courts. The civic pride of the medieval cities was often further expressed in great popular religious festivals while wealth, learning, and power were institutionalized in foundations, libraries, and schools.

To a tragic degree this aspect of the Arab cultural heritage was destroyed by the invasions of the Mongols and the Turks, in which such great urban centers as Baghdad, Aleppo, and Damascus were virtually obliterated and by the centuries of waste and neglect which brought floods, famine, and pestilence in their wake. Baghdad, which in the twelfth century had a population of nearly a million—or five times that which Paris was to achieve two centuries later—was sacked and massacred in 1258. When this happened, culture, which in Iraq in Islamic times was always an urban phenomenon, withered like a plant in the scorching blast of a desert summer. Unlike the plant, the culture was not deeply rooted in the soil and little survived for the refreshing nourishment of subsequent, peaceful centuries. Moreover, when centralized control over the vast and complex irrigation system was ended, great tracts of land were ruined. Irrigation and drainage ditches were allowed to fill with silt, the desert broke in to the black lands, and much of the best land turned into a swamp. With its rural base sapped, the urban structure of Iraq did not again reach the scale of its medieval days until this century.

Yet, by the end of the eighteenth century urban life was beginning to recover, and some cities, such as Aleppo and Damascus, though small by modern terms, had again developed relatively high standards of cultural and commercial life. Damascus was described by a French visitor in 1833 as "a vast factory town comparable to Lyon." And the merchants of even such small seaports as Jiddah were able to buy and sell shiploads of merchandise from Zanzibar, India, and the Red Sea ports. Little towns like Gaza derived their importance in part from the fact that the caravan routes passed through them and they were trading centers for the bedouin.

The point is that a real urban society existed. It offered both an urban government and a satisfying community life, based upon villagelike neighborhoods and laced together by religious foundations, brotherhoods, and guilds. Life was sufficiently organized to encourage cultural and educational development, and so to keep alive the forms of Islamic culture.

The three levels of Arab society, the nomadic, the village, and the city, though separated in important ways culturally, politically, and geographically, historically have been in other ways dependent upon one another. The bedouin furnished meat, wool, and transportation to the villagers who raised the grain that sustained the bedouin in bad years and the urban people always as well as the cotton and silk which were fashioned in the cities and sent out again on the backs of bedouin camels. These patterns of life interacted and for all their differences were accepted. As we shall see, it was in part the dislocation of this pattern which has been a prominent feature of society in our times. For today, in the Arab countries as in most society, the urban areas are growing rapidly in numbers and in power at the expense of both the steppe and the sown cultures. Cairo today has a larger population than all of Egypt had in 1800 and Beirut has grown from about 10,000 in 1830 to half a million in 1963. As industry develops relative to agriculture this trend will continue.

The "frontier" between desert and sown land, as we have seen, is a highly determining factor in the structure of the Arab world. Another of the "frontiers" of Middle Eastern Arab society is religion. Before the advent of Islam some Arabs had become Christians and Jews, but most of the nomads were pagans with rudimentary cults of gods and goddesses often symbolized by stones. As we shall see, Islam became a great codifier of society, giving not only law but also highly specific rules and mores, and a unifier of society in that it set forth principles that transcended the boundaries of clan, tribal, village, and regional strife. Islam also tried to transcend religious differences by marking out the rights and duties not only of its own citizens, the Muslims, but also of the members of other religions. More than other great religions, notably medieval Christianity, Islam was highly successful in extending the perimeters of tolerance. One measure of this fact is that for many centuries after the conquest the peoples of the new empire of Islam retained their separate languages and religions. Conversion to Islam is still far from complete in the Arab lands and as late as the last century many whose descendants now regard themselves as Arabs spoke other languages.

In the Arabic community are many who are not today Muslim while among the Muslim community are several sects and many non-Arabs. Historically these differences were abetted by the Muslim rulers who allowed each community, as distinguished by religion, to rule itself in matters of personal status, taxation, and internal security. Western powers have often been associated with these minority groups. The Italians and Greeks had their own nationals in several of the Arab countries; the French protected the Catholic community; and tsarist Russia aided the Orthodox community. Great Britain traditionally aided the Druze and the Jews, and private American groups helped to create and then foster Protestants. So the existence of minority communities has import both in domestic and international terms.

Egypt has nearly four million Copts. The word Copt is a corruption of the Greek word for Egyptian; the Copts are the remnant of Hellenized ancient Egypt. Today, they share with other Egyptians the Arabic language but remain monophysite Christians under an unbroken line of 116 patriarchs since the Council of Chalcedon in A.D. 451. Like minorities elsewhere, the sect was often used by, and lent themselves to use by, alien rulers who knew that the Copts, while having detailed knowledge of the country, could never threaten their rule. Thus, the Copts tended to become identified as a clerical class, although many are peasants, and to be tarred with the brush of governmental tyranny and alien privilege. As late as the end of World War I almost half of the Egyptian civil service was Coptic.

Egypt also has had large communities of Jews, Greeks, and Italians, although all three have declined greatly in recent years. They benefited to such an extent from alien patronage that hardly any members of these communities could be brought to an Egyptian court for any offense and virtually all were able to escape taxes and other obligations. Quite naturally they were resented, often bitterly, by the less fortunate natives. As a British satirical writer once said, in every wave of nationalist violence it was the Greek grocers who laid down their lives for Britian. The Greek grocer was the usurer of the typical Egyptian village. Alexandria was largely a Greek city until quite recently. The Italians aroused less public ire but have suffered in the generally antiforeign feelings which followed the coming of independence.

The Jews have suffered proportionally as violence and hatred between Egypt and Israel have increased. As early as the 1930's, when Zionism became strong in the Palestine Mandate, there were anti-Jewish demonstrations, and when Israel defeated Egypt in 1948–49, public feeling increased in violence. The Egyptian government took various steps to control the animosity but when, in 1956, Israel attacked Egypt, it openly encouraged emigration.

Lebanon, on the contrary, as a vast natural fortress of steep valley sides and rocky crags, has been historically a refuge of minorities. Indeed, Lebanon has no true majority. In a population of about two million about 6 percent are Armenian, and 0.5 percent are Jews. Of the rest, the Arabs, the latest estimates give this breakdown: 7 percent Druze, members of a heritical offshoot of Islam, 18 percent Shii or non-Orthodox Muslim, 20 percent Sunni or Orthodox Muslim, 38 percent Uniate Christian, 16 percent Orthodox Christian and 1 percent Protestant. These subdivisions are so woven into the "confessional" system of Lebanese political and administrative life as to enable each community effectively to defend itself today as, behind the walls of villages and the rocks of steep mountain sides, it could traditionally.

In Jordan about 2 percent of the population of one and one-half million are Circassians whose ancestors in the last century migrated from the Caucasus to escape the Russians, and 1 percent are Armenians who came for similar reasons. Nine percent of the people are Christian, mostly living in what used to be the mandate of Palestine on the west bank of the Jordan River, and all the rest are Orthodox Muslims.

Of the roughly seven million Iraqis over 75 percent are Arabic speaking and about 20 percent Kurdish and Turkoman. The Arabs are divided into the Sunnis and the somewhat more numerous Shiis while the Kurds and Turkomans are mostly Sunnis. Iraq, like Lebanon, has no true majority: religiously, the Sunnis are preponderant but are divided ethnically and linguistically between Arabs and Kurds while ethnically and linguistically the Arabs form the majority but are divided religiously and culturally between Sunnis and Shiis. Other minorities include the Chaldeans, Armenians, Jews, Yezidis (popularly called "Devil Worshipers"), and Assyrians, each in small numbers.

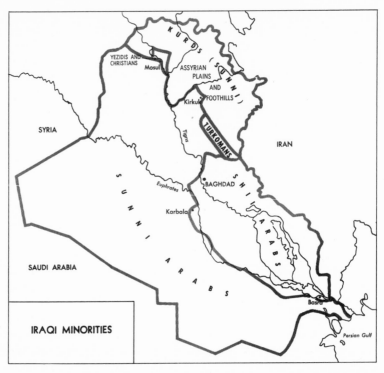

IRAQI MINORITIES

Syria, with a population of five million, is basically Sunni Muslim but contains 13 percent Christian, 11 percent Alawi, 3 percent Druze, and 1 percent Ismaili minorities.

Alone among the Arab areas, the Arabian Peninsula is comparatively devoid of minorities. North and south Arabic differ somewhat, but they are in their written form the same language, and almost everyone who now lives in the peninsula is today Muslim. Yemen did have a large Jewish minority and was once ruled by Jewish kings; but in recent centuries it has been ruled by an imam who represented the Zaidi branch of Shii Islam. Otherwise, the people of the peninsula are primarily Sunni Muslims.

The total population of the Arab Middle East has exploded in the last century. The birth rate, apparently, has always been high but it was canceled in large part by a very high rate of infant mortality and by famine and plague. Centuries ago the Arabs of the desert, aware that the settled areas were sources of disease, strove to remain in the cleaner air of the desert, but drought and famine drove them in tidal pulsations toward the urban centers. Hunger accounts for some of the most graphic and tragic pieces of Arabic literature. The peasants usually managed to eat but their economy hovered barely above mere subsistence. It was partly for this reason that they resisted growing nonfood crops like cotton. For the food they grew they paid a heavy toll in their exposure to malaria, bilharzia—the snail-borne disease associated with irrigation—and dysentary.

There are no accurate population statistics even now for most of the Arab countries—figures for Saudi Arabia over the last decade have varied from two to ten million—but reasonable estimates in the third decade of the nineteenth century give the basis for an informed guess that there were then about six million Arabs in the Middle East of whom half lived in Egypt. Today, Egypt's population is nearing 30 million and, increasing at 3 percent yearly, will double in a quarter of a century. It is clear that this extremely rapid rate of growth places the most serious pressure on the economies of the Arab countries which will require enormous investment of capital and skill to enable them to feed their people. But not only are the actual numbers of people increasing, the minimum scale of living for which they are prepared to settle is also rising. Thus, in political and economic terms the difference between 1830 and 1965 is not just six million compared to roughly fifty-two million but six million at a certain living standard and fifty-two million at a living standard several times as high. Today, economies must not only feed and clothe but furnish medical care, education, consumer goods, industrial plants, roads, dams, and, unfortunately, highly sophisticated and highly expensive weapons for large armies.

In most natural resources other than oil the Middle East is poor. Even where minerals exist, they either are difficult of access or are not present in usable combinations. For example, Egypt has iron deposits but no coal; Jordan has phosphate rock but no power with which to process it. The whole area is deficient in timber. Therefore, most industry is still primarily engaged in processing agricultural products.

Oil is the great exception to generalizations about the Middle East. Here, Middle Eastern Arab resources are tremendous. Kuwait, the golden land of the Middle East, with an area of 6000 square miles or roughly the size of Connecticut and a population of a third of a million of whom only about half are native, has about a quarter of the world's oil reserves. Saudi Arabia has roughly 16 percent and Iraq 8 percent. Other parts of the Arab Middle East account for an additional roughly 3 percent of proved reserves.

As Europe has recovered from World War II and the whole world has taken to wheels and wings, the oil industry and the oil-producing countries have prospered. The Arabs now draw nearly one billion dollars yearly from royalties on their oil. But, tragically for the economic impact of this flow of capital, oil is primarily to be found in those areas of the Middle East least suited for human habitation and where nature has provided little else in which men could invest. It is only recently that the Arabs have found ways in which the income from petroleum could be put to work effectively in the Arab area rather than causing a boom in the real estate markets of Cairo, Beirut, and Lausanne.

From the point of view of outsiders, the Arab Middle East contains assets of great world importance. The Suez Canal, which yields about $150 million dollars yearly in revenue to Egypt, is of enormous value to international commerce and industry. In 1963, 209 million tons of cargo in some 20,000 ships passed through the canal. But even before the canal was dug, Egypt was a transit point in international commerce and communication. In the Middle Ages Egypt waxed rich on this trade. Its later poverty was in part a consequence of one of the great blockades of all time, the seizure of control over the mouth of the Red Sea, to close off Venetian-Egyptian commerce, which was the consequence of the Portuguese sailor Vasco da Gama's great feat in rounding the Cape of Good Hope in 1498. For both Napoleon and the British,

Egypt seemed a key to Europe's control over India. Finally, the existence of the canal was a major causative factor in the Anglo-French invasion of Egypt in November 1956.

And, in this age of air travel, the airspace over and the landing and transit facilities in the several Arab countries, but most importantly in Lebanon and Egypt, are of the greatest importance in international relations. Thus, for themselves, for their assets, and for their very weaknesses, the Arabs will command the attention of the great powers in our time.

PART TWO   FOUR LEGACIES FROM THE ARAB PAST

II. The Ancient Arabs: The Code of Honor

Like most peoples, the Arabs cherish a memory of times of glory, halcyon days when the world paused to allow men to aspire to the fullness of their bravery, strength, and refinement, and which, ever after, set a banner on the pinnacle of their achievement and a seal on their aspirations. Ancient song and story; in its content and form of expression, forms the core of a classical tradition, the quarry of artistic endeavor, and the repository of national ethic. The Arabs call these *Aiyām'u-'Arab* or "the Days of the Arabs." For all those who speak and relish the richness of the Arabic language and who call themselves Arab, the Days of the Arabs are an ideal past.

Such a period in Western civilization was the Age of Pericles, or, in a slightly different form, the England of the Arthurian Legends. Americans, even with our short history and varigated backgrounds, have already begun to make of the early years of the Republic—or of the Wild West—an idealized past in which men stood straighter, strove more nobly, and reached more surely for glory.

An idealized past, even one with which a person can identify only by great stretch of imagination, is a mirror for the present. However dimly it may be related to a real past, it provides a clear and bright picture of the aspirations and values of the present. What then has come down to modern Arabs from this dim, distant, and wild past?

The traditions and values of the ancient Arabs are not simply of antiquarian interest. Ancient Arabic poetry is today the syllabus of linguistic and literary study in every Arab school. Poetry to the Arabs is what folk stories, drama, legend, and epic are to the West. Few indeed are the Arabs, even those who are illiterate, who have not memorized hundreds of lines of poetry, and few are the political discussions, social gatherings, or entertainments in which poetry does not figure prominently. On its poetry Arabic civilization has lavished all of the inventive genius which in other cultures has been spread over the whole range of the arts. Study, memorization, and repetition of ancient Arabic poetry tie the modern age to previous ages and on this string is hung that sense of continuity which makes those who live in the modern Middle Eastern Arab states think of themselves as Arab. It is not only a living tradition, it is the essence of tradition.

By their British and French rulers and by many Western visitors, the modern bedouin nomads, and so by extension ancient Arabs, were regarded as the "good Arabs," a wild, childlike people, indolent perhaps and unproductive of social well-being, but whose courage and simplicity one could admire in contrast to the superficially Westernized, devious, difficult "town Arabs." Others, including their Turkish governors under the Ottoman Empire, have thought of the bedouin as gypsies, a people wandering aimlessly through the deserts, or pirates who, living in the vast inner sand sea of the Middle East, raided and plundered the coast and then retired, out of reach, to their distant "islands" and "fishing grounds." Arab philosophers have thought of the bedouin in terms similar to the eighteenth century European philosophers' "Natural Man"—the bedouin were the simple, pristine, children of God, uncorrupted and untamed by civilization, a bloodbank of new vigor for jaded urban society.

These attitudes have led, of course, to different policies. The British attempted to police the bedouin while protecting them from the city Arabs. Transjordan was to be their state, and in Iraq they were to have a strong voice in parliament. The French were less protective but, if anything, more appreciative of *la civilisation du désert*. The Turks generally sought to destroy the bedouin as others have sought to destroy pirates. Punitive expeditions were tried repeatedly but succeeded only against the settled or semi-nomadic tribes, who, having invested in lands and houses, could be caught. The true nomads simply moved away from the slow Turkish infantry or struck back by isolating Turkish garrisons. Few were those wise enough to lure the bedouin to settle so that they might be controlled.

The attitude of the urban Arabs themselves was and still is ambivalent. The Arabs glory in the traditions and art of the bedouin as ancient Arabs, and nobility is claimed by descent from the bedouin. Historically to say of a student of Arabic that he studied with the bedouin was to accord him the best of credentials. Classical Arabic was the language of the bedouin of the Arabian highlands. Yet, the bedouin are feared and even hated, for if they have infused new vigor into society they have also drained off the old life and have overthrown existing orders of society. Today in the Arab World there is no government which can be said to be sympathetic with the bedouin. All seek to convert him into a settled peasant and all have upset the administrative arrangements which set him apart from other citizens.

Actually, nomadism has been in decline for at least a half a century. Settled peoples have not needed the meat and wool of the bedouin camels, for they could get them elsewhere cheaper. They have found cheaper and faster means of transport. And, with the use of the airplane and the truck with a machine gun mounted on top, they could prevent the nomads from raiding one another and the settled lands as never before. As the high commissioner of Iraq wrote in 1924 in his report to the League of Nations, "now, almost before the would-be rebel has formulated his plans, the droning of the aeroplanes is heard overhead." Always bedouin life has been fragile; now the delicate balance of conditions which sustained it have been upset. The bedouin, like the knight and the cowboy, is rapidly passing from the scene, but like all heroic figures he leaves behind a legend which dwarfs reality.

As we have seen, the harsh realities of desert life shaped bedouin society and thought. The bedouin never lived under government, and even their own tribes were loose federations in which every man was an equal. The shaikh was little more than a respected arbiter and generous host, never a ruler to his people. Burckhardt, one of the great observers of bedouin life, wrote in *Notes on Bedouins and Wahabys*, "the shaikh has no actual authority over the individuals of his tribe; he may, however, by his personal qualities obtain considerable influence. His commands would be treated with contempt; but deference is paid to his advice . . . thus the Bedouin truly says that he acknowledges no master . . . and in fact, the most powerful chief dares not inflict a trifling punishment on the poorest man of his tribe."

But, if the desert gives scope for such democracy, it also puts a heavy premium on social cohesion. Life in the desert is and must be a team effort. The clan—for which Arabic, as it has for most things, has many names—or qawm is the group of kindred which lives, herds animals, fights, and makes peace together. The qawm was the effective social unit—it was, in reality, the nation-state of the bedouin. No larger or more elaborate social gathering had more than transitory existence and none had real authority over the clan. Since there was no "international" law and no supraclan institutions, the identity and protection of the individual were derived from membership in a clan. It was the certainty that a man's clan would protect him where possible and exact retaliation when he was harmed that gave him security of property and person.

Pride in folk and boasting of their qualities is one of the common features of the Arabic poem. The poet finds many ways to enhance the reputation of his folk, detailing their bravery, their wisdom, their generosity. As an-Nabighah sang,

. . . a people are they whose might in battle shall never fail
When goes forth their host to war, above them in circles wheel
    battalions of eagles, pointing the path to battalions more:
Their friendship is old and tried—fast comrades in foray, bred to
    look unafraid on blood, as hounds to the chase well trained . . .
Of steeds in the spear-play skilled, with lips for the fight drawn back,
    their bodies with wounds all scarred, some bleeding and some half-
    healed.

And down leap the riders where the battle is strait and stern and spring in the face of Death like stallions amid the herd;

Between them they give and take deep draughts of the wine of Doom as their hands ply the white swords, thin and keen in the smiting-edge.

In them no defect is found, save only that in their swords are notches a many, gained from smiting of host on host.

(translated by Lyall)

Behind the boast of his folk is the poet's implied and, at the end of the poem, explicit boast of his own virtues.

Most of the poet's virtues could be shown in performance of the duties of the tribe but the ultimate in personal bravery was to pit oneself against all mankind and all nature. If a man were expelled by his qawm he was literally an outlaw against whom the hand of every man was turned, living as Hobbes said in "continuall feare and danger of violent death." Since the ideal of rugged individualism always clashed with that of corporate sub-ordination, some Arabs, including some of the greatest of the poets, were expelled from their clans and tried to "go it alone" by feats of almost superhuman endurance. As the greatest of these outlaw poets, Shanfara, sang,

By your life, the earth is not so narrow that a man cannot find elbow room,

As long as he uses his wits and by desire or fear travels in night's black gloom.

The poet tells his folk to begone for he has chosen wolves for his qawm, since wolves do not break confidence and live by a sterner code than fickle men. He fears nothing as, accompanied by his three companions—a stout heart, a glistening sword, and a long singing bow—he moves through deserts so awesome that before them even riding camels panic and in weather so hellish in the "dog days" of summer that the very mirages melt and vipers writhe on the stones, "prolonging my hunger so long that it is the *hunger* I kill and I become unmindful of it." But the outlaw-poet wants his audience to know that he does not punish himself for

masochistic reasons. "Were it not to avoid a shameful action, no
drinking bout or feast would be found without my being there."

But a proud and bitter soul will not uphold me in the face of wrong,
except as I plot my vengeance.

I am the master of patience draping its gown over the heart of a wolf
and tenacity I wear for sandals.

Such stark and unbending glorification of egotism, violence, and
hatred led to lives that were often, as Hobbes put it of *his* man
in nature, "solitary, poore, nasty, brutish and short."

Yet there are mitigating features. First, the option always remained open, even at terrifying personal sacrifice, for the individual to save his own honor even at the expense of loss of his
folk. In this direction lay heroism and poetic ennoblement. In
more normal circumstances a family quarrel could be ended by a
split of the qawm into two parts, each of which could live normally, or by the grafting of the weaker group onto another clan
within the same tribe much as one might migrate and become
naturalized in another nation. In this direction lay salvation.

Westerners—and most Arabs—may find the content of this
poetry of bravery, as the Arabs called it, objectionable, but its
grand gesture, its eloquence, the flow of its language, cannot but
sway men's emotions. No one who has watched an Arabic audience can fail to have noticed the way in which linguistic virtu-
osity hypnotizes the people. It is this which has given to the radio
station in our own time such extraordinary influence throughout
the Arab World and which allows even vitriolic and vile propaganda to be accepted, if well done.

Ironically, even in the poems which express hatred of one man
for others or one folk for another, and which are, therefore,
divisive propaganda at its most effective, there is a force for cultural unity. Over the years, as names and events were forgotten,
the poems lost their political sting and came to be a common heritage of all Arabs. It was, indeed, the sharing of the classical literature which provided the common cultural experience of the
ancient Arabs.

The contrary sentiment to a rugged individualism bordering on suicide is the intense emotional attachment to one's clansmen, right or wrong, and the personal acceptance of responsibility for any and all of their acts. The Arabic word for the sentiment which bound together the clan is the same as the modern word for nationalism, *qawmiyah*. In one of the most widely quoted poems in Arabic, this sentiment is summed up by a bedouin poet of the clan of Ghaziyah. The clansmen have been on a raid and foolishly stop their retreat before they are out of reach of their enemies. The poet Duraid bin Simma, having warned them and realizing their folly will probably cost him his life, stays to fight for, as he said,

When they spurned me, I was still with them, having seen their folly and my own imprudence

For what am I apart from Ghaziyah—if the clan goes astray, so I,

And if Ghaziyah is rightly guided, I too am rightly guided.

Then he fought the

Fight of a man who nurses his brother with his own person, knowing that man is not immortal.

Failure to protect one's kinsmen or, if they are killed or wronged, to retaliate against those who inflicted a wrong would destroy the meager protection the individual could find in desert tribal life. It was the categorical imperative of bedouin life and honor. To fail or shirk was a cowardly action which stained the individual and his kindred with the "stain of shame." Only the blood of the enemy could wash away this stain. And virtually every Arabic poem has some reference to the fear of blame for not acting as a man should.

This duty was incumbent upon a clan not only for its own members but also for those they undertook to protect. Annoyance at the "protected stranger" often showed through the lines of the poems. As Urwa bin Ward sang:

God curse the starving thief who concealed by the blackness of night steals behind the tents to suck the marrow bones in the refuse heap.

Who counts as the riches of his lot to be every night where he can demand hospitality from a luckier friend.

But each poet boasts of his folk's generosity and protectiveness toward the guests or dependents. And no more bitter reproach could be made of a qawm than that it had failed in this duty. In the earliest of all known Arabic poems, the Basus Cycle, the poetess taunts her protectors by warning a friend that she is in "the encampment of such a folk that even when a wolf attacks he always seizes *my* lamb." Her protector, insulted beyond all compare, prepared to take vengeance on those who have harmed her after begging mankind not to blame him for "My protected one, know you one and all, is of the closest of kin." And so, like the Trojan War, began, poetically at least, a war of honor. For the Arab, said one of the greatest of Arab poets, must be a "spring pasture to the protected strangers." This is one of the deepest of obligations which has been rooted in Arabic civilization and nurtured by the tradition embodied in Arabic poetry.

The wise man is not foolhardy. Patience, cunning, and reserve are so much the attributes of the perfect man that they even spill into Islamic thought, Indeed, in the Koran God is described as the "best of the Plotters" (iii.54). But the final and greatest quality of the perfect man is generosity. The arbitrator is "one above the fray, possessed of such a generosity as leads him to aid others to show their generosity."

Generosity is not a virtue among the weak. For them the proper road is retaliation which should lead to the status quo ante. Other ways, however, could create a new balance of power. If the wrongdoer offered to pay recompense, the wronged could, after a decent interval, accept, and peace could be made. The strong, on the other hand, could be generous and could make peace without loss of face. One of the seven "Golden Odes" of ancient Arabia celebrates the peacemaker, who by his personal generosity and wisdom manages to stop war between two clans.

. . . If we set our hands to Peace, base it broad and firm by the giving of gifts and fair words of friendship, all will be well.

"Yea, glory ye gained . . . the highest—God guide you right! who gains without blame a treasure of glory, how great is he!"

(Translated by Lyall)

Otherwise war to the knife was not only sanctioned but demanded by the social ethic. Even if it meant death, no man could with honor or pride shirk his duty of retaliating, goaded as he was by his womenfolk and the very ghost of the slain and wracked by a "burning fever"—"Hearts are cured of rancour-sickness, whether men against us war, or we carry death among them: dying, slaying, healing comes."

To Western tastes some of the value system embodied in classical Arabic poetry is not appealing. The boasts of the poets, the thirst for vengeance, the hunger for fame, and the fascination for the wounding of the foe, though not unfamiliar to readers of classical Greek literature, are not attractive. But to understand their impact on modern Arabic thought is vital to an understanding of politics in the Arab Middle East. For the imperative of preserving or achieving dignity, the fear of reproach as being unworthy or impotent people, and finally, the importance of the form of action and the word of communication as equal to or surpassing that of the content, greatly influences Arab political behavior. To outsiders who would understand, whether condoning or opposing, this is the beginning of knowledge.

III. Islam: The Regulation of Society

Islam never made peace with bedouin society. In the Koran the bedouin Arab is scorned as one who, failing to believe in the religion, merely submits to the outward power of the religious state. However, Islam was born in an Arabia deeply colored by the values, the presence, and the literature of the bedouin Arabs. And Islam defined itself in the framework of a corporate, tribal society. The wonder is not that Islam was so influenced by Arabian experience but rather that Muslims were able so to elaborate the structure they inherited as to form one of the great religious civilizations of human history.

The historical role of Muhammad, the society of early Islam, and the Islamic creed are here set forth in bare outline. But this bears to the civilization of Islam the relationship of a skeleton to a man: omitted are the nerves, brain, heart, and flesh, an account of which would fill more than this volume. In short compass, this chapter will attempt to show the structure of the skeleton and to suggest the richness of the whole.

Muhammad, the Messenger of God who delivered the Koran to the Arabs in Arabic, as the Koran explains, was born in the commercial city of Mecca about A.D. 570. Around his life has grown an immense literature of fact and fiction, devotion and scorn, conjecture and artifice. But from the Koran and the Traditions related by his early followers we know that he was born into a poor branch of Mecca's ruling oligarchy and was an orphan from his early youth. When about twenty-five, he married a wealthy widow whose business agent he had become. With her capital he acquired some status in the community while engaging in the caravan trade with Yemen and the Levant.

Then, apparently quite suddenly, when he was about forty, Muhammad had a vision of the Angel Gabriel who ordered him to "Recite in the Name of the Lord." The stunned and frightened Muhammad is said to have stammered, "But what shall I recite?" After an interval in which he received no further visions, he transmitted to his people, in an unending stream until his death in 632, what has been collected by his followers as the Koran.

For his contemporaries as for later, non-Muslim writers, Muhammad has proved to be a difficult and complex figure. To some Western medieval writers he appeared as a satanic adventurer who sought to undermine Christendom or, to the more fanciful, a "fallen" cardinal who, having been passed over for the Papacy, set out to create his own religion. Modern writers have portrayed him as an epileptic, a sufferer from hysteria, a self-deceiving spiritualist, a madman, or a dupe of the Devil. The pagan oligarchs of his own city were unconcerned with precise labels. To them, he was a troublemaker who was upsetting the pagan religion on which was based the prosperity of Mecca.

For himself, Muhammad claimed no superhuman attributes except one: he was the messenger through whom God's Word—the same Word as that delivered by previous prophets, both Christian and Jewish, to their peoples in their languages in former times—was to be taken in Arabic to the Arabs. He admitted that he could perform no miracles although Jesus, with God's permission, had; though Islam specifically denies the divinity of Jesus, it does ascribe to him an exalted place in Creation. But God intended, the Muslims hold, that Muhammad, in his time and in his language and among his people, should be the leader of men to the Highroad of the Virtuous.

After some initial success in converting members of the community of Mecca, although few among the citizens of the oligarchy, Muhammad reached what appeared to be a dead end in his mission: with the popular support he had he was at once too weak to defend himself and win more converts to his faith and too strong to be tolerated by the defenders of the pagan cults which intertwined Meccan commercial practice and political structure. Meccan prosperity was conditional upon pan-Arab recognition of the city's special status as a sanctuary in which no fighting could take place and of the "Forbidden" months when men could trade freely throughout Arabia without fear of raid or vendetta. The fact that the new religion would upset this balance was apparent both to the rulers and the ruled—the one viewed it as sedition and the other as a rallying point for opposition to their oppressers. Probably it was not lost upon the oligarchs of Mecca either that to accept Islam meant accepting the primacy of its prophet.

The fact that Muhammad was tolerated at all was due to the requirement of Arab society that his clansmen protect him. Then in 619 the clan found a way to expel him as one who behaved disreputably toward his fellows. In that year in quick succession died Muhammad's first (then his only) wife and an uncle who though a pagan had been his main support. When Muhammad was asked if his uncle was in the Islamic Heaven as a virtuous man or in its Hell as a pagan, he replied "in Hell." He was immediately repudiated by his clan and became an outlaw, exposed to the fury of the Meccans. In desperation he fled from Mecca to find a safer haven.

First, Muhammad took his message to the nearby town of Taif which, like Mecca, was prosperous, well-organized, and conservative. Like Mecca it had a pagan pantheon intimately associated with its trade. Poor soil it was for the seed of Islam. As a Meccan, Muhammad was able to command an audience of Taif's chief men but, as the Victorian scholar Sir William Muir imagined, "the disproportion to the outward eye between the magnitude of the prophet's claims and his present solitary condition turned fear into contempt." The men of Taif set their slaves and street urchins against Muhammad, stoned him, and literally ran him out of town. Bloody, exhausted, and shaken, Muhammad returned to a hostile Mecca where he lived in seclusion for over a year, until, feeling that "his thorn had been cut," another Meccan gave him protection and succor.

But others had heard of his mission. To Mecca came men of many of the Arabian towns and tribes to trade, to experience the delights of a market town, to exchange information, and. to listen to the soothsayers, poets, and storytellers. Mecca was the intellectual and cultural, as well as the commercial, market of Arabia. Under the "peace" of the Meccan gods men who would have fought—would have *had* to have fought on sight—elsewhere were able to mingle freely. In such a situation Muhammad met some of the men of the northern Arabian town then called Yathrib and later (and now) called Medina.

Medina, unlike Taif and Mecca, was agricultural. Moreover it had no pantheon, and, inhabited by a Jewish or Judaized Arab community, it was familiar with monotheism. More important, Medina had no organized corporate life, being less a town than a collection of hamlets, midway between a bedouin encampment and a city. Like the former it lacked a government to settle differences and enforce security but like the town it so constricted its members that they could not escape from one another as could nomads. Hostility could be settled neither by official pressure as in Mecca nor by movement as in the desert. In Medina a perpetual civil war threatened the very life of the community. The situation, in fact, had so far degenerated a few years before Muhammad's mission that in an orgy of destruction the rival clans had hacked down one another's trees and almost ruined the economy.

In this circumstance it was natural that the town should seek a neutral arbitrator to settle their differences. This, it seems, was what they sought in Muhammad. The fact that Muhammad was a Meccan lent prestige to his name and that he was a man of religion gave him a moral stance above the partisan politics of Medina. Whereas both Mecca and Taif felt endangered by a new creed, Medina welcomed any solution to its war and agreed to obey Muhammad "in all that is right."

Muhammad, with the painful memory of his Taif adventure

fresh in mind, carefully negotiated for over a year on what his status would be and sent ahead, by small parties, about 150 of his followers to form, as it were, his qawm in Medina. It was as a prophet armed that he was to enter the city. Glad to be rid of him, the people of Mecca did nothing to halt this migration until the very end when they decided to take no chances on the future by assassinating him. At the last minute Muhammad slipped away and rode northward to his new home. This was the Hijra, the "Flight," from which the Islamic calendar is dated.

Upon entering Medina, Muhammad faced the initial problem of winning an immediate peace; then he had to settle his followers; and finally he had to secure his own power. All of these tasks he approached within the political traditions of Arabia. The pattern which emerged is expressed in a document called the "Constitution of Medina," dating from the second year after the Hijra.

With a flash of brilliance, Muhammad established his people as a part of the economy of Medina by arranging for each immigrant to be adopted as a "brother" by some member of the community. Like most things Muhammad did, this was to linger through Islamic history as a social ideal—all Muslims are supposed to be brothers and to assist one another in personal as well as institutional ways.

The central problem, however, was to get the warring clans of Medina to sink their differences in some larger social organization. The theoretical unit larger than the clan in Arabic society was the tribe, but among the nomads, due to the nature of the desert economy, the tribe rarely had actual existence. Its "chief" had no real power and was merely the most respected clan shaikh. But within the tribe it was possible to negotiate an end to hostilities, through the payment of "bloodmoney," whereas against foreigners the settling of hostilities was far more difficult. Therefore, it was both natural and reasonable that Muhammad should think of the city in terms analogous to a tribe. And, indeed, the community he set out to create in Medina was to have the same essential qualities.

Like the Arab tribe, the new community of Islam laid upon its members obligations for the defense of the whole. The "believers and adherents" were to struggle together and jointly to pay blood money or ransom. If an outsider harmed a member of the community, in a way parallel again to tribal society, the entire force of the community was brought to bear against him—"the Believers to a man will be against him." The community of believers was enjoined never to abandon one crushed by debts, and jointly to oppose those sowing sedition. Believers, the "clansmen of Islam," were ordered never to kill believers or to help others against believers. Like the tribe, the Islamic community could grant protection, for "the protection of God is one," and the weakest Muslim could impose this obligation upon all his brothers. As in the tribe, so in the Islamic community, foreigners could seek protection and succor. And as befit the new basis of society, religion, in a way parallel to the old basis, kinship, not only men of different kindred but also those of different religions could be so protected. The Jewish clans of Medina were confirmed in their customary rights, property, and practices, but, since they did not fight in the militia of the community, they were obliged to contribute to the defense of the whole through taxation. Lastly, the community was bound to act together; the clans were prevented from making a separate peace and had to accept responsibility for the acts of all.

Muhammad had profited from his one major failure by learning that in order to establish the religion of God in a moral society he needed political power. In a corporate society this could only be "tribal," and the tribe is the essence of the early Islamic community. The boundaries of Muhammad's tribe, however, were religious rather than genealogical.

It was the Koran which was to set the moral tone and the way, or sunna, of the community. This again was not an alien thought in Arabia. As the pre-Islamic poet Labid, in one of the *Golden Odes*, sang, "And we are of a clan whose forefathers laid down for them a sunna since each qawm has its sunna and its imams." Whereas the tribe had no fixed abode, Islam, being based on a town, did. Muhammad, borrowing from his native city, institutionalized Medina as a sanctuary in which no fighting could take place. Theoretically, throughout Islamic history the *Daru'l-Islam* or the abode of Islam has been a place of peace in distinction to other areas which were the abode of war. In this abode of peace lived Muslims and men of other religions and men of many clans.

When Muhammad died eleven years after the Hijra, in A.D. 632, he had barely had time to draft the outlines of his conception of the community. As we shall see, he appointed no successor—indeed, there could be no successor as the Messenger of God—to govern the community. Few of his followers understood his concept. To the "adherents," those who formed the bulk of the new "religious tribe," Muhammad had been a sort of paramount chief to whom, as a person, they submitted, and whose death freed them from all obligation. The true believers were few and, without Muhammad, without a guide. Consequently, it appeared that like all empires based on a tribal structure, Islam would not survive the Messenger's death.

Islam started as a community and only much later became a system of thought. This sequence, markedly different from the history of Christianity, has deeply colored the system itself. Muslim theologians and jurists have worked from precedent—the Traditions of the Prophet (*Hadith*)—as much as from the Book. From the beginning they were as much concerned with the regulation of man in earthly society as with the preparation of man for Divine Judgment.

The sunna, or "way," of Islam is based upon the society which Muhammad created in Medina. In this code, men are separated from one another by their religions. Each is entitled, within certain bounds, to practice his own faith, but Islam is recognized as the proper religion for Arabs. And though all three of the then-known monotheistic religions are theoretically the same, as the religion of Abraham, both the Jews and the Christians are said to have corrupted what they received from God. Muslims hold that the Jews have distorted their texts and altered various practices

(Islam is closer to the less Orthodox Jewish sects) and that the Christians have committed the sin of associating Jesus with God, who is Alone, One, and Unapproachable. To correct these mistakes and also to take His message to a new people, the Arabs, God sent Islam.

Concerned as Islam was with precise definitions and with the practical administration and moral tone of the Medina community, we should expect to find, and do find, explicit and full treatment in the Koran of such affairs as property rights, inheritance, marriage, divorce, punishment of theft and adultery, treatment of slaves and orphans, commercial practices, food, drink, games, and bribery.

Islam envisaged no division of Church and State. To be precise, it foresaw no Church at all. Society, if not a State per se, encompassed all aspects of man's proper life. Indeed, in early Islam those functions we call "religious" play a utilitarian part—in a new society fighting for its life against external enemies and beset by internal divisions, even the ceremonial of public prayer had a disciplinary quality not different from the drill of new recruits in an army. But Islam went beyond simply laying down the rules of society by addressing itself to the method of living the correct life in all of its detail.

Formally, the religion of Islam was extremely simple. To be a Muslim, a man must affirm the Unity of God and the Prophecy of Muhammad, saying, "there is no god but God and Muhammad is His messenger." Beyond that, the latitude of action or inaction is wide. Muslims are supposed to pray in a prescribed manner, give alms in a certain amount, fast during the daylight hours of the Holy Month, perform the pilgrimage at least once, and "strive in the way of God."

These are the "pillars" of the faith. To convert these into the elaborate, formal civilization of Islam, as the subsequent centuries were to know it, was the work of generations of scholars, theologians, and jurists who, mining the lodes of the Koran and the Traditions, fabricated from this simple ore an elaborate structure. Their task, difficult enough in a changing and growing society, was complicated by the gaps, alterations, and conflicts within the materials they worked. Since Islam, like Christianity, is divided into many sects, it is well to understand something of this early source of difference.

The 6000 verses which have come to us as the Koran were not written down in the lifetime of Muhammad. It was the fact that many of those who had memorized the verses were being killed in warfare that led Muhammad's successors to collect his messages. Naturally, there were different renditions. Several of the more famous were collected into "rival" Korans, which began to spread throughout the Islamic world. Individual versions tended to become associated with regional or tribal groupings. Ultimately this situation became so dangerous that a single authorized codex was prepared and all other copies were ordered destroyed.

However, Arabic writing at that period, like early notations in Western music, allowed considerable interpretation; the letters were, in fact, prompters for those who knew the text. Not only were vowels not written (so that, for example, the first part of this sentence would read "nt nl wr vwls nt wrttn") but no distinction was made between a number of consonants (for example between n, t, th, y, and b). Therefore, a single line could have more than one meaning. Thus, within the official text a number of different interpretations were equally orthodox. In fact, in a typical commentary on the Koran one finds after most verses, "but so-and-so reads it thus and another reads it thus."

Later, the issue was further complicated when various religious thinkers and, indeed, whole sects within the family of Islam suggested that the text of the Koran itself was subject to an inner meaning and required allegorical interpretation.

So complex was this problem to become, even early in Islam, that the religion developed not a priesthood but a legal profession who specialized in the application of Koranic law to social problems. This body of jurists and scholars of the Law has remained the cardinal organizational cadre of Islam to the present day.

The absence of a priesthood, holy men, and saints in Islam was felt early in its history. The religion, in the limited sense of man's relationship to the godhead, was in primitive, Orthodox Islam—as it is today in such puritanical sects as the Wahhabis of Arabia

—an austere, stark, and cold system. Between man and the all-powerful, unrelenting God-Judge was a vast gulf, across which no man could help another, since not even Muhammad was an intercessor. Nor was the religion satisfyingly visible. It began by destroying the visible signs of pagan cults and was even hostile to the sensual representation of religious subjects. A patch of desert was as "holy" or acceptable to God as a place of prayer as the most beautiful and elaborate mosque.

It is not surprising, therefore, that early in Islam men sought softer, warmer, and shorter ways to reach God. As Islam spread to areas which had known other religions, elements of sensualism, sainthood, and ecstasy were injected into it. The early followers of Muhammad were accorded a position not unlike that of the Apostles. Locally revered good men achieved locally recognized sainthood and their graves became places of pilgrimage—often, indeed, these places were associated with the gods of former religions. The intercession of such figures was devoutly sought despite the formal anathema of Islam. Ultimately, a religious art grew, although this never flourished among the Arabs, and great care in the design of religious buildings brought about an architecture comparable to Gothic Europe. Finally, the faith received a symbol in some ways akin to the Crucifixion when the grandson of Muhammad was killed on the battlefield against a government which many regarded as oppressive and secular. Those who opposed that government, who came to be called the Shiis or Partisans, seized upon the death of Husain, Muhammad's grandson, as the emotional nucleus of their political rebellion against the Orthodox State.

But the Shiis, like the Orthodox or Sunni Muslims, became deeply divided amongst themselves over points of dogma and interpretation. Some of the Shiis actually merge their imams with the godhead, ascribing to them, in inherited succession, the spirit of God. Others express in a religious medium their political, social, or economic differences from the rulers in a theocracy. Thus it is that many of the conquered people who were treated as second-class citizens in the new Islamic empire expressed their resentment against the Establishment by espousing unorthodox religious beliefs. Even Orthodox Islam, coping with the multifarious problems of a vastly expanded society and drawing on various sources, developed four distinct schools of law.

The greatest of the merits of Islam is that it has been able to retain the simplicity of its beginnings, so that to be or become a Muslim is easy, while being flexible enough to embrace a wide variety of practice, to accommodate dissent, and even to submit to total reinterpretation. For this flexibility a price has been paid. The religion has never made possible the weaving of the strands of society into a social fabric capable of clothing in one garment the whole Islamic world.

In Islam, as in tribal life, geographical division and separate historical experience gave additional scope for diversity. It is for this reason that the Arabs hark to language—the language of the Koran and of the poets—as the immutable base of their dream of nationhood.

IV. Conquests and the Caliphate: Glorious Yesterdays

When in A.D. 622 Muhammad moved his Meccan followers and fled himself from the hostility of the Meccans to Medina, he set the stage for the growth of the Islamic community. What distinguished the move to Medina from the abortive venture in Taif was that Muhammad went as a Prophet armed with the nucleus of a state. The fact that he had his own partisans raised him above the position of a neutral arbitrator and gave him the balance of power in the community. With his Book—and his sword—Muhammad was able to fuse the natives of Medina, who were composed of two Arab and several Jewish tribes, with his own followers to make a new and much larger tribe whose membership was defined not by kinship but by religion. Within the group no fighting was allowed and the hand of every man was turned against the common external enemy, but the enemy always had the option of joining the group, as believers in Islam or as adherents who accepted its suzerainty.

In this arrangement was a powerful stimulus to growth since the energies of the groups of members, formerly balanced one against another, were now turned outward. The community of Islam was spurred to action and given certainty of victory by the messianic force of God's favor to their leader. But the proof of divine grace was the conquest of Mecca. Muhammad realized that he must prevail over Mecca, the chief city of western Arabia, or fail in his mission.

To humble Mecca was not easy since the Meccans were rich, numerous, and experienced; but they were divided internally and lacked the fervor—and the lean hunger—of the new rival. Moreover, Mecca, depending as it did on the caravan trade, was vulnerable to blockade. As a former merchant himself, Muhammad began his "campaigns" with a thrust at Mecca's lifeline by attempting to intercept a caravan. The raid failed, however, when bedouin tribes allied to Mecca gave warning. It thus became evident that though the strategy was correct, its first tactical step must be to subdue and bring within the Islamic community the tribes who controlled the desert.

A normal tribal group, the clan, was small. When the groups it encountered were also small it could survive. Muhammad, however, had found a way to combine a number of clans into a large unit. Since no fighting was allowed within this unit, all its warlike energies were turned outward. Thus, it brought overwhelming force to bear on each clan it battled. The old balance of power had been upset. The tribe attacked was unable to combine with other tribes, since its only means of achieving a limited degree of political cohesion was based on real or imagined kinship, and alone it could not stand against the larger Islamic community while facing other, traditional tribal enemies. Only by submitting could it save itself, and, having submitted, it had to renounce the use of its force against other members of the Islamic Community and so its power was added to that directed outward against other tribes. In this way a large if ephemeral tribal "empire" was rapidly created. And, finally after several encounters, Mecca itself submitted to Muhammad in A.D. 630. The prestige thus gained and the addition of the most sophisticated and able men in Arabia in turn brought in to at least nominal submission tribes from all over the peninsula.

The tribes, however necessary as a force against external enemies, were always regarded with great suspicion by Muhammad and the early Muslims, who were, after all, urban Arabs. Tribesmen at best were lukewarm adherents rather than true believers (Koran xlix. 14) and had to be taught civilized manners toward the Messenger (Koran xlix. 1–5) and treated severely if they got out of line. More economical than trying constantly to suppress the tribes was to give them a target for their warlike energies. Only in this way could they be made loyal members of the Islamic community. Thus, shortly before his death in A.D. 632, Muhammad had planned a foray into Palestine.

Muhammad's death presented the community with what might have been a mortal crisis. So completely had his mission captured the imagination of his inner group of followers, the true believers, that some could not accept the fact of his death. Muhammad himself had made no provision for his succession. He had established no formal organization of statehood or of religion; only in his person was the state manifest to believers and adherents alike. The only "office" held by anyone in the community was leadership of public prayer in the absence or sickness of Muhammad. It was this office which was seized upon by Muhammad's inner circle and imposed upon the rest of the community. And it is from this humble beginning that the caliphate (caliph meaning successor) derives.

To the tribes, however, this innovation was unacceptable; in their eyes Muhammad's death dissolved all bonds of allegiance. Throughout Arabia the empire, like a mirage, vanished, as the tribes, in the religious terminology of later Muslims, "apostatized." The caliph appeared to have inherited a memory. So strong was the hold of Muhammad over his inner circle that the caliph nevertheless honored Muhammad's last command by dispatching the small remnant of the Muslim army into Palestine on a raid. It was with great difficulty that Medina withstood attacking bedouin until the army returned with booty and boasts of successes yet to come. The nearer bedouin once again leaped aboard the bandwagon of success, wealth, and glory and as before were turned against the other tribes in what became the bloodiest and most repressive war in Arabian history. So successful were the flying columns of cavalry scouring Arabia that they fused, almost imperceptibly, into an army of conquest. Their leader, Khalid ibn al-Walid, nicknamed the "Sword of God," was one of the great generals of all time.

To understand what happened next, it is important to realize that the two great Middle Eastern empires of that era, Byzantium or Eastern Rome and Sassanian Iran, had fought one another to an exhausted standstill. In A.D. 611 the Persians had invaded Syria and Palestine and in 614 had captured Jerusalem. Returning to the attack, the Byzantine forces slowly won back their lost ground, took repressive measures against the pro-Sassanian Jewish community, and tried, vainly, to enforce the Orthodox faith among the monophysite Christians who prevailed in Syria and Palestine. Both empires were exhausted, faced financial crises, and were rent by internal schisms. To economize, the Byzantines stopped paying subsidies to the Christian Arab tribes who had guarded the steppe lands of Syria and Jordan. This may have been the crucial factor in the Muslim Arab success.

In 633 the caliph launched probes of tribal forces northward into Byzantine territory; in the following year his great general marched northward in Iraq and, turning westward, rode straight across the Great Syrian Desert for 500 miles, appearing suddenly outside the walls of Damascus. After looting Damascus this army and the other Arab tribal groups fought several brief battles with Byzantine forces, until in July of 636 on the Yarmuk River in what is now Jordan they met and destroyed the assembled Byzantine forces led by the emperor.

What had started as a punitive expedition became a raid, and the raid became a war of conquest. Spurred on by the very shock of their success and by the tales of glory and booty, a torrent of tribes poured out of Arabia. In the words of Sir William Muir, "It was the scent of war that now turned the sullen temper of the Arab tribes into eager loyalty: for thus the brigand spirit of the Bedawi was brought into unison with the newborn fire of Islam. The call to battle reverberated throughout the land, and was answered eagerly . . . warrior after warrior, column after column, whole tribes in endless succession with their women and children, issued forth to fight. And ever, at the marvellous tale of cities conquered; of rapine rich beyond compute; of maidens parted on the very field of battle 'to every man a damsel or two'; and at the sight of the royal fifth [the caliph's share] fresh tribes arose and went. Onward and still onward, like swarms from the hive, or flights of locusts darkening the land, tribe after tribe issued forth and hastening northward, spread in great masses to the East and to the West."*

The defeated Byzantine forces fell back upon the seacoast, abandoning the hinterland to the Arabs. The caliph himself came to Jerusalem in 637 to make peace and organize the new province. In the chronicles he is described as riding a white camel, dressed in worn and torn robes, as he came to pray at the place where Muhammad dreamed he had ascended to Heaven and to which the early Muslims had directed their prayers, as modern Arabs do to Mecca. As in Arabia, so in the new empire, the "People of the Book," the Christians and Jews, were given the status of protected clients and allowed to continue to practice their religions, to manage their internal community affairs, and to avoid military service by payment of a tax.

The Muslims, who regarded Islam as the religion of the Arabs and who wanted revenue more than soldiers, put little effort in an attempt to convert anyone to their religion. Meanwhile, a world was waiting to be won. In the same year as the caliph's visit to Jerusalem an Arab army defeated the forces of the Sassanian emperor and captured his capital of Ctesiphon near modern Baghdad. Now all Persia was open before them. Shortly thereafter, another Arab general convinced the caliph to let him conquer Egypt. He is related as saying "its people are playthings, its soil is gold and it belongs to those strong enough to take it." With a force of Yemenite cavalry the general defeated the first Byzantine garrison he met. Reinforced and aided by the local Coptic Christian community he then captured Babylon, near modern Cairo, and laid seige to Alexandria, which surrendered in 642. By 669 the Arabs had created a navy and had attacked Cyprus; six years later this force was able to destroy the bulk of the Byzantine fleet of 500 ships. Meanwhile, Arab armies were plunging deep into Anatolia to the north and eastward into Afghanistan.

The Caliph Omar, the second caliph, was assassinated by a Persian slave in 644. Once again the young Islamic state was left

* *The Caliphate, Its Rise, Decline and Fall* (Edinburgh, 1915), p. 43.

without a designated successor. This time the powerful Meccan oligarchy, which had chafed under the puritanical rule of the first two caliphs as it watched others reap the spoils of the conquests, managed to get one of its own number, Uthman of the Umayyad clan, elected caliph. Quick to profit from their new position, the old oligarchy reached out to gather the fruits of power and majesty from the vast new empire.

The empire itself was the jerry-built creation of expedience. The tribal armies, interested in loot rather than in rule, would have melted away had they not been gathered into cantonments or garrisons and paid a share of the booty. The garrisons, Kufa, Basra, Qum (in Iran), Old Cairo, and Qairawan (in Tunisia), rapidly grew into towns and cities as the local people flocked to them and settled to sell goods and services to the soldiers in the exchange for their newly won riches. But the gathering, conversion, and transportation of the caliph's fifth of the booty, the payment of the army, and the administration of taxes and governmental expenditures were vast new undertakings. The inner core of Muhammad's followers were not fitted by experience for these tasks; alone among the Arabs, the oligarchy of Mecca was. Eagerly they sought to reap this worldwide harvest. For their private gain, they were immensely aided by the fact that there were no universal laws or customary practices and little thought of ethics. In most parts of the new empire the old practice and often the old civil servants were maintained, with only such changes as were necessary to accommodate a different ruling group in the place of the Byzantine or Sassanian overlords. For men of wit, and the Meccans were certainly that, the interstices in the several conflicting tax systems opened onto enormous fortunes.

Resentment grew against the old Meccan oligarchy, the late comers to Islam, the men who had driven the Prophet from their city and who only submitted when they were beaten, and yet who now reaped the Muslim harvest. The resentment came to rest upon the third caliph who, though personally a good and pious man, was an "agent" of the Meccans. Not only Arabs grew resentful but also the conquered, who found in the rich and pompous Meccans a target for their hostility against the victors. So, while Islam rolled from one brilliant victory to another, internally it was wracked by dissension and corruption. Finally, in 656, after a campaign of extensive public criticism of his rule, the caliph was murdered by a group of Arabs from the mutinous army in Egypt.

Never again were the Arabs to be united. As universal as the discontent had been, it had no internal cohesion. Ali, son-in-law and cousin of Muhammad, was proclaimed caliph by those who had murdered Uthman, but he had to fight for his title, first against the other members of the "old guard" of Islam, including a widow of the Prophet, and next against the entrenched relatives of the slain caliph. Even his own followers were split into mutually hostile groups so that he could never direct his force against his major rivals. Finally after a sequence of pitched battles, truces, and conferences, Ali himself was murdered by a fellow Muslim in 661 in his new capital of Kufa. His reign was brief, but his name and memory linger on as the spiritual leader of the movement of dissent in Islam, the Shiis.

The provincial governor of Syria who defeated Ali and became caliph was the nephew of the Umayyad Caliph Uthman. With the forces of discontent against the Umayyads scattered and defeated, he set about unabashedly to found a dynasty which was little concerned with Islam. Under his successors this Arab kingdom held sway until 750 from Syria; after a brief hiatus it managed to re-establish itself in Spain where it lasted until 1030. The Umayyads were great patrons of the Arab poets and laid heavy emphasis on the bedouin virtues of hardihood, chivalry, and enjoyment of life within a code of honor. Little did they care for the spiritual life in Islam. Yet, their armies won for Islam its vast empire. They attacked Constantinople itself in 669, and blockaded it from 673 to 678. Their armies thrust eastward into Afghanistan, taking Kabul in 664, and northward across the Oxus to take Bukhara in 674 and Samarkand in 676. To the west they took Carthage, in modern Tunisia, in 698. From 708 to 715, Arab armies plunged deep into India and in 711 began the invasion of Spain. In 717 they tried again to seize Constantinople and invaded France. By 733 they had conquered Georgia in the Caucasus and in 738 reached their highwater mark at the battle of Tours or Poitiers in France. At that time their empire was probably the largest yet known in history.

But the Umayyads were never able to find an acceptable foundation for their empire. The real bases of their power were the Arab tribes of Syria, but these were so scattered over the vast empire that the government ultimately had to hire mercenary armies of Armenians. The Arab forces, moreover, were split by tribal and ultimately geographic interests. The conquered peoples, attracted by Islam but repelled by the Arab government, were drawn to movements of protest within Islam.

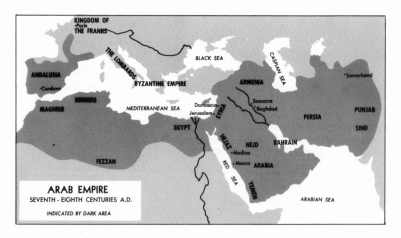

Finally, in 747 a revolt broke out in eastern Iran. Picking up adherents, the insurgents turned it into a full-scale revolutionary war in which they defeated the Umayyads and killed the caliph. For a while it was not clear in whose name this revolt had been fought, but after some months another branch of the Prophet's family, called, after his uncle Abbas, the Abbasids, emerged as leaders of the victorious forces of revolution.

The Abbasid revolution has often been portrayed as a Persian reaction to Arab rule. There is much truth in this. The revolt began in Khorasan, or eastern Iran, and many of its partisans were Persian converts to Islam, but the new ruling house, the bulk of the army, the language, and the religion were Arab. What had changed was the political matrix: the new dynasty could not impose itself upon the empire as an Arab kingdom. The Abbasids had to find a new base of authority and build a new structure of power. The Arab warrior caste was deposed from its privileged position because it was no longer strong enough to justify that position. In an attempt to find a replacement for the cohesive force of the tribal confederations and the Meccan oligarchy, the rulers allowed a new class of scribes to become a bureaucracy. The easterners, both Arabs and Arabized Persians, infused into the government elements of Oriental magnificence and mystery. The armies became less and less Arab and more like those of the Sassanian Empire, comprised in large part of contingents of mercenaries and foreigners. Yet emphasis on Islam, in the ruling group still defined as Orthodox or Sunni Islam, was heightened, for it had acquired a new popularity among the citizens of the empire.

The vast size of the empire influenced its politics and economic life. The richness of its far-flung provinces and the relative peace and stability they enjoyed in early Abbasid times supplied ample wherewithal for a brilliant and cultured urban civilization in the new metropolis of Baghdad which became the capital of the empire in 762. Apparently the original idea had been to lay out a garrison and administrative center, but rapidly a city collected around these and in the ninth century Baghdad had become perhaps the largest city in the world outside of China.

The world of the "Good Caliph Harun ar-Rashid" as it has come to the West in the *Thousand and One Nights* is a part of the treasure of legends of both East and West. In many ways it does mark the height of Islamic pomp and circumstance. But precisely because history is here so incrusted by the jeweled glitter of legend and fancy, it has exercised a powerful attraction on later ages of Arabs. So hypnotic, indeed, has this become as to immobilize the many for whom its greatness, learning, and wealth could never be matched. Arabs have found an escape from subsequent weakness, ignorance, and poverty in daydreams of this past instead of galvanizing themselves for efforts in their own times. Even today, the typical Arabic history book is a "heroic harangue, as a prominent modern Arab-American historian has written, in which "modern historians have addressed themselves almost exclusively to the glorious aspects of Arab and Islamic history, depicting them in bright colors and skipping over the many dark spots and inglorious episodes [or] to a mere listing of personalities, theories, works which were translated into European languages, Western scholars who were influenced by them, and orientalists who sang their praises."* This makes it useful to know both the myth and the reality.

The myth is perhaps best spelled out in the dozens of stories in the *Thousand and One Nights* or in Hollywood movies—enjoying record-breaking runs in many Arab cinemas—which rightly depict the Arab Empire as the bright light of civilization during the European Dark Ages. The Arabic contribution to world culture was not solely associated with the Abbasid caliphate but even more with successor governments and with the rival caliphates in Egypt and Spain, but the nationalist myth of Arab grandeur makes few distinctions, so here it will be treated as a whole.

The major contribution made by the Arabs was in keeping alive, during the long period of European ignorance, the substance and some of the spirit of inquiry which had been the gift of classical civilization. Translations from Greek and other languages into Arabic were actually begun under the Umayyads but were officially encouraged by the Abbasid government. Moreover, the Islamic men of learning were able to draw upon other civilizations they encountered. From the Indians they got their system of numbers—an innovation which made possible mathematics as we know it—and from China that great tool of our civilization, paper. The concept of zero; basic work on optics, in which the classical notion of Euclid and Ptolemy that the eye emitted a beam of light was upset; advanced work in mathematics, including the development of algebra, geometry, and trigonometry; and significant contributions in astronomy came from the

* Nabih Amin Faris in *Middle East Journal*, 8(1954):157–159.

members and clients of the Muslim-Arab Empire. The fact that many of the contributors were neither Arab nor Muslim is a great tribute to the tolerance and receptivity of that civilization. This great contribution was to be transmitted to and to stimulate Europe at a time in which, hungering for knowledge, it emerged into the beginnings of the Renaissance. Indeed, from the recapture by the Christians of Toledo in 1085 Muslim learning was available to all who wished to study it in Europe. The names of such of its philosophers, scientists, and doctors as ar-Razi (d. 925), Ibn Sina (d. 1037) and al-Biruni (d. 1048) fill medieval texts. But in the Islamic world itself from about the twelfth century onward the increasing power of the Orthodox religious leaders contributed to a gradual intellectual paralysis. As its scholarly lights dimmed, a Dark Age came to Islam, as it had to Europe.

At the time of Harun ar-Rashid the central administration of the state was in the capable hands of a family known as the Barmakids, who also figure prominently in the *Thousand and One Nights* as the boon companions of Harun. This family, to whom much of the stability and richness of the empire was owing, was descended from a Buddhist temple guardian in the city of Balkh. For reasons which are so obscure as themselves to be sources of many legends, after seventeen years Harun dismissed the Barmakids and confiscated their wealth. Thereafter, his reign was a disaster. Upon Harun's death in 829 the empire, at his instructions, was divided between his two sons. The result of this division— in which one got the army and the other the capital—was a civil war which so weakened the central authority as to accelerate the process of disintegration. Province after province peeled off from the central core.

Within itself the caliphate ever had great capabilities for growth and equal susceptibility to destruction; what it always lacked was a basis of stability. Never had it managed to integrate its rural base into its civilization; ever was it exploitive of its resources. Neglect and decay are fatal to a system of irrigation, which was the wealth of Iraq and Egypt, and ruinous taxation makes refugees of productive peasants. Both were features of Abbasid rule. One of the more quaint and yet horrifying records of the Abbasid caliphate is the *Tabletalk of a Mesopotamian Judge*, but it is by no means unique in retailing the frivolous way the ruling elite squandered the resources of the empire.

The very success of the empire in conquering so much of the known world undermined it in two ways. First, so vast were the expanses of territory to be covered and so slow the means of communication, that decentralization of power began almost from the inception of the empire. And second, the *élan* of the empire could not be sustained: neither the original quest for loot nor the opposition to rival world empires sufficed. Looting had to be stopped if the government was to function, and Byzantium, the other side in the "Cold War" of that era, was too distant to pose a threat credible and immediate enough to cause men to rally around their flag. Rather, politics was played on less grand stages as provincial governors, petty officials, and army commanders performed vivisection on the body politic.

Within the ruling group itself sufficient man power was lacking to staff the bureaucracy and the army. The bureaucracy, the virtual creation of the Barmakid family, improved and diffused by study of Persian court ritual, managed to develop a degree of a tradition of the service but not sufficient to survive in a basically hostile environment which lacked the public and governmental forces necessary both to sustain and to tame a bureaucracy. The army was always a problem. As the opportunities for conquests were dissipated in building an empire, other means had to be found to employ the army's energies. The Arabs increasingly withdrew from the military or were thrust away from it by suspicious caliphs, and were replaced by praetorians of many nations. As long as these contingents balanced and checked one another peace could be maintained, but outside of sheer force there were no balancing factors. So, as we shall see, those hired to act as the guardians of the state became its tyrants.

V. The Alien Empires: Arab Exclusion from Rule

The Arabs were always a small minority in their vast empire, as they are today in the world of Islam, and even this small minority was rent by schisms. Tribe opposed tribe, one geographical area contested another, and Arabs were attracted not only to different religions but also to different sects within Islam. Moreover, these various religions and political groups attracted non-Arabs as their adherents and partisans. Thus, the exercise of centralized authority became more and more difficult as the establishment of a principle of allegiance and identity, which most people today seek in nationality, became impossible. More immediately significant, lack of political consensus produced such turmoil as to induce the caliphs to seek politically neutral agents of power. It was thus that the last Umayyad caliph, Marwan II, came to rely upon Armenian mercenaries and the early Abbasids created separate guards regiments of "foreigners" from eastern Persia, Central Asia, and North Africa.

As they found their way to power in the military and civil bureaucracy blocked, the original elite, the Muslim Arabs, began a process of withdrawal. In some provinces, notably in north Syria, Arabs remained supreme, but this was the exception. Elsewhere, tribal groups returned to nomadism, and urban Arabs began to detach themselves from the politico-military functions of the state to specialize, almost as a caste, in the legal-religious aspects of Islamic society. These divisions—the politico-military and legal-religious—come the closest to matching the division of

Church and State in Western society. Thus, long before the fall of Baghdad the exercise of authority passed out of Arab hands and was not to return for many centuries.

The principal disadvantage of the alien bodyguards of the early Abbasids was that they tended to become Arabized too quickly and involved themselves in Baghdad politics. This was partly because among the "foreigners" of eastern Iran and North Africa were many Arabs. This "conflict of interest" made these regiments dangerous, or at least compromised, in a system in which the caliph sought to hold the balance of power between rival groups in his capital. It was the Caliph Mutasim (833–842) who took the fateful step of creating a praetorian guard of truly alien Turkomans from the lands beyond the Oxus River in Central Asia. Prior to Mutasim's time some Turkomans had been in the guard, but under him the guard as a whole, including its commanders, became Turkoman.

Troubles with the Baghdad mob and plots within the other regiments of the guard caused the Caliph Mutasim to move from Baghdad to Samarra where he established the new capital in 836. This city, a sort of Arab Versailles, was laid out on a vast scale with separate quarters for the divisions of the army. The caliph's hope was that there he would be safe from the Arab politics of Baghdad. His hope was realized but at the cost of upsetting the delicate balance of power on which his freedom of action was contingent. Isolated in the magnificence of Samarra, with its vast gardens, palaces, and a mosque three times the size of St. Peter's Cathedral, the caliph was at the mercy of his guardsmen. The outward magnificence contrasted violently, suddenly, and tragically with the near collapse of the caliphate. The Caliph Mutawakkil was murdered in 861. Then, in rapid succession came—and went—four caliphs, mere puppets of the Turkish generals, who inspired the satirical poem

> A caliph in a cage, between [Generals] Wasif and Bugha,
>   Who says what they say to him, just like a parrot echoes.
> Kha-li-fa-tun fi qa-fa-sin baina Wa-sif wa Bu-gha
>   Ya-qu-lu ma qa-la la-hu ka ma ta-qu-lu al-ba-ba-gha.

Mutawakkil's first successor was poisoned in six months, the second and the third were stabbed and the fourth was killed in battle against his guard. During this decade of chaos the outer provinces of the empire defected. In the south of Iraq, the home province, black slaves, originally from Zanzibar, who worked the salt deposits revolted and set up a revolutionary state. In Egypt the Turkish governor began to lay the foundations of what became an empire within the larger Abbasid empire, and in Iran the Saffarids carved out another kingdom. Meanwhile, the Arab tribes, who had even in the time of Harun been "bad neighbors" to the caliphate, espoused dissident religious movements under whose banners they were to sack Basra in 923, Kufa in 926, and Mecca in 930.

In Spain, at about the same time, a similar train of events had been set in motion. Abdur Rahman, a grandson of the tenth Umayyad caliph of Damascus, had established himself in Cordova in 755, and his descendants managed to recapture in Spain something of the grandeur of the Umayyads. Abdur Rahman III (912–961) carried Spanish Islam to its apogee and assumed the title of caliph in 929. Like the Abbasids, he brought in slaves and mercenaries to overawe his fellow countrymen; the main difference was that in Spain it was the *Saqalibah* or Slavs who were the praetorians.

In Egypt the governors since 858 had been Turks. The greatest of them, Ahmad ibn Tulun, who ruled Egypt from 868–884, best remembered for the great mosque he built in Cairo, was a sort of shogun, ruling Egypt, Syria, and much of Anatolia under the nominal suzerainty of the Abbasid caliph in Baghdad. Following him, Egypt was ruled by other Turks, an Abyssinian, and a motley crowd of rival bands of mercenaries, slave warriors, and bureaucrats who jostled one another for power and revenues. None was strong enough to win or establish a dynasty. But their rivalries so disrupted the life of the country as to attract the aggressive attention of the Arab-Berber dynasty of the Fatimids who had risen to power in North Africa.

After an initial failure in 914 the Fatimids conquered Egypt in 969. Laying out their capital under the guidance of the astrologers when Mars (al-Qahirah) was in the ascendant, they named it Cairo (al-Qahirah), and proclaimed a new era of Egyptian power and prestige. Legend has it that when the fourth Fatimid, the conqueror of Egypt, was questioned on his claim to be a descendant of Fatimah, the daughter of the Prophet Muhammad, he assembled the learned men and jurists of Egypt, unsheathed his sword, and said, "here is my pedigree."

Unlike the other Arab-Muslim dynasties, the Umayyads and the Abbasids, the Fatimids were bolstered by a religious movement, the Ismailis, an offshoot of Shii Islam. This gave them wide influence throughout the Middle East, and at one time they appeared on the point of absorbing the Abbasid caliphate, but it raised against them powerful counterforces of Orthodox Muslims. It was not the Fatimid religious mission but Egypt's rich Nile Valley and strategic central location in East-West trade that carried the new dynasty into a brief golden age. Their great mosque-university al-Azhar, founded in 970, still embellishes Cairo and stands today as the oldest university in the world.

But the Fatimids, however much they were favored by their location, the richness of Egypt, and their religious mission, were unable to consolidate a base of authority. Like the Spanish Umayyads and the Iraqi Abbasids they were forced to rely upon alien mercenary troops to whom they gradually lost power. By the time the fourteenth Fatimid caliph died in 1171 the Fatimid empire had lost its former grandeur.

In Baghdad, meanwhile, the caliphate had, after the bitter and tragic period of praetorian violence, managed to restore some of its former power. But, as in the later Roman Empire, the cost was great. From 870 to 908 the empire was reconquered, rebels destroyed, and tribute reassessed, but the effort virtually exhausted the dynasty and again the praetorian guard intervened, extorting and pillaging the citizenry, so that by the third decade of the tenth century the empire had virtually collapsed financially. Province after province broke away and refused to pay its tribute—it has been estimated that the revenue for the year 900 was about 3–4 percent of that of a century before. Men of influence in the bureaucracy and army commanders carved out estates for themselves even in the home province of Iraq and evaded all taxes. Smaller owners and men of little influence, on whom the remainder of the taxes had to fall, were ruined, abandoned their lands, or made over their titles to those rich enough to defend them. Lacking real power, the central government needed more, not less, revenue to buy allies and friends; moreover, it proved incapable of deflating the bloated administrative structure which had grown, sporelike, through all of the changes of Abbasid fortune. Even the imperial court, now ruling only a memory of an empire, continued to live on a lavish scale. It was as though the Abbasids could pretend to rule an empire only so long as they sat in an imperial court—even if it were supported only by a single, misgoverned, impoverished province.

In their desperation the Abbasids created yet new pieces of bureaucracy with the frank and honest names of the "Office of Bribes" and the "Office of Confiscations." Judging from the chronicles, these were staffed by the hardest-working bureaucrats in Baghdad. Increasingly, as money became difficult to get, officials came to be paid for their services in land or, if their assignments were of limited tenure, in rights to the revenue of certain estates for given periods of time. This, apparently, was the origin of the system of fiefs which was later to become common.

Finally, in 945, a Persian dynasty of Shiis, the Buwaihids, put an end to the pitiful pretence that was the caliphate. Under the new ruler, self-styled as *sultan* or holder of temporal power, the caliph became little more than a court functionary to be brought out on ceremonial occasions and discarded when troublesome or tiresome. At one point three former caliphs who had been blinded (and thus made legally unfit to hold office) by order of the sultan were alive in Baghdad, and one had to beg in the streets.

Only in Mosul (from 929–991) and Aleppo (944–1003) had an Arab dynasty, the Hamdanids, who were charged with guarding the Byzantine marches, managed to survive. But, ultimately, they too succumbed. As their great poet laureate al-Mutanabbi sang,

Men from their kings alone their worth derive
But Arabs ruled by aliens cannot thrive:
Boors without culture, without noble fame,
Who know not loyalty and honour's name.
Go where thou wilt, thou seest in every land
Folk driven like cattle by a servile band.*

In their turn the Buwaihids fought amongst themselves, and by the end of the eleventh century anarchy again prevailed throughout their empire.

Meanwhile, at the other side of the Asian land mass, in China, the Turkomans played a similar role in the affairs of the late Tang Dynasty. It was a Turkish general who ended the Tang Dynasty in 907 and Turkish officers who established the "Five Dynasties" which preceded the Sung. The re-establishment of a strong, centralized rule in China in 960 closed the northeastern frontier to further Turkish tribal incursions. Blocked by the Chinese and by a Mongol dynasty, the Liao or Ch'i-tan, bands of Turkoman tribesmen turned westward.

What distinguished the Turkish incursions of this period was that they came not as individuals to serve in the praetorian guards of Arab rulers, but in tribes, under their own leaders, knowing that they could not return. One of these groups, now known by the name of their chieftain Seljuk, was moving ever westward, bringing a new future to the Islamic Middle East. By 1040 the grandson of Seljuk had conquered eastern Iran, and in 1055 he captured Baghdad. Gathering Turkish bands as he went, the Seljuk Sultan Alp Arslan invaded Anatolia and in the battle of Manzikert in 1071 defeated and captured the Byzantine emperor. Anatolia was now open to Turkish migration and settlement. His successor, Sultan Malik Shah, and the famous vizier, Nizamu'l-Mulk, brought the Seljuk empire to the crest of its power and completed the conversion of what had been a money economy in the Middle East into one based on fiefs in land.

In Egypt at this time the Fatimid caliphate was dying out, and Syria was divided between several petty states. The Middle

* Translated by R. Nicholson in *Literary History of the Arabs* (Cambridge University Press, Cambridge and New York, 1953).

Eastern Islamic world was suffering, on the political level, from that sense of confusion and drift which is symptomatic of physical and emotional decay of civilizations. It was at this time, in 1096, that the First Crusade was launched against the Muslims in the Holy Land.

After a long march through the Balkans, the Crusaders were urged rapidly forward by anxious and mistrusting Byzantine officials. As they moved down the Levant coast, the Crusaders were relatively unopposed and were able to capture each town on their route. Finally, on the evening of June 7, 1099, they encamped before "Jerusalem the Golden."

The native Christians, perhaps having heard of the treatment of their cousins along the coast by these crude barbarians, who were interested in little but loot and cared not a whit for the religion of its former owner, were not pleased to see the Crusaders. But the Fatimid governor of Jerusalem took no chances on the enlightened self-interest of his Christian subjects or their loyalty to his empire and expelled them from the city. The Jews and Muslims resisted the invaders and after the Crusaders broke into the city were massacred. Most of the Jews were burned alive in their chief synagogue, in which they had taken refuge. Even those Jews and Muslims who surrendered were cut down in an orgy of blood, plunder, and religious ecstacy.

The state founded by the Crusaders, gradually tamed and softened by the balmy climate and easy ways of Palestine, lived, as it were, in the schisms of the Islamic world. With Syria divided between Aleppo and Damascus and Egypt under a weak and decayed regime, the Crusaders could survive. No sooner, however, were the Muslims to gain even a semblance of unity than the Crusaders were expelled. This was the work of the great Kurdish leader Saladin, who in 1171 put an end to the Fatimid caliphate, assumed all power, and set out to reunite Egypt and Syria. In 1187 he was able to muster just enough strength—and no more—to reconquer Jerusalem and most of Palestine. Upon his death in 1193, however, his state was shattered.

Again, the scene must shift far beyond the Arab lands to Central Asia where Genghis Khan (1155–1227) was putting together the most powerful military empire the world had ever seen. In 1215 the Mongol armies invaded China and took Yenching (modern Peiping), in 1219 they advanced into Korea, and in 1221 made their first raids into Russia and invaded Iran. The death of Genghis Khan temporarily slowed the Mongol advance, but soon Mongol armies were masters of most of Asia. In 1238 they took Moscow and two years later Kiev. A grandson of Genghis, Hulagu Khan, resumed the westward march in the Middle East and in 1258 captured Baghdad, killed the last, the thirty-seventh Abbasid caliph, and abolished the caliphate. Pushing still westward, the Mongols reached Palestine where in 1260 they were finally stopped by forces of the Turkish "slave-rulers," the Mamluks, who had been established in Cairo after the death of the last of Saladin's heirs in 1260.

By this time the rapid turnover of masters had long since ceased to concern the subject Arab population. Deprived of their old military functions, excluded from authority, mere servants of those who exercised rule, the Arabs turned increasing to the preservation of the institutions of Islam. For Islam itself this was an era of external expansion. Muslim traders spread Islam deep into Africa and eastward into south and southeast Asia. Even the Mongols, who had wiped out the remains of the political power of the Arab Muslims, were converted in large numbers, so that Islam became in the full sense a world religion. But in the realm of Islamic learning, as in Europe during the Dark Ages, scholars devoted themselves to the task of preserving the pale glow of a great civilization with little hope of rekindling its fire or adding to the former blaze, never daring to experiment or tamper for fear of snuffing out what little remained.

Further devastation, pestilence, and flood followed the sack of Baghdad in 1285. The remnants of the city population shrank within its walls. The peasants tried desperately to avoid contact with all outside their villages. Only the bedouin, who had already withdrawn from the empire, remained virtually untouched. The dreary chronicle of this period would net us little. Men clung to niches as we have imagined some might in the aftermath of nuclear war, desperately trying to survive, not daring to hope to live as they or their fathers had in former times. Then, in 1400–01 Tamerlane led another invasion of the Arab Middle East in which he sacked Baghdad, Aleppo, and Damascus. As the English historian Stephen Longrigg has written, "If the scenes and losses were less dreadful than those of the ruin of the Khalifate, it was that Baghdad in 1401 had not the same pride to be humbled, the same materials for atrocity." Part of Tamerlane's spoils in Damascus were the learned men and artisans whom he took back to his Central Asian capital and so dealt yet another blow to the civilization of the Middle East.

In Anatolia the petty states left by the decay of the Seljuk Empire struggled with Byzantium and with one another; gradually one of them, the House of Osman, the Ottomans, prevailed over the others and began to grow. In 1361 the Ottomans seized Adrianople and then moved into the Balkans. Their plan to capture Constantinople in the last years of the fourteenth century was delayed as they tried to ward off the attacks of Tamerlane who in 1402 captured the Ottoman sultan. But this was only a temporary setback. Finally in 1453 the Ottomans had recovered and were able to take Constantinople. For half a century their attentions were turned to Europe, but in 1514 Sultan Salim took Tabriz in a war with the Persian Empire. The problem of securing his flanks led him to conquer Kurdistan in the next year, and the following year his forces clashed near Aleppo with the Turko-Circassian Mamluk forces of Egypt. The great victory of the Ottomans encouraged them to seize Cairo, which they did in 1517. Rapidly they spread over the whole Middle East. A Turkish fleet was in the Persian Gulf in 1529. And in 1533, having just failed in their second attempt to seize Vienna, Ottoman forces took Baghdad.

Initially, the Turks made few efforts to change what they found. Often they confirmed the governments, as they did in the Lebanon, or merely imposed a chief functionary over the existing structure as they did in Egypt. Even when they sought changes, the great distances and slow communications of the empire made for a large degree of local autonomy. By the end of the sixteenth century the empire was in its more central parts a kingdom but further afield more of a federation, as local chieftains, the "lords of the valleys," exercised the functions of government while paying allegiance to the sultan. The vast desert and steppe lands, of course, were never effectively a part of the empire. And frontier provinces were often under a state of seige. Baghdad, which had been reconquered by Persia, was again beseiged, sacked, and massacred in 1630. By 1704 Baghdad had recovered sufficiently to become the seat of a dynasty of pashas who were, for all practical purposes, independent. In Egypt, meanwhile, the Ottoman pasha had become little more than a figurehead; real power was in the hands of the landed Turkish aristocracy, the Mamluks. What is now Israel, Lebanon, Jordan, and part of Syria became in the middle of the eighteenth century an autonomous state, which in 1775 came under the rule of a Bosnian adventurer named Ahmad Jazzar, whose importance in Western history is that he was to give Napoleon one of his few defeats.

All over this vast expanse of empire the common people, tribesmen, peasants, and townsmen, lived their lives much as they always had. In religious brotherhoods, craft guilds, neighborhood associations, village councils, and tribal kinship, they found meaningful social life. Economically, they needed little as their standards of life and their expectations were minimal. Matters of their personal status, even transactions in land, taxes, and religious and civic expression, were governed by custom and legal codes which had little or no relationship to secular government. Their judges and religious leaders were not dependent upon their governors either for appointments to office or for salaries. Between the government and the people was a gulf defined not alone by language, culture, and temperament but in that the spheres of life were different. So total had this withdrawal become that it resembled a caste system: Turks were governors; Arabs were governed. Turks were warriors; Arabs were peasants or men of Islamic learning. In the colorful analogy to be drawn from Turkish terminology, the Turks were the shepherds and the Arabs the flocks.

PART THREE   THE IMPACT OF THE WEST

VI. First Encounters: Point Counterpoint

Toward the end of the eighteenth century the Arab areas of the Middle East, although under the suzerainty of the Ottoman Empire, were in fact ruled by local dynasties or alien slave, military bureaucracies. The Arab population was not only small—with perhaps two million in Egypt and two million each in the Levant and the Arabian peninsula—but widely scattered and economically, administratively, and culturally isolated from all but near neighbors. Groups of towns, villages, and nearby clans of nomads or semi-nomads tended to cluster together as autarkic units. Few towns were large, but many which later became insignificant were in this period important trade centers. Even such widely scattered towns as Sidon, Kuwait, Jiddah, and Mokha carried on a wide-ranging and relatively prosperous trade. In some of the larger cities—Cairo, Aleppo, Damascus—as well as in a number of towns, medieval industrial crafts were practiced on a large scale.

Where men were favored by nature, as in the mountains of Lebanon, Palestine, Syria, and the north of Iraq and in the deserts of Arabia, they achieved a considerable degree of autonomy and freedom. Mount Lebanon, the most protected of these areas, not only had a high degree of village self-government, with secure land tenure, but an established and officially recognized "national" government which, at times, even carried on a separate foreign policy. Baron de Boislecomte, traveling about 1830, noted in his *Mission* that in many places the "cultivated valleys, separated from one another by the mountains and the great stretches of desert, form themselves into small republics." Writing of the bedouin "nations" in the Great Syrian Desert, Burckhardt observed that they were for all practical purposes autonomous states.

Bedouin tribes covered much of the land that is now agricultural. In the summer, for example, the valleys of Lebanon and Palestine and areas virtually within the shadow of the walls of Aleppo and Baghdad, were dotted with bedouin tents. In fact, as has been suggested above, a true picture of the Middle East at this period can be depicted in analogy to the sea: the agricultural areas and oases were the coast and islands in a vast sandy desert. Only occasionally could the people of the settled areas "go to sea," but the bedouin—merchantmen, privateers, fishermen—came and went at will. The sand sea was their natural element and in it they were safe from government tax collectors. Only rarely and temporarily could they be brought to heel by the forces of the government; in fact, they often are recorded as raiding and plundering the armed forces of the government whose valuable weapons were more targets than shields.

Between the tribes and the urban government, as between the upper and nether grindstone, was the peasant, accessible and defenseless, himself a domesticated animal, humbly submitting to the shears of the tax collector and the "brotherhood" extortion of the nomad. Where he could not defend himself, in the great river deltas of Egypt and Iraq or on the Syrian steppe lands, he paid the bill for both the town and the desert. Few families lived their entire lives in a single village. Great areas of agricultural lands had been abandoned and the so-called "frontier of settlement" had receded toward more protected areas. The Frenchman C. F. Volney remarked in his *Voyages*, "the peasant lives therefore in great distress; but at least he does not enrich his tyrant and the avarice of despotism is its own punishment."

Wherever possible towns were walled, and every man was a part-time soldier. Travel was expensive since each town, jealous of its autonomy and needing funds to pay taxes and hire guards, charged customs duties—in some cases little different from ransom—on entrants. Where the governor was strong, as in the city of Acre, he was really an autonomous prince although nominally an official of the empire. If he took a short-sighted view of his position he merely gathered as much treasure as he could, paid out to the empire or his overlords as little as possible, and retired to Constantinople. Jean Joseph Poujoulat, recounting his visit to Gaza, observed that the pashas looked upon themselves as travelers, camping out in their posts, never bothering to invest or repair. But this was not always the case. The pashas of the walled city of Acre encouraged the production of goods, both agricultural and industrial, which they monopolized, and taxed but tolerated the foreign merchant communities who settled in their midst. In some respects, Acre resembled a medieval Italian city-state.

With travel insecure and expensive, men moved mainly in caravans after careful preparation and along established routes. Some of these caravans were vast affairs. From Damascus, a city of 100,000, the Mecca caravan of 2000 camels departed once a year with 40,000 pilgrims; the Baghdad caravan of roughly a thousand camels made two or three round trips yearly. Ten to twelve thousand pilgrims yearly visited Jerusalem, then a city of 20,000.

Also because of the expense of travel, men tried to satisfy their wants locally. It is surprising to read the long lists of manufacturing "factories" of such little villages as Gaza, Dair al-Qamar, Homs, and Zubair. The important fact, however, is not the *scale* of economic life but the fact that for centuries men had accommodated to it and had found in it a satisfying pattern. Woven into their commerce, social organization, military service, and family life were their religious beliefs and their expectations from life. In a man's family, clan, or neighborhood was the seat of his loyalty. City dwellers found in trade and religious guilds what tribal life gave to the bedouin, a social matrix for individual life. Desires were limited because horizons were narrow. Weapons had changed little in centuries and they were usually inherited from relatives or made locally; the principal luxury item of clothing was the Kashmiri shawl and this too lasted at least one lifetime. Agricultural implements were made by the farmers—the hoe and the "stick plow" were the whole range—while those of the artisan in the town required little more investment of time and resources. Food was not more exotic or expensive. The staples were cracked wheat, vegetables, and yogurt. Meat was a luxury for the agricultural and urban population.

The elements of society interacted and met one another's requirements. The bedouin provided the villager with a market for his crops and sold him animal products; the towns brought the products of bedouin and peasant, fashioned them into leather, soap, cloth, and luxuries, and sent them out to the world on the backs of bedouin camels. The economic machine was a simple one which by modern standards was slow and inefficient, but it worked. The breakdown of this machine, even if it is to be or in some instances has been replaced by a vastly superior though much more complex and expensive one, is what is ascribed to the "impact of the West."

European contacts with the Middle East had never totally ceased in the Middle Ages. Venice and Genoa, even in decline, maintained merchants' "factories" along the Levant and Egyptian coasts. The Portuguese, reaching the Indian Ocean in the sixteenth century, rapidly established similar factories on the Persian Gulf. Gradually, as the British and French aspired to world empires, they too created, took over, or inherited centers of trade and influence. Even the most remote areas of the empire were visited by the traveler and the merchant. The French monopoly port of Marseilles and the British East India Company developed vested interests in the politics of the area for not only was trade with and within the Middle East of importance, but the Middle East was the road to India.

In France plans for the conquest of Egypt had been discussed since the reign of Louis XIV. Behind them were motives more often romantic than practical, but Egypt did offer a shorter route to India than the Cape of Good Hope. This became of great moment to the French government when, in the last years of the eighteenth century, it entered a mortal struggle with the British

Empire. Not only, it was thought, was Egypt capable of becoming the granary of France and a market for French goods, but from the port of Suez a French army could reach India in six weeks. This idea was first discussed by Napoleon in his correspondence with the Directory in the summer of 1797. With his customary dispatch he was ready to depart the following spring.

On July 1, 1798, a French army of 38,000 men disembarked from an armada of 280 ships off Alexandria. In a few hours Alexandria fell to the French force. The Egypt he found must have come as something of a shock to Napoleon. The population, living in the midst of the relics of ancient grandeur, was small and poor. It was, to the advantage of the French, divided into several, compartmented sections. The rulers, nominally Ottoman Turks but in practice the Turko-Circassian Mamluks, spoke a different language from the native population. The natives themselves were divided by religion, class, and education. The peasants, cut off alike from Islamic learning and from political experience, were, like the peasants of the rest of the Middle East, more objects than actors. The Copts, "Franks," Greeks, and Jews were the scribes, merchants, and tax collectors. And the literate, educated, Arabic-speaking Muslims tended to all matters of personal status and law. It was to them that Napoleon was to address his impassioned, nationalistic pleas for understanding and support. "People of Egypt, you are told that I come to destroy your religion. Do not believe it. Reply that I come to restore your rights, punish the usurpers and that I respect, more than the Mamluks, God, his Prophet and the Quran . . . Tell the people that we are friends of True Muslims. Is it not we who have destroyed the Pope who wanted to make war on Muslims? Is it not we who have destroyed the Knights of Malta because they believed that God wanted them to make war on the Muslims? Is it not we who have been throughout the centuries the friends of the Sultan (may God grant him favor) and the enemy of his enemies?" All Egyptians, Napoleon proclaimed, "are called upon to fill all the posts; the wisest, best educated and most virtuous will govern and the people will be happy."

In the Egypt of that time these were such outlandish notions as simply to be incomprehensible to the Egyptians. Indeed, even generations later the notion that the Egyptians were peasants, that rule was not their function or calling but rather was that of the Turks, was firmly held by very large numbers of people. The habit of centuries of foreign rule had deeply scored the Egyptian character. This withdrawal from politics was to be incomprehensible to Napoleon throughout his stay in Egypt.

Much more startling and evident was the ease with which Napoleon marched to Cairo with his large, disciplined, and modern force and in the famous Battle of the Pyramids, on July 21, in the space of an afternoon, utterly destroyed the colorful, dashing medieval army of the Mamluks. The next day the French army entered Cairo.

For Napoleon Egypt was a way station on the road of Alexander the Great to the Orient, but, realizing the necessity of consolidating this forward base, he entrusted to the Commission des Sciences et Arts the task of organizing an administration, surveying the country, regulating taxes and expenditures, in short, of performing all of the functions of a military government. For the most part the personnel and practices of the past were retained by the government; the major innovation, and the major failure, was Napoleon's attempt to enlist in the service of the government a council of native Egyptians. On October 21 the population of Cairo, led by the very people whose favor Napoleon had courted, the native Muslim, Arabic-speaking Egyptians, rose in revolt to throw out the French. Though they failed, they did shatter the liberation image of the French occupation.

Like most of the strong rulers of Egypt before him, Napoleon realized the importance to the security of Egypt of control over the Levant coast, and so early in 1799 he set out on the expedition to conquer Palestine and Syria and perhaps to open the route to the East. At the walled fortress-city of Acre he was handicapped by an English naval blockade and the outbreak of the plague. After an unsuccessful, fever-ridden seige, Napoleon turned back to Egypt in which, since it now was a jumping-off place to nowhere, he quickly lost interest. After one more major battle against an Anglo-Turkish force, in which he demonstrated again the tremendous superiority of his army, Napoleon left Egypt on August 23.

Napoleon's invasion, and the long-range threat it posed to British interests in India, marked a great turning point in the history of the Middle East. The impact, however, was initially less in the Arab East itself—changes there have been greatly exaggerated by writers caught up in the romantic image of Napoleon and provided with superb propaganda in the publications of the expedition—than in the policies of the great powers. The French, pushed out militarily from the East, never lost their aspirations to play a major role in the East. The Ottoman government, surprised by the tremendous superiority of modern armies, accelerated its own programs of modernization and of the reimposition of authority over its huge but anomalous empire. Lastly, and more importantly, the British, frightened by the possible loss of their Indian empire, redoubled their efforts to drive the French out of India and, by a deep involvement in the affairs of the Middle East, to block any future moves from Europe toward southern Asia. A British army assisted in the expulsion of the French from Egypt in 1801, and in the Persian Gulf, Iraq, Mount Lebanon, and Egypt itself the English presence, whether the consul, the merchant, or the traveler, began to be felt.

The major if somewhat delayed impact of Napoleon's expedition was that made on one of the great figures of the nineteenth century, Mehmet Ali Pasha, a Turkish soldier of fortune who had nearly lost his life fighting the French.

Mehmet Ali Pasha, born in the Macedonian port town of Kavalla in 1769, the son of a police officer, orphaned young, a man whose energy was matched only by his ambition, was fond of remarking, "I was born in the same year as Napoleon in the land of Alexander." Throughout Mehmet Ali's life Napoleon and the expedition to Egypt were to exercise a profound influence on him. Like Napoleon he was a foreigner in the country he was to make his own; like Napoleon he was to win a vast empire; like

Napoleon he was a superb opportunist. He realized, as few in the East in his time, wherein lay the real strength of the French, and his life was spent in attempting to acquire the modernization, the industrial and materials base, and the organization which had made a Napoleon possible.

By 1805 Mehmet Ali emerged as the leader of the most powerful faction within the Ottoman forces in Egypt and was able to seize power. He had his seizure of power ratified locally in Egypt rather than from the Ottoman Empire, by an assemblage of notables in Cairo—itself rather an unusual move—and then negotiated with the empire as to how his position could be confirmed. Confirmation as governor came in 1806. But the political situation was still very unstable in Egypt, where rivals watched as hungry wolves the leader of their pack. The attempted British invasion of Egypt in 1807, which ended disastrously for the British at the Battle of Rosetta, came at a dangerous point for Mehmet Ali and his "victory" was not of his design or execution but was due to peasant xenophobia, poor British planning, and thirst.

In this period the necessity for reform in Egypt was recognized by everyone. Napoleon's military force had so easily destroyed the flower of Mamluk cavalry as to produce a profound impression on the whole Middle East. The Mamluk beys themselves, particularly the two who emerged as Mehmet Ali's major opponents in these years, aped French uniforms, had their troops drilled in French style, and tried very hard, insofar as they knew how, to look French, to behave like they had seen the French behave. The first Ottoman governor against whom Mehmet Ali contended for power, Khusrev Pasha, who was later to be grand vizier, enlisted French officers to train a Sudanese regiment on the French system. So it took no unique insight on the part of Mehmet Ali to realize where the new road of power lay. Each contender for power recognized that if he were to survive in the kind of situation which had been created by Napoleon's challenge to Egypt, he must create a modern army. Mehmet Ali won partly by his reforms and largely by luck. But, having won, he knew he must go on.

In 1815 he tried to introduce into Egypt the *Nizam Jadid*, the new-style army. But there was such opposition on the part of his own army that he was forced to drop this program, and it was not until a lengthy war in Arabia against the Wahhabis had virtually killed off the veterans of his existing force that he was able to undertake the imposition of a modernized military system. It happened that just about the time the political situation was ready in Egypt for the introduction of this system, a former French army officer, then a captain, by the name of Sève, who subsequently became known as Sulaiman Pasha, arrived in Egypt and offered his services.

Mehmet Ali ordered Sève to introduce into Egypt several schools for the training of soldiers on the French system. At first these schools were largely made up of Turkish and Mamluk young men. Subsequently, Sudanese were enlisted in the Egyptian army, and ultimately, apparently at the suggestion of a French adviser, Egyptian peasants, for the first time in many centuries, were conscripted into the army.

The wars of Mehmet Ali made further and further demands for a larger and larger military machine. By 1833 there were about 190,000 men in the Egyptian army and auxiliary forces, and by 1839 one out of every ten Egyptians was in one way or another involved in the army.

It was the genius of Mehmet Ali that he recognized that it was not simply a matter of numbers, or of the drill, or the style of uniforms, or equipment of troops which made power in the new sense. It was rather the control over the *means of production* both of modern weapons and of modern soldiers which differentiated him from his rivals. He recognized that he could not rely on Europe for either but had to open schools to train soldiers and factories to equip them. Therefore he set out to build in Egypt factories to produce guns, ammunitions, and uniforms; arsenals to equip the army and the fleet; and ultimately shipyards to produce the fleet itself. The production of these things required not only a handful of technicians who could be hired in Europe, but also an intricate bureaucracy, a large number of literate, qualified,

capable people, to run and organize all of the myriad services that
a modern government required.

Mehmet Ali began quite early in his career to train his people
abroad. In 1809 the first man was sent from Egypt to Europe for
training, and in almost every year thereafter a new mission of
students would be sent abroad. Very few of these were sent for
what we would call "higher education"; most were sent for rudimentary technical training. Workers were sent to Italy to learn
about the textile industry; others were sent to learn how to
manufacture guns and equipment. Others were sent to military
schools to learn not only tactics but engineering, medicine, and
logistics. Although he apparently had not intended to do so,
Mehmet Ali created a new generation, which was to come to the
fore in Egypt after his death, of men who had begun to learn
about the inner nature of European civilization.

Perhaps the most famous of these men was one who was sent
to Europe not as a student but as the imam, or chaplain, of a
group of students in 1824. This was Rifaa Rafi, who was born
in the little Egyptian town of Tahta, where his father had been
a fairly wealthy local landlord. So struck was Rifaa with the new
world he discovered that while in Paris he set about writing a
book which was intended to explain to the Egyptians what life
was like in France. This book, called *The Journey* and published
in 1834, went through three Arabic editions and a Turkish edition
and was the most widely read of any book produced in the Middle East in the first half of the nineteenth century. It and that
great classic of European description E. W. Lane's *Manners and
Customs of the Modern Egyptians* present the most fascinating
contrast of the intellectual contact between Europe and the Middle East produced in the nineteenth century.

When each Egyptian student returned from Europe, he was
placed in the Citadel in Cairo and told to translate the textbook
that he had been studying in France. So, somewhat casually, individual students made available to their confreres the works
upon which they had relied during their European exposure.
Ultimately, a special bureau was set up to translate a great corpus

of European literature into Arabic. And it was this work which laid the intellectual foundations of subsequent Egyptian history.

The third aspect of Mehmet Ali's creation of power in Egypt lay in the field of economics. He recognized that it was necessary for the government to centralize agricultural, financial, industrial, and commercial control just as it had centralized military and political control. This was not the result of a sudden decision to undertake a new program. It was not comparable with the sort of decisions made for governmental activity in five-year or seven-year plans common in the Middle East today but came about as a purely pragmatic solution to a problem. Mehmet Ali had effectively eliminated his rivals, one by one, and finally in 1811 had massacred the Mamluk opponents of his regime and confiscated a great deal of their property. In 1816 he formalized the trend in centralization by subsuming land rights over all of Egypt. What these rights had amounted to was administrative control over a given area of land. The holder of this right (*iltizam*) would agree to pay to the central government a specified sum of money yearly in return for which he would be allowed to tax the people who lived on the land. He did not himself own, *de jure*, the land. The land was theoretically owned by the Empire. What Mehmet Ali did in broad outline was to take fiscal control over the land to himself and subdivide the rights to use the land among other people—in the main, peasants—who after 1816 produced crops for and paid taxes directly to the government.

Similarly, in the realm of urban finance, commerce, and industry, Mehmet Ali established a monopoly in 1816. Anyone desiring to buy Egyptian produce had to do so through a government agency. Ultimately, Mehmet Ali came to recognize that the government must undertake the stimulation of industrial growth. For this purpose the government sent industrial workers and students to Europe for training, hired European industrial workers and technicians to come to Egypt, furnished capital and raw materials, set production goals, purchased all finished goods, and paid the operating costs of the industry Mehmet Ali thought Egypt needed.

In Egypt in the 1820's, as in America at a later date, the textile industry formed the major thrust of the industrial transformation. Between 1818 and 1828 thirty cotton textile factories were opened. Additional woolen factories were built to provide uniforms for the army. This is a development which continued in Egypt, and as late as 1952 textiles accounted for 36 percent of the workers in establishments of ten or more workers. Other industries lagged far behind textiles as Egypt lacked iron and coal. Here again there is continuity: in 1952 mining and manufacturing, of which textiles and food processing accounted for the bulk, still amounted to only 8 percent of the gross national product.

But in the time of Mehmet Ali as later, noneconomic factors caused the government to industrialize. In the 1820's and 1830's the Egyptian military machine, with about 130,000 men under arms, required the manufacture of artillery, small arms, powder, and other munitions. The growing navy demanded and got a rapid acceleration in the manufacture of naval vessels and stores in Alexandria. Troops and those who supported them had to be fed and supplied, so sugar refineries, dye works, glass-blowing factories, tanneries, paper mills, and chemical works were set up throughout the country.

All of these factories were supervised, financed, and controlled by the government. Many were under the immediate jurisdiction of foreign technicians but even in them Egyptians or other Orientals were trained to fill, ultimately, all the jobs. All of the personnel, including the directors, were government employees. The products were marketed by the government and all raw materials were procured by the government. Perhaps this government monopoly was necessary, as the growing and already far larger industries of Europe could swamp the area with their cheaper products, but the system, as the perceptive Egyptian writer Moustafa Fahmy has pointed out, did not permit the entry of a single capitalist or entrepreneur into industrial or, at times and in certain fields, commercial activity. This was to have profound social, economic, and political implications in later times.

In order to train the new personnel required by the government for its bureaucracy and its various other technical and military activities, Mehmet Ali also began a new venture or, more correctly, series of new adventures in education. Ultimately, over 10,000 students were enrolled in various government institutions, where they were given lodging, food, and stipends at a total yearly expenditure of approximately £150,000 or 5 percent of the then gross national product of Egypt.

In the enrollments one can see the obviously utilitarian aims. A school of languages, to train translators, was opened for 225 students; a school of secretarial service for clerks was opened for 300; a polytechnic institute had 300 pupils; artillery and medical schools had 300 each; a school for infantry officers enrolled 800; and a veterinary medical school, to minister to the cavalry, absorbed 120 young men. Upon graduation each young man was immediately taken into government service. Uniformly, and this was to remain a feature of the system until recently, education led directly to service in the government.

The number of salaried, permanent workers in factories reached approximately 30,000 in the 1830's and over a quarter of a million others worked in smaller establishments, or at their homes, on the government account. It has been estimated that between 1816 and 1850 the total number of industrial workers was at least 400,000.

At this same time rapid transformations were in process in Syria, which came under Egyptian rule in 1832. The population of the Syrian hinterland and coast was 1.3 million, of whom half were urban. In this area as in Egypt, commerce had always been an element in the economic life but relatively a secondary element. Following the French Revolution and during the French invasion of Egypt the violent and greedy rule of the Ottoman pashas based in Acre and Sidon caused a sharp decline in the international trade of the Levant. The French trading establishments were closed, the British had not at that time interested themselves in the Levant, and the American effort was then minor. On the eve of the Egyptian invasion even the British consul could not establish himself in Damascus so restrictive and zenophobic were its people. The people, as mentioned above, were content with the small world they knew and feared outsiders would destroy it. They grew, built, or inherited most of what they needed; and what little they got from outside was mainly from the Far East rather than from the West.

The effect of the Egyptian invasion of 1832 was to "open" the Levant to Western influence. This is a process which the author has described in detail in a recent book.* Here it is useful to point out that a change in tastes and technology distinguished the Egyptian period, as old ways, old tools, and old weapons were quickly judged to be outmoded. Cheap Western goods, the products of the new and booming industry of Europe, flowed into the Syrian market. Syrian handicraft industry was doomed. In the one year of 1833 an estimated 10,000 workers, mainly in textiles, were thrown out of work in Damascus and Aleppo. The smaller towns, which had to some degree specialized in particular local products, could no longer market their goods. Even the old caravan trade was hurt as clothing styles changed. The people of Damascus who would not allow the entry of one British official in 1830 were patronizing 107 shops retailing British goods in 1838. Even the great tribal groups in the deserts were affected as they found they could buy their headdresses and gowns from factories at Birmingham at less cost than they could weave them. Within a few years even the chief moneylenders of Damascus and other towns were British. The flood gates, once opened by the Egyptians, were never again closed.

In Syria, as in Egypt, the army was the principal agent fostering change. The soldiers were major purchasers. Officers were important investors. For the first time in Syrian history since Byzantine times the government, that is the army, undertook public works projects and gave security to the roads thereby encouraging trade and travel. As a direct result the Levant began to be tied to the world market on a massive scale and to acquire a taste for the goods and disquieting new ideas of the West. As the British agent John Bowring wrote in 1839, "The soldiery be-

* *The Opening of South Lebanon* (Cambridge, Mass., 1963).

came protectors instead of destroyers of property; they formed part of a structure of social improvement, which, with some attendant evils, brought an incomparably great portion of benefits. The effect of this better organization has been immense. Even in the populous parts of Egypt, before the time of Mahomet Ali, there was little security for life or property; in the Desert, none whatever . . . the Desert has been made as safe and secure as the high road of the Nile."

It is difficult to say what might have happened in Syria—or in Egypt itself—had Egyptian rule in Syria continued. This was not to be. At the height of his powers, after a series of campaigns that had taken his armies into Africa to conquer the Sudan, into Europe to attempt to retain Greece in the Ottoman Empire, and into Asia where they had conquered Arabia, Palestine, Lebanon, Syria, and half of Anatolia, Mehmet Ali had routed the forces of the Ottoman army and assumed control over the Ottoman fleet. The major Western powers were increasingly alarmed that the threat posed by Mehmet Ali to the empire would force the sultan into the arms of Russia. The English realized that they must weaken Mehmet Ali to get the sultan, and his prized Straits, away from the Russian grasp. Specifically, they must get the Egyptians out of Syria. Moreover, industrial England was actively in quest of markets and the restrictive practices of Mehmet Ali were frustrating British commerce. Mehmet Ali refused to allow the Commercial Code of 1838—which, having been negotiated with a weakened sultan, was extremely favorable to foreigners—to be applied in Egyptian-controlled areas, rightly seeing in it the ruin of Egyptian industry and the denationalization of commerce. "Monopoly," in free-trade England, was almost as damning a word as "Communism" is today. So, when the Egyptians had made themselves thoroughly unpopular and were in the midst of a civil war, the British assisted the sultan in driving them out of Syria, and forced Mehmet Ali to reduce his standing armed forces from over 130,000 to 18,000. With the *raison d'être* of the reform program removed, Mehmet Ali lost interest in the sweeping changes he had set in motion.

VII. The High Cost of Modernization: Coming of the West

The residual effects of Mehmet Ali's rule, both in Syria and in Egypt, were to be felt strongly by future generations. Mehmet Ali had created, albeit for his own limited purposes, the first of the successive groups of "new men" who were to come forward in Arab society over the next century.

What Mehmet Ali did was to unleash forces of economic change which had long-term but slowly maturing social consequences. He once referred to himself as "the armed missionary of European civilization in Arabia," trying to accomplish there what England was doing in India and what France was to try in Algeria. But Egypt lacked the power to control the process of change or to replace the older institutions of society with new ones.

In 1824 Damascus alone had bought twice as much from the Orient (brought by the Baghdad caravan) as all Syria bought from Europe. When Egypt opened the Levant to Western trade, this situation changed drastically: by 1838 urban men were wearing fezes imported from France and drinking from glass made in Bohemia. By 1854 the French and Austrian steamers, plying the coastal Levant towns, had in the words of the British consul "annihilated the local carrying trade." New ideas from the West changed clothing styles, so that the key luxury import from the East, the Kashmiri shawl, went out of fashion. By 1857 the old Baghdad-Damascus caravan was finished. Routes of trade were either forgotten or reversed: Aleppo traditionally had got its coffee from Yemen but began to get it from Santo Domingo via France; pepper, which had come to Beirut from the East via Baghdad, was, after the advent of steam, sent to Baghdad via Beirut.

Specialization in the produce of the area led to entry into the world markets. This in turn led to the necessity of cultivating certain kinds of crops and of processing these in a way suitable for European use. Silk, long the staple export of Lebanon, had been reeled by hand, but by 1850 the requirements of the European industry had brought a drastic change in methods. Silk thread reeled by hand fetched only a quarter as much as silk reeled by steam power. This opened a new market for European investors who constructed large-scale filatures in Lebanon. Cotton, which was introduced on a national scale by Mehmet Ali in Egypt in 1831, was likewise affected by the European market. The short-staple cotton of Syria was useful only for producing wicks, while that of Egypt commanded a wider market.

However, cotton and other large-scale crops were affected by the vagaries of the world market. The Crimean War caused a rapid rise in prices but the return of peace in 1856 caused a fall of 50 percent in prices of cotton and other local produce in the Middle East. In 1860 the United States supplied over 80 percent of the cotton used in European industry; thus, when the outbreak of the Civil War cut the source of supply, a "famine" was caused in textile mills, which were the heart of British industry. In the year 1861–62 the price of raw cotton quadrupled and attention was attracted to alternate sources of supply, of which Egypt was the most promising. British purchases from Egypt increased from £8 to £22 million between 1861 and 1865. Such smart operators as Ismail Pasha, who was to become khedive of Egypt in 1866, made their fortunes in this period (Ismail is reputed personally to have made £1 million). But the slump which followed ruined many who had overinvested in lands and equipment.

Thus, the units of society began to change both absolutely and relatively. The bedouin alone held out, relatively unaffected by the slow pace of the new social revolution. But incursions into the nomad's sanctuary were made. Relentlessly the line of settlement was pushed out into the steppe and modernized armies became more efficient in hunting him down.

British and French consular dispatches of the 1840's and 1850's are filled with references to Ottoman punitive expeditions against the bedouin. Since the Ottoman administrators regarded the bedouin as pirates, they tried to drive them back into the desert, cut them off from trade with the towns, and where possible to kill them. Fairly typical of their efforts was a campaign in 1864. It was, wrote the British consul in Aleppo, "successful as far as regards the numerous tribes of settled Arabs, all of which have confirmed their submission to the authorities and consented to pay their annual taxes. The [nomadic] Anezi tribes, however, are during this season in the plains of Nejd or Central Arabia whither they withdraw regularly for the winter." The Ottoman policy, in short, was similar to the American policy toward the Indians, but whereas the Americans were a numerous and pioneer people, backed by a mobile army, the Ottoman government was represented by tax-collecting pashas with small and usually immobile military forces. Their proper target was the land-bound peasant, not the elusive nomad. It was only as the bedouin could be induced to settle and invest in immovable objects that they could be controlled.

Settlement of the bedouin had been one of the most interesting aspects of the Egyptian occupation of Syria. The Egyptians had a large and relatively mobile army which could overwhelm the nomads if necessary, but continual warfare was expensive. Moreover the Egyptians needed more agricultural production. So the Egyptian governor hit upon the solution of inducing tribes to settle. Purchase of land was made extremely easy, bedouin and peasants were assisted with government loans, and a ready market existed for the produce. In this way a great deal of land was brought into cultivation on the Syrian steppe. But following the Egyptian withdrawal the market for agricultural produce declined. A return to government exploitive practices induced many peasants to abandon their newly acquired lands and return to nomadic life. The British consul in Damascus reported the complete failure of the policy of settlement of the tribes when, in 1863, he noted that the bedouin "are being pursued by the Government troops in every direction without any reason other than they are nomadic tribes." It was not until the able and wise Ottoman Governor Midhat Pasha went to Baghdad in 1869 that the policy of inducing settlement was again tried and with some more success.

In Lebanon one of the principal effects of the Egyptian occupation had been the upset in the traditional relationship between the Christians and the Muslims and Druze. Lebanon, set apart by its mountains from the surrounding areas, had always been able to live an independent life. The position there of the Christians and other minorities was always stronger than that of their confreres in other areas. But at least in the southern half of Lebanon the Christians were second-class citizens in 1830. Often they were the clients and peasants of the Druze warrior class. Favored by a tolerant or even superficially pro-Christian Egyptian government, the Christians of Lebanon emerged in 1840 as landlords and creditors of their former masters. The Druze attempted when the Egyptians were driven out to regain their former possessions but were thwarted not only by the Christians, against whom they probably could have won a war, but by the European powers who undertook either to protect the Christians (in the case of France) or to hold the peace (as in the case of Great Britain). When the Christians invaded a Druze area, they were defeated, but the British and French stopped the Druze from following up their advantages. When Druze shaikhs tried to collect rents from their properties, their agents were killed by townsmen whose arms were conveyed to them by priests under French diplomatic protection. Indeed, the first Ottoman governor referred to the "innumerable French Missionaries . . . [as] the Pope's Light Irregular Cavalry Established in Lebanon, who under the garb of priests were in fact political Agents and Pertubators of the Public Peace."

Friction between the Christian and Druze communities invited outside intervention and led to a series of crises which culminated in the 1860–61 civil war during which the French sent a military expedition to restore the peace. Finally in 1864 Lebanon's unique character was enshrined in a *reglement organique* which acknowledged Lebanese autonomy under a Christian governor appointed by the Ottoman sultan but approved by the great powers. This was the formalization of Lebanon as a Christian and Western-oriented enclave which it has been to this day.

Foreign religious activity in the Middle East was facilitated by the organization of non-Muslim subjects of the Ottoman Empire into self-governing millets or "nations" on the basis of religion. Most of these had long existed. The separation from the rest of society and the relative internal cohesion engendered both by a common concern in community affairs and the existence of a single hierarchy or ethnarchy, which controlled not only matters of personal status but also the rate of taxation, made each millet a receptive partner for foreign political, missionary, and economic activity.

Lebanon—a land protected by its mountainous chain, relatively isolated from the East but open by sea to the West, whose population included religious minorities with a long tradition of contacts with the West—was an ideal place for early Western Christian missionary activity. The first American missionaries came to Lebanon in 1823, but it was not until 1831 that the mission was firmly established. Faced as they were by hostile Christians in long-established churches (until 1871 the Protestants were hampered by not being recognized as a separate millet with their own institutions), and unable to make overt efforts to convert Muslims, the Americans turned to educational activities. To succeed in these, they had to learn Arabic. Having done this, they were able to establish ties with local men of letters, some of whom became converts and in cooperation with whom they translated numbers of Western books and the New Testament. Gradually, they spread a network of schools over the Middle East and in 1866 founded the Syrian Protestant College, now known as the American University of Beirut. The French opened the Jesuit Université St. Joseph, and by the eve of the First World War the Levant coast had over three hundred foreign schools educating more than twenty-five thousand students.

Foreign intervention in the life of the Middle East characterized the second half of the nineteenth century. Whereas in 1830 a British consul had been unable to enter the city of Damascus, in 1840 another British consul actually picked the man who was to be governor of Lebanon. British consuls intervened even in the most minute political affairs of remote areas. For example, in 1854 in the port of Beirut a native and a foreign ship collided. No court then constituted could try the case. It was the British consul not the Ottoman governor whose powers were adjudged most nearly able to meet the requirements of the situation, and he constituted a mixed commission to assess damages and responsibility.

The commercial code of 1838 gave to European merchants great advantages over their native competitors, and they used these with the full support of their governments. The "capitulations" removed them from the jurisdiction of local courts. Capitulations had long existed. Originally, they were granted by the Byzantine Empire to encourage trade by allowing merchants to follow their own customs and laws while temporarily residing in the empire. This fit easily with the Islamic notion that nations or groups of people with a common religion should have corporate institutions of their own. The Ottoman rulers granted this privilege to the French in 1535, to the Austrians in 1567, and to the English in 1592. However, in the decline of the empire the capitulations became both a symptom and a cause of the denegration of Ottoman sovereignty. By the middle of the nineteenth century all foreigners enjoyed more privileges than do modern diplomats.

Foreigners on criminal charges could appeal their cases to courts in their native lands; even when their crimes involved natives, the local government was powerless to punish them. So flagrant were the abuses possible under this system that it was to be regarded as one of the great triumphs of Egyptian nationalism to get the great powers to recognize and participate in the creation and functioning of "mixed courts," in which Egyptian judges, though a permanent minority, could have a voice in the decision of cases involving their countrymen with Europeans. It was not until 1937 that Egypt was able to get the capitulations abolished.

The great stimulus to European investment in the Middle East in the nineteenth century was, of course, the huge Suez Canal project. This was the lifework of Ferdinand de Lesseps, who in 1854 was able to convince the Egyptian governor to grant him a concession to dig a canal to link the Mediterranean with the Red Sea. Lesseps was as ruthless, shameless, patient, and brilliant an entrepreneur as lived in a century of Morgans, Guggenheims, Rockefellers, and Rothschilds. The terms under which he began his operations in Egypt were almost the antithesis of those under which modern concessionaires work: The Egyptian governor was to purchase over half of the stock of Lesseps' company, but the stock gave him few rights and was held under various restrictions. Egypt was to get 15 percent of the net profits of the company but was to furnish a labor force of nearly 20,000 men to dig the canal. Then, as the company needed new sources of revenue, the Egyptian treasury was literally plundered of "untold amounts . . . for indemnities, fraudulent and semi-fraudulent claims, exorbitant prices to purveyors and contractors, and all manner of bribes designed to buy cheap honours or simply respite from harassment," writes Professor David Landes. In 1869 Lesseps was especially hard pressed for money, and this, in Landes words,

forced the ingenious entrepreneur to find other pretexts for an assault on the treasury. He found them without delay (the company cashbox did not admit of procrastination) in a catch-all of rubbish that was either no longer of use to the company or never belonged to it in the first place. By agreement of July 1869, the canal sold to the Egyptian government those barracks, hospitals and other structures built to serve during construction and no longer required; a stone quarry that the company had been *allowed* to exploit for purposes of building and maintaining the waterway . . . divers other imaginary "rights"; and, most important for Egypt, a renunciation by the company of any further claims . . . The Egyptian government paid 30 million francs for the package. Since it had no cash, it abandoned its rights to interest and dividends on its shares in the company for a period of twenty-five years. Lesseps in turn issued at 260 francs 120,000 assignment bonds covering the detached coupons; the gross yield to the company on the transaction was therefore almost 60 millions, while the purchasers of the assignments could hope for a total of about 110 million francs in interest alone during the period in question. As though this were insufficient, the Egyptian government also agreed to share with the company the proceeds of future sales of improved land along the canal, in spite of the fact that the Emperor's arbitration had specifically enjoined the company from seeking any profit from this source.*

The governor of Egypt, Ismail, made the opening of the canal in 1869 an occasion for Egypt to gain a sort of diplomatic recognition of independence from the Ottoman Empire. At vast expense he prepared a gala ceremony for the crowned heads of Europe, built palaces to accommodate them during their visits to Egypt, and commissioned Verdi to write an opera extolling the grandeur of Egypt—thereby giving us *Aïda*.

To meet the financial obligations he had undertaken, to buy his autonomy from the Ottoman Empire, and to satisfy his own wishes for luxury and for the development of Egypt, Ismail began contracting ever larger loans from the great European banking firms. It was this, wrote the later British proconsul Lord Cromer, that brought the British in control of Egypt. When Said Pasha died in 1863, the external debt of Egypt was £3.3 million; thirteen years later the debt totaled £94 million. Lord Cromer, who rarely minced words, wrote that "for all practical purposes it may be said that the whole of the borrowed money, except £16,000,000 spent on the Suez Canal, was squandered."

However, a contemporary English author, J. Seymour Keay, in a widely sold pamphlet called *Spoiling the Egyptians, A Tale of Shame*, and later historians have pointed out that of the vast debt, "only about 45,500,000 [pounds] were even nominally received" and on some loans the rate of interest was over 26 percent; indeed, one loan of £9 million was paid over to the Egyptians in defaulted bonds. Typical of the debts contracted was one in 1865 for £3 million. The Egyptians received £2.2 million and had to repay £4.1 million plus various fees and penalties. European sharp practice in Egypt was paralleled by European treatment of the Ottoman Empire, which between 1854 and 1875 borrowed the equivalent of $900 million of which it actually received not much more than $600 million.

* *Bankers and Pashas* (Cambridge, Mass., 1958), p. 316.

Ismail did "waste" a great deal of money—the festivities at the opening of the Suez Canal, for example, cost £1.3 million—but his big outlays were to the Ottoman Empire, an obligation forced upon him by the fact that Europe had refused to allow Egypt to become independent, to the European creditors whose pressures he could not resist once he was caught in the web of usury, and for the development of Egypt. During his reign the new basis of the Egyptian economy was laid. Apart from the Suez Canal Ismail Pasha constructed over 8000 miles of canals, 900 miles of railroads, 5000 miles of telegraphs, 430 bridges, the harbor of Alexandria, mills, factories, and lighthouses and reclaimed about 1.25 million acres of land. During this period Egypt's exports tripled in value.

By 1875 Egypt had sold its shares in the Suez Canal through the offices of Rothschild to Disraeli's government for a mere £4 million and had ceded to its creditors control over the collection of taxes and duties in large parts of the Egyptian economy. By 1877 about two thirds of the revenues of the Egyptian government were devoted to the debt, and Egypt was in effect, placed in receivership by its European creditors and their governments. Finally in 1879 Ismail was deposed at the instigation of the European powers and replaced by a weak and vacillating ruler who could be little more than a front for the Europeans who controlled Egypt.

As a part of the economy drive the new governor allowed an international liquidation convention to force him to issue a "liquidation law." Then he cut the pay of the native officers, newcomers to high command, in the Egyptian army. This brought on a rebellion led by a triumvirate of officers—the first Egyptians to rise to the rank of colonel—of whom the principal was Arabi Pasha. In 1882, to maintain his throne, the discredited ruler called upon the great powers and both Great Britain and France sent warships to Alexandria. On July 11 the British bombarded Alexandria, while the French withdrew. In September a British force invaded Egypt by way of the Suez Canal, routed the Egyptian troops at the battle of Tal al-Kabir, captured Cairo, and arrested Arabi Pasha.

Retrospectively Arabi Pasha has been magnified as a great national figure who tried to protect the independence of Egypt and who sought to enhance the position of the native Egyptians in the face of a corrupt, alien aristocracy. But in his own time Arabi was not a popular man; his limited intelligence and lofty pride were not solid foundations for national independence and the Egyptian people had not yet firmly grasped the concept of nationalism. In large part nationalism was to be a by-product of the British occupation.

The British seizure of power in Egypt was almost embarrassingly easy. The official reason for it, the bankruptcy of Egypt, could not be satisfied by an early withdrawal. Thus, though Britain immediately announced that it was planning to withdraw, British officials set about the reorganization of the country. Once involved in this program they found it more and more difficult to leave. The last British troops did not, in fact, leave until 1956.

The underlying reason for Britain's interest in Egypt was the one which took Napoleon there—Egypt dominated the route to India. It might, indeed, be argued that the construction of the Suez Canal made inevitable in an age of unblushing imperialism, as Mehmet Ali had predicted it would, the occupation of Egypt by some one or a consortium of European powers. It should be noted that 80 percent of the ships using the Suez Canal in 1882 were British. Thus it was that when the two immediate causes of the invasion were satisfied—Arabi was overthrown and the finances of the country restored, as they were by 1890—the British remained in Egypt. There was always some compelling reason to stay a bit longer. As Lord Cromer put it, "England did not want to possess Egypt, but it was essential to British interests that the country should not fall into the hands of any other European power . . . British diplomacy, which may at times have been mistaken, but which was certainly honest, did its best to throw off the Egyptian burden. But circumstances were too strong to be arrested by diplomatic action."

Having acquired a position in Egypt and built a cadre of able administrators there, Britain was inexorably drawn into all of the Middle Eastern affairs which had been the traditional concerns of rulers of Egypt. The affairs of the Sudan could not be neglected, so an Anglo-Egyptian force reconquered it from its native ruler in 1898 and established in it a new administration. The affairs of the Levant coast and Arabia, to which thousands of Egyptians went yearly on pilgrimage, became the concerns of the British. As a buffer to Egypt, the British government required the Ottoman Empire to cede the Sinai Peninsula to Egypt in 1906. During the First World War these area-wide concerns forced the British government to take a commanding role in the whole Middle East even at the expense of a partial estrangement from its principal wartime ally, France. The occupation of Egypt, then, may be said to have begun the political phase of the impact of the West while it set a seal on the first efforts of the people of the Middle East to find their own way into the modern era.

The "impact of the West," whether the result of actions by Europeans or by modernizing Middle Easterners, resulted more in the destruction of institutions and old balances between resources and expectations than in the creation of new institutions and balances. But, of course, it was long before intellectuals in the Middle East were able to formulate their fears of this disruption. Essentially the question posed to those who would protect their way of life was how to recoup the strength of the East in order to protect it from the West.

Answers to that question could be found in many ways. There was some flickering interest in "love of homeland," as expressed in the *wataniyat* poetry of the middle of the nineteenth century, but this amounted to little. In Egypt at least, Islam seemed to be the best rallying point and found two able spokesmen in Jamal ad-Din al-Afghani, who spent the years 1871–1879 in Egypt, and Muhammad Abdu, who eventually became grand mufti of Egypt before his death in 1905.

Jamal ad-Din, who was born near Kabul, Afghanistan, in 1839, briefly served as prime minister of Afghanistan until the amir under whom he served was forced out by British pressure. He traveled widely in the Islamic world and thought he had found in Islam itself and in the community of the Islamic peoples the best hope of the East to defend itself. During his stay in Egypt, Jamal inspired a new generation of Egyptians with his interpretation of Islam and so gained the disfavor of the British and their Egyptian friends. In September 1879 the new pro-British khedive expelled Jamal from Egypt, as one of the first acts of his government.

Some of those associated with Jamal took part in the Arabi rising in 1881–82, and his foremost student, Muhammad Abdu, joined Jamal in Paris, where he was living in exile. In 1884 the two began publication of a weekly newspaper in Arabic called *al-Urwah al-Wuthqah* (the Unbreakable Bond) in which they urged Muslims everywhere to unite to save themselves from Western domination. The paper was short-lived, issuing only eighteen numbers, and was banned in Egypt and India. Nevertheless it had a profound influence on a generation which had begun to search for a means of identification and defense.

Secular nationalism was more difficult to project into popular concern. The government and all political figures were men of the well-to-do classes of the city, were cut off from the life of the people in the countryside, and were themselves too caught up in the process of modernization and Westernization to oppose it effectively. Indeed, such seemed to be the case all over Asia. To the Egyptians it came as a major shock to learn of modernizing Japan and particularly of its victory over Russia in 1905. Thus it was natural that the principal leader of the secular nationalist movement at the turn of the century in Egypt should have written a book called *The Rising Sun*.

Still, this was rather intellectual and esoteric fare. The average Egyptian peasant had benefited from British rule, and whether his benefit was due to investments made by the Khedive Ismail in the 1870's or to honest government under Lord Cromer in the 1890's mattered little. It was not until the 1906 Denshawai incident that public opinion was crystallized against the British on a mass emotional basis. The incident itself was small, resulting from a dispute between British officers and villagers during a

pigeon shoot near the village of Denshawai, but the violent, un-
fair, and bullying response, in which the British-controlled government sentenced three Egyptians to be hanged and others to
be flogged and thrown into prison, shattered the mask of benevolence to reveal the face of imperial power. The Egyptians were
never again able to focus on the benevolence, despite the best
efforts of the British to play down their power. This new aspect
of imperialism was to captivate Egyptian thought and lead them
to revolt in 1920.

Though it was Egypt that was the main threat to British interests in the area in 1800 and the main base of British activity in
the Middle East at the end of the century, Britain's major holding in Asia was India, and it was India that set the stamp on
British endeavor throughout the Middle East. This concern
tended to draw British activity into areas other than those of
even long-term interest to Egypt or to the maintenance of the
Egyptian–Red Sea route to India.

From the time of Napoleon the British were obsessed with the
thought that another European power—first France, then Russia,
then Germany, and then Russia again—might use the Euphrates
River–Persian Gulf route to attack India. This concept was
most clearly stated in the House of Lords in 1911 when Lord
Curzon said, "the Gulf is part of the maritime frontier of India,
and . . . in the politics of the Gulf are involved the security, integrity and peace of India itself." But as early as 1798 the British
Secretary of War wrote that "Bonaparte will, as much as possible
avoid the dangers of the Sea, which is not his element, but . . .
by marching to Aleppo, cross the Euphrates, and following the
example of Alexander, by following the River Euphrates and the
Tigris, and descending to the Persian Gulf will march on India."
The walls of Acre and the Royal Navy blockade stopped Napoleon but the memory of the real or imagined danger remained
fresh in the minds of successive British and British Indian statesmen.

Moreover, communications were vital to the retention of control over the Indian empire. Before the advent of steam the Red

Sea was regarded as a dangerous route, and the Isthmus of Suez was until 1882 in the hands of a potentially hostile or untrustworthy power. The route around Africa was excessively long for the carrying of intelligence reports and government communications. A governor general of India complained in 1800 that "in the present year I was nearly *seven months* without receiving one line of authentic intelligence from England . . . Speedy, authentic, and regular intelligence from Europe is essential to the conduct of the trade and government of this empire."

An alternative and rapid route was, therefore, what in modern policy pronouncements would be labeled a "vital national interest." Usually such a communication route was available on the Tatar post of the Ottoman Empire, but it was unreliable and was often subject to interference by agents of other European powers. Therefore, it was early realized that Britain must create its own service, the "British Dromedary Post," protected by the agents and consuls established at Basra (in 1764) and Baghdad (in 1798). One undertaking led to the next as the very mechanics of the problems of communications drew the British deeper into Middle Eastern affairs. The Persian Gulf, although cleared of European rivals by the seizure of Hormuz in 1622, was still endangered by the pirates of Muscat. Indeed, these pirates raided India and the eastern African coast as far south as Zanzibar. After several expeditions the British established complete control over the gulf by 1820, suppressed piracy, and entered into treaty relations with the shaikhs of the "Pirate" (renamed "Trucial") Coast.

The desire to improve this route, and fear of Russian penetration, led the British government to send Lt. Francis Chesney to explore the Euphrates River with a view to establishing on it a steamboat service in 1830. In 1834 Chesney had two steamers on the river. Though the plan he had conceived did not prove feasible, it left behind a private company which operated a steamer on the Tigris River between Basra and Baghdad and provided the basis of British commercial penetration and development in Iraq.

If steamers were not practical, the advent of the railroad seemed to offer renewed hope. The desert route itself was still in use by camel riders as late as 1886. A Euphrates valley railroad scheme was first discussed in 1840, but the British government lost interest. By 1888 Constantinople was linked by rail to Europe. France, the principal banker of the empire after 1854, also led the way in railroad development; by 1914 French investors had 500 million francs in Ottoman railroads. But as early as 1872 an Austrian engineer, serving as a consultant to the Ottoman sultan, had recommended that a rail net link Basra with the capital. As the land was then sparsely populated, and such a project was not economically feasible, the engineer suggested that two million Germans be settled along the route to develop the resources of the empire. Although relatively latecomers to Turkey, the Germans plunged rapidly ahead. Several German authors urged that ancient Babylonia was a proper area of German colonization; expansion of trade was vigorously fostered; and through military missions, Germany entered deeply into the affairs of the Ottoman Empire.

The actual concession to build a railway was given by the sultan in 1899 to a German company. By the outbreak of the war in 1914, 1200 miles from Constantinople to Baghdad were completed. In 1901 the Germans began the construction of the railway from Damascus south to the Hejaz, to take pilgrims to Mecca. Everywhere the Germans seemed to be pushing southward. After 1890 German trade increased dramatically, and by 1910 it ranked just behind that of England and India.

The British felt secure south of Basra where they had agreements with the native rulers not to deal with foreign governments. In 1869 the first of these had been negotiated with the Trucial shaikhdoms. Similar agreements were made with Bahrein in 1880 and Muscat and Qatar in 1891. In 1898 the British used their position to deny to the French a coaling station in Muscat. In 1899 the British and the Shaikh of Kuwait agreed to prevent other foreign influence there. So, when a visiting German ship arrived shortly thereafter in Kuwait, the shaikh did not receive its captain, and when in 1900 a commission arrived to survey Kuwait as a possible terminus for a railway, it was turned back.

The British interest could have been accomplished by holding the line at Kuwait except for two developments which drew the British deeper into Iraq. The first was the discovery of huge deposits of oil in Persia (Iran) to the east of Abadan in 1907. The increasing production from this field stimulated interest in possible fields in Iraq—who had not heard of the "fiery Furnace" —on which the British secured a concession on the eve of the First World War. The conversion of the Royal Navy to oil-powered ships and the rapid development of Persian oil led the British government to purchase control of the oil company operating in Persia just six days prior to the outbreak of the war. So important was this to become that Disraeli was to say that "the Allies floated to victory on a wave of oil."

The second development was the growth of a belief in Europe that "Babylonia" could become the farm of Europe and a residence for the surplus and hungry population of India. The English expert on irrigation Sir William Wilcocks wrote glowingly in 1910 of the possibilities of agriculture in the Tigris-Euphrates valley to meet the wheat and cotton requirements of England and India. A few years later he wrote that "the delta of the two rivers would attain a fertility of which history has no record." A popular book of the period was J. T. Parfit's *Mesopotamia: Key to the Future*. And a senior British official, reflecting on this Garden of Eden, wrote that "there is no doubt that the land is the richest in the world."

VIII. The First World War: Midwife of Nationalism

The years before the First World War were filled with contests between the European powers, principally Britain, France, and Germany, for concessions and points of influence, but this rivalry in the Middle East had little to do with the actual outbreak of the war. Until the eve of the war itself the Middle Eastern issues seemed on the road to accommodation, particularly in the new oil industry, through the development of international consortia. Indeed, the Anglo-German Turkish Petroleum Company received its concession in Iraq as late as June 28, 1914. Like the causes so most of the events of the war were acted in other theaters. Here, four aspects of the war are of lasting concern, however: the situation on the eve of the war; the course of the war in the two separate and contrasting Arab theaters, the Arabian Peninsula–Syrian area and Iraq; the wartime arrangements, promises, and declarations of the participants which have left such a strong imprint on subsequent history; and the immediate aftermath of the war.

But first a word of caution. The First World War ended one era and began another. It began half a century ago, yet even today a satisfying perspective is difficult to achieve, so embedded are the events of those years in the politics of our own times. And even if a clear and logical perspective is achieved, it will be profoundly unreal. A too-precise systematization of events and pronouncements results in a pattern which, though true in hindsight, distorts the context in which each decision was taken and each event occurred. In the midst of that vast and protracted crisis, the events were confused, the future obscure, and the actors imperfectly informed. It is, therefore, difficult and necessary to keep in mind but separate both the events and their subsequent implication.

It is now fashionable to inveigh against the Ottoman Empire as the corrupt, tyrannical, "sick man" of Europe, which lived by exploiting the sullen, resentful, and uniformly hostile non-Turkish population of Asia, and thwarted all progress in the East. The facts are otherwise. The government of the empire, with few resources in trained people or a developed economy, chronically insolvent, and hard pressed by foes and well-wishers alike, was able to control inexpensively a vast, heterogeneous area—a feat beyond the capacities of its richer successors—while retaining the *essential* loyalty of the several nations who were its subjects. The secret of its success was its toleration of *other* loyalties. To see what happened in the Arab areas, at least, it is useful to understand what these loyalties were and what they were not.

There was, first of all, no clear sense of territorial loyalty. The empire was divided into administrative districts, but these were in no sense nation-states and were not separated from one another by frontiers, linguistic barriers, or marketing patterns. Only Egypt, over which a British protectorate was declared in December 1914, had a discrete identity. There was no "Syria" or "Iraq" except in a geographic sense, as one might refer to an American Midwest or to the eastern seaboard. The "Syrian" moved easily to Baghdad, Mecca, or Cairo and felt no more alien in any one than an American from Kansas City would in Los Angeles.

Such loyalties as transcended the family, clan, and tribe centered mainly on one's religious "nation" or millet, and this concept had no geographic expression. Members of the several Christian millets were scattered all over the empire as were the Jews. The millet system did not divide Turks from Arabs and

Kurds as most of each group were Muslims. And, by extension, the millet of the Muslims was the empire itself.

Dissatisfaction with this conception of a polyglot, multinational, universal empire had grown gradually except in the Balkans, where it was accelerated in the nineteenth century as the Greeks (from 1821–27), the Bulgarians (in 1879), the Rumanians (in 1881), and others won recognition of their distinct nationalities. But even in the Balkans nationalism was often equated with religion—the Bulgarians, for example, won recognition in 1870 for a separate national church to distinguish themselves from the Greeks.

It was the Armenians who brought into the heartland of the empire, Anatolia, the notion of nationalism in the new, ethnic sense in the last years of the nineteenth century. This, in turn, stimulated the Turkish element in the empire to probe its own historical legacy for what came to be called Turkism. This new sense of particularism was a part of the drive in the Young Turk revolution of 1908. As the Young Turks assumed power they forced upon the empire their Turkishness in a way never before attempted by an Ottoman government. School systems throughout the empire began to teach in Turkish and to emphasize the virtues of the Turks. This new exclusiveness of the Turks compelled the Arabs to seek for themselves an identity which was different from Ottoman and different from Muslim.

From about 1890 onward Egypt was the cultural center of the Arabic-speaking Middle East. There, of course, *the* national enemy was the West as represented by Great Britain. Most Egyptians who sought a means of defense against this enemy turned to Islam as represented in part by the Ottoman sultan-caliph. Unaffected by the growth of *Turkism*, since the British posed a barrier between the Ottoman Turkish suzerain and their administration and school system, the Egyptians followed a different drummer than did the literate, vigorous, and modernizing Arabs of the Levant and Iraq, who were in contact with the new Turkish administration.

What the Syrians and Iraqis found exciting was that in Beirut, particularly at the American University, a sort of literary revival of Arabic was in process. This literary revival had meager origins and was of small influence. Much has been written to make it seem otherwise, but the intellectual archaeology of nationalist writers always makes rather pitiful reading for the dispassionate foreigner. Even the most friendly foreign observers have found little Arab nationalism before the advent of the Young Turks. However, the core of such a movement was there and its elements were clear. The major stimulus came from ideas of Europe and America, and religion was excluded as a prime factor since the Turks were also Muslim while many of the best Arab thinkers were Christian. It was to the rich, pre-Islamic heritage of the Arabic language itself that these Arabs turned for the basis of national identity.

In 1905 a young Syrian Christian Arab, who subsequently published a book in French called *Le Rèveil de la Nation Arabe*, issued a manifesto deploring the alien rule of the Arabs. "Encouraged by our servility, the Turks pretend to preserve the remaining independent tribes of the Arab nation. [But they plan to dominate all Arab lands] where they wish to construct railways . . . And what is even more degrading, they plan to do it with our money and our labor so that we ourselves will forge the chains of our own servitude." But, although the author claimed to speak for a vast network of secret organizations throughout the Middle East, few were interested.

In the first blush of the excitement of the Young Turk revolution of 1908 the Arabs had cooperated and even formed "Ottoman Arab" organizations to participate. When the Young Turks suppressed this form of organization, the Arabs retreated first to "literary" societies and then to secret societies. These, though very small in number, attracted the younger, active, literate Arab element in the Ottoman civil and military service. But the Arabs had no spokesman. None among their group had a "national" reputation, and, of course, no one transcended the religious barrier which divided their community. An early manifesto reflects this problem: "Muslim Arabs, this despotic state is not Muslim.

Christian and Jewish Arabs, unite with your Muslim brothers. Those who say that they prefer the Turks-without-faith to you are imposters and enemies of our race." Ultimately, however, it was to a quasi-religious official of the empire, the sharif of Mecca, to whom the Arabs turned for leadership. But even if the young Arabs could have agreed among themselves on their ultimate objective, which they could not, they had little of any substance to offer the sharif, that cautious and skilled figure who had lived most of his sixty years under the close supervision of the sultan's police. It was not the Arabs but the British who tempted him to act on a grander stage.

We have seen how the impact of the West altered the traditional social relationships and created new aspirations in the more advanced parts of the Ottoman Empire. It would be a mistake, however, to exaggerate the size and influence of the groups who, on the eve of the First World War, had already been led to sedition by these changes. Nevertheless, some overtures to outside powers had been made. In 1913 a group of Arabs toured the European capitals to seek support for reforms in the empire, a tactic used by the Armenians before them, while another group visited Cairo to suggest that the British annex Syria. More important, Amir Abdullah, a son of the sharif of Mecca and a man whose name figures prominently in subsequent Arab history until his assassination in 1951, contacted Lord Kitchener in Cairo and laid the foundation of subsequent British-Arab negotiations.

These negotiations, and others with the French, led the Turks to warn their military governor in Syria, on the outbreak of the war, that "the news from Syria points to general disturbance in the country and great activity on the part of the revolutionary Arabs." This intelligence was confirmed when the papers of the French consulate were seized in Damascus.

What distinguished this surge of resentment against the empire was the fact that the outbreak of a world war provided the opportunity for a revolt sparked by the growth of both Arab and Turkish national consciousness. Yet, it is notable that many Arabs continued to be loyal to the empire and to serve in its armed forces throughout the war.

The outbreak of the war in Europe in August 1914 was not immediately followed by war in the Middle East. It was not until November 5 that Great Britain and France declared war on Turkey. Great Britain then annexed Cyprus and on December 18, after nearly deciding on annexation, proclaimed a protectorate over Egypt. But already in October, before the declaration of war, British troops from India had landed at the little port of Fao, at the Tigris-Euphrates delta in Iraq, to safeguard Persian oil. And in return for assistance from the shaikh of Kuwait, Great Britain recognized his independence under British protection from the Ottoman Empire on November 3.

The British and French governments were profoundly worried at that time about the effect on the large Muslim populations in India and North Africa of the proclamation of a holy war by the sultan-caliph of the Ottoman Empire. Pan-Islam was then credited by Europeans with great popular appeal and the dangers of a massive Muslim revolt, in the midst of the war, were never far from the minds of the British policy planners. On November 14 the sultan-caliph did, in fact, issue a call to holy war but the sharif of Mecca, who should have joined in the appeal, kept his silence. The British now hoped that the sharif could be persuaded to espouse the Allied cause, which would undoubtedly end the threat of a Muslim revolt. This was the basic aim behind the correspondence between the British government on the one hand and on the other the sharif of Mecca, the so-called Husain-McMahon Correspondence, which set the terms upon which some of the Arabs entered the war on the Allied side.

It is important to remember that the First World War was a hard and bitter contest, fought over vast distances by huge armies from many nations, and that the issue was in doubt until almost the very end. The battle plans for Europe had been conceived in great detail years before the war, but the fighting brought a revolution in military tactics. Early in the war the British considered making the Middle East a major front, to attempt to bring the Balkan states into the war on the Allied side. Had this been done, not only Middle Eastern history but also the course of Russian history might have been profoundly changed. In a

sort of compromise, in April 1915, a British invasion force landed
at Gallipoli, but the Turks held firm. Russia remained effectively
cut off from Allied assistance. It seems possible, from what is
now known, that had this force landed on the Syrian coast, a
native uprising might have assisted it to bring the war in the
East to a more speedy close. The Turkish military governor, who
should have known, later wrote that after finding in the French
consular records evidence of Arab plans to revolt he had quickly
shifted the local Arab units in the Turkish army away from
Syria. He was, he said, "certain that to the executions [of Arabs
suspected of nationalist sedition in 1915 and 1916] alone do we
owe the fact that there was no rising in Syria."

In the history of what was rather than what might have been,
Syria did not revolt and the Turkish armies on all fronts fought
determinedly and bravely. In February 1915 a Turkish force
reached the Suez Canal and in the same month pro-Turkish
tribesmen in western Iran cut the oil pipeline from the fields to
the port; the threat thus posed at both ends of the British holdings in the Middle East required the British to garrison large
armed forces in the Middle East throughout the war. In August
1915 the British army in southern Iraq attempted to push northward, to capture Baghdad, and so to relieve the pressure on the
oil fields. Just south of Baghdad, however, they ran into a strong
Turkish force which turned them back with heavy losses and
ran them to ground in the town of Kut in December. There,
after a seige of four months, in which the attempts to relieve the
beseiged garrison cost the British over 7000 casualties, the 13,309
men of the garrison surrendered. It was not until March 1917,
after a bitter struggle in which 40 percent of the 40,000 attacking British and Indian soldiers were casualties, that Baghdad was
taken. On the Egyptian front, likewise, the fighting was hard.
The British would not agree to American suggestions to urge
the Turks to make an honorable peace. It was December 1917
before the British took Jerusalem and October 1918 when they
took Damascus.

Of course, at the beginning of the war the British could not
have known how hard-fought it would be, but prudence alone

would have encouraged them to seek all the local support they could muster. And thus it was that on October 31, 1914, the British government offered Sharif Husain of Mecca a conditional guarantee of independence.

As a result of these factors—probable Turkish might, supposed Muslim restiveness, and actual Russian hunger—the Allies, led by Britain, entered into a series of agreements of a "tactical" nature to contribute to victory. Within two years Britain had made three major (and several lesser) commitments or proclamations of intent. To one of these the Arab allies were to rally as the fount of their rights in the Middle East. To another Zionists pinned their hopes; and on yet a third the French based their claims to realize their traditional desires for a French enclave in the Levant.

First in point of time came the letters exchanged between the Arab Sharif Husain of Mecca, who was then an official in the Ottoman administration, and the British high commissioner of Egypt, Sir Henry McMahon. This is the Husain-McMahon correspondence, which contains the terms upon which the Arabs revolted and entered the war on the Allied side.

In the first letter in the series of eight, dated July 14, 1915, Sharif Husain demanded British recognition of the independence of the "Arab countries" in an area now divided between Syria, Iraq, Jordan, Israel, Saudi Arabia, and a part of Turkey. These demands were countered in a letter from McMahon, dated October 24, 1915, which excluded as not "purely Arab" the districts of Mersin and Alexandretta and portions of Syria lying to the west of the districts of Damascus, Homs, Hama, and Aleppo. The British also reserved their position, established by treaty, with other Arab chiefs and in Basra and Baghdad. Further restrictions were made in the series of letters to protect the interests of France. The last letter was dated January 30, 1916, and the Arab Revolt began on June 5, 1916.

The Husain-McMahon Correspondence has been the object of detailed and searching criticism. The letters were not officially published until 1939, when a special Anglo-Arab committee was set up to evaluate its importance to Palestine. The existence of the exchange was known, however, and the terms had been printed in part in 1919, in the Paris newspaper *Le Temps;* but, in spite of the subsequent urging of Earl Grey, who was Foreign Minister during this period, the British government refused for twenty strife-torn years to publish the full text.

At the close of war a dispute arose over the phrase excluding from the area promised to the Arabs the land to the west of the "districts" (*wilayat;* the Arabic plural) of Aleppo, Hama, Homs, and Damascus. The later British contention was that *wilayat* meant here both "town" in the cases of Aleppo, Hama, and Homs and the Turkish administrative district known as a vilayet in the case of Damascus. If the word means the same in all four instances, then it must mean only town or township, since the towns of Hama and Homs were in the same vilayet and only the sea is to the west of the vilayet of Aleppo. West of the district of Damascus is Mount Lebanon. If by the *wilayah* (the Arabic singular) of Damascus was meant the whole of the vilayet of Syria, then excluded from the Arab area was the whole Levant coast including Palestine. Summing up the British government opinion in 1939, the Lord Chancellor said he had

been impressed by some of the arguments brought forward in regard to the exclusion of Palestine under the phrase "portions of Syria lying to the west of the districts of Damascus, Homs, Hama and Aleppo." He considers that the Arab point of view as regards this aspect of the question has been shown to have greater force than has appeared hitherto, although he does not agree that it is impossible to regard Palestine as covered by the phrase.

The vilayet of Baghdad was, likewise, left until the end of the war for disposition. Distinct from the British pledge were agreements with other Arab chiefs. These included Kuwait, the Idrisi Sayyid of Sabya in Asir and the Amir Ibn Saud of Riyadh, who later founded the Kingdom of Saudi Arabia.

At the same time, in Europe, negotiations were begun with France to clarify postwar aims. These were spelled out in an agreement, known for its drafters as the Sykes-Picot Agreement, in which the parts of the Middle East here under consideration were divided into five parts: (1) the Levant Coast which the French claimed; (2) the Syrian hinterland which the French would assist (the word used is *soutenir*); (3) a zone in Palestine which would be internationalized; (4) British-protected Arab areas of Transjordan and much of Iraq; and (5) British-controlled areas of Baghdad and Basra.

The Arabs had heard of the agreement by way of diplomatic hints before, but it was not until the Bolshevik government published the Russian Foreign Office Archives late in 1917 that the Arabs knew the full extent of the agreements. This information was obligingly passed by the German General Staff to the Turks, who relayed it, with an offer of a separate peace, to Husain. To his credit, Husain turned the message over to his British ally with a request for an explanation. In reply the British informed him that the Sykes-Picot Agreement was merely a series of exchanges of views which in any case no longer represented the situation because of the Russian withdrawal from the war. It was, however, put into effect at the end of the war in Syria.

The second, and much more important, European agreement was the Balfour Declaration of November 2, 1917. During the subsequent thirty years this was to the Zionists what the Husain-McMahon correspondence was to the Arabs: the final rallying point in the struggle for supremacy over British policy on Palestine. The declaration is disarmingly simple and delicately balanced in phraseology; is described as an "expression of sympathy"; and is only sixty-eight words long. Yet, it was the result of months of discussion in the British cabinet and was carefully and deliberately constructed to thread the thinnest rail on the fence of political indecision. Like the pledges to the Arabs, it must be seen in context.

The key figure among the group of advocates of Zionism in England, Chaim Weizmann, supported by the Secretary of the War Cabinet on Middle Eastern Affairs, Mark Sykes, and others, made a concerted effort to convince the government of the value to Britain of a pro-Zionist declaration. Their efforts could not have come at a more favorable moment. In the first place, European Jewry was naturally suspicious of the Entente, for the same reason that the Turks were hostile to it: tsarist Russia was a member. To the Turks, Russia was the aggressor par excellence; and to the Jews, it was the land of the pogrom. Russian oppression had displaced many East European Jews—including Weizmann himself—and sent them into the West, where some had reached positions of influence. Thus, to a considerable extent Great Britain and France labored under the bad reputation of their ally. Germany, on the other hand, then had perhaps the best record in Europe of treatment of the Jews. There Jews found not mere toleration but acceptance. Many Jews had achieved national prominence, and the Jewish community as a whole was more assimilated than in almost any other European country. Germany had not yet had her pogroms or even her Dreyfus case. When World War I broke out, the Zionist Organization declared itself neutral but retained an office in Germany.

The Russian Revolution somewhat reversed the situation in Russia by bringing a number of Jews into key positions. The strong sentiment in Russia for leaving the war was an important element in the Revolution, and both the British Foreign Office and the German General Staff thought that Jews in Russia were leaders of this move. To encourage this feeling and to win over those who wavered, the Germans put pressure on their Turkish ally to grant concessions to Jews wanting to colonize Palestine. Turkey delayed, perhaps fearing to antagonize those Arabs who had remained on her side in the war, but eventually, as her armies were being pushed out of Palestine, granted the Zionists a concession there similar to the Balfour Declaration.

At the time the Germans were making a determined effort to win Jewish support, Britain was worried both about keeping Russia in the war and about American neutrality. In both cases British statesmen came to the conclusion that Jewish support could greatly aid British policy. As early as March 1916 Lord Grey had suggested to the Russian and French governments the utility of a pro-Zionist arrangement on Palestine to "bring over to our side the Jewish forces in America, the East and elsewhere which are now largely, if not preponderately, hostile to us." Mark Sykes was alarmed by the American position and thought pro-German Jews to be the cause. And Prime Minister Lloyd George noted that "their [the Jews'] aid in this respect [financial affairs] would have a special value when the Allies had almost exhausted the gold and marketable securities available for American purchases." Consequently, Lord Robert Cecil encouraged the English Zionists to request a British-Jewish Palestine. It thus would appear likely that the Balfour Declaration is rightly to be regarded as a declaration *through* rather than *to* English Jews, many of whom were opposed to Zionism. The real audiences were in Russia, Germany, and America. To inform them of the Balfour Declaration millions of leaflets were dropped by air, circulated by hand, and printed in the press. In the Middle East, however, the declaration was withheld by military censorship until May 1, 1919, when it was read in Nablus, Palestine, by Allenby's successor.

The Declaration reads as follows:

I [Balfour] have much pleasure in conveying to you [Lord Rothschild] on behalf of His Majesty's Government the following declaration of sympathy with Jewish Zionist aspirations, which has been submitted to and approved by the Cabinet:

"His Majesty's Government view with favour the establishment in Palestine of a National Home for the Jewish People, and will use their best endeavors to facilitate the achievement of this object, it being clearly understood that nothing shall be done which may prejudice the civil and religious rights of existing non-Jewish communities in Palestine, or the rights and political status enjoyed by Jews in any other country."

I should be grateful if you would bring this declaration to the knowledge of the Zionist Federation.

In this form the declaration was approved, before issue, by President Wilson and subsequently was endorsed by the French and Italian governments. It was reaffirmed at the San Remo Conference in 1920, was written into the Mandate instrument for Palestine and so passed by the Council of the League of Nations, was unanimously passed by both Houses of the American Congress, and was approved by the Vatican. In 1922 the British Colonial Office declared it to be the basis of policy in Palestine and as such "not susceptible to change."

It was to prove a most difficult sentence to divide by a comma.

Among the less famous Allied commitments are the following.

1) The proclamation of General Maude (also written by Sir Mark Sykes) upon the capture of Baghdad, in which the British government set out its aim in grand but imprecise phrases, "that the Arab race may rise once more to greatness and renown amongst the peoples of the earth and that it shall bind itself to this end in unity and concord . . . Therefore, I am commanded to invite you, through your Nobles and Elders and Representatives, to participate in the management of your civil affairs in collaboration with the Political Representatives of Great Britain who accompany the British Army so that you may unite with your kinsmen in the North, East, South and West in realizing the aspirations of your race."

2) In January 1918 the British government ordered Commander Hogarth to deliver a message to Sharif (then King) Husain which stated that "The Entente Powers are determined that the Arab race shall be given full opportunity of once again forming a nation in the world. This can only be achieved by the Arabs themselves uniting, and Great Britain and her Allies will pursue a policy with this ultimate unity in view." Continuing, the message embodied some of the language of the Balfour Declaration and urged the Arabs to consider that "the friendship of world Jewry to the Arab cause is equivalent to support in all States where Jews have a political influence. The leaders of the movement are determined to bring about the success of Zionism by friendship and cooperation with the Arabs, and such an offer is not one to be lightly thrown aside."

3) The June 1918 "Declaration to the Seven" was a statement on British policy addressed to seven Syrian Arab leaders then living in Cairo. It affirmed that British policy was to "recognize the complete and sovereign independence of the Arabs" inhabiting areas free before the war and those liberated by Arabs during the war "and support them in their struggle for freedom." In regard to areas liberated by the Allies, the declaration reaffirmed the proclamations issued at Baghdad and Jerusalem by the occupying armies which stated that "It is the wish and desire of His Maj-

esty's Government that the future government of these regions should be based on the principle of the consent of the governed and this policy has and will continue to have the support of His Majesty's Government."

4) Sir Edmund (later Field Marshal Lord) Allenby officially assured Amir Faisal, the Arab leader in Syria, that all military government arrangements were provisional and would not prejudice a final settlement. "I reminded the Amir Faisal that the Allies were in honour bound to endeavour to reach a settlement in accordance with the wishes of the peoples concerned and urged him to place his trust whole-heartedly in their good faith."

5) A joint Anglo-French Declaration of November 7, 1918, affirmed a policy for "the establishment of national governments and administrations deriving their authority from the initiative and free choice of the indigenous populations . . . Far from wishing to impose on the populations of these regions any particular institutions they are only concerned to ensure by their support and by adequate assistance the regular working of Governments and administrations freely chosen by the populations themselves."

These pronouncements were, with official encouragement, given extremely wide distribution in the press and on handbills. It seems highly probable in retrospect that without this official encouragement the population would have settled for far less, but with encouragement their aspirations soared.

It is easy to exaggerate the part played by the Arabs in the war. The glittering romance of Lawrence of Arabia is far more real to most people—both Arab and non-Arab—than is the murky reality of the war. If the Allies had landed at a Levant port instead of Gallipoli, the Arabs of Syria *might* have risen in revolt. But the British did not. As a result the Syrians suffered through the war in hunger and disease but did little to win their freedom.

In the desert the Amir Faisal's Arab army did isolate Yemen, capture most of Arabia, and harass the Turkish supply lines in what is now Saudi Arabia, Jordan, and Syria. By British consent they captured Damascus. (This was in accord with General Allenby's interpretation of the Sykes-Picot and Husain-McMahon agreements.) But probably the most important contribution made by the Arabs was as Muslims in deflecting the threat of a religiously inspired insurrection against the Allies on the part of their huge Muslim colonial populations.

When the war ended, there was a profound contrast between British-occupied Iraq, where the population was hostile and still quite pro-Turkish or at least anti-Western; Syria, where an Arab government had been installed at least nominally by Arab arms; and Palestine and Lebanon, where foreign armies of occupation were greeted as liberators by the inhabitants.

In the East the war came to an end with the Armistice of Mudros on October 30, 1918. Subsequently, however, the British forced the Turks to evacuate Mosul, in north Iraq, which they still held. The armistice was ultimately formalized in the Treaty of Lausanne which was signed on July 24, 1923.

The war in the East had been costly. Typhus, smallpox, and starvation had taken a heavy toll in the areas long under blockade. The British had committed almost 1.5 million men and had spent about £750 million (of which £6 million were used to subsidize the Arab Revolt). The French had relatively little part in the war in the East but had, of course, borne the brunt of the war in Europe and, at the end, demanded that their rights under the Sykes-Picot Agreement be honored on this basis. The British were not eager and the Arabs were strongly opposed, but it was a French naval unit which occupied Beirut and its hinterland.

In Iraq, little of value could be drawn from Ottoman precedent for the empire had vanished, records were packed and taken away, and the administrative personnel was gone forever. Necessity was the mother of the new government. The job of supporting an army makes harsh and immediate demands. Shortage of shipping space made it imperative to grow produce, especially cereals, locally. India, then facing another famine, could feed its army in Iraq only with the greatest difficulty, and every ton of shipping space that could be saved was vital. So the occupation force was immediately faced with nonmilitary demands in a situation in which it had the assistance of neither local personnel nor guides. If necessity was the mother, India was the father. Since the British forces came from India, it was not only natural but inevitable that British India would become the exemplar of Iraq. Large numbers of Indian laborers and clerks from the civil service and soldiers from the army were brought into Iraq. Moreover, the officers of the army and civil service were either directly trained in the Indian service or inspired by men who were. Many of these made distinguished careers for themselves and played a key role in the events over the next two generations.

In Egypt the war had brought prosperity and, at last, independence from the Ottoman Empire in name as well as in fact. Egypt became the farm for vast armies in Europe and the Middle East, and the peasants grew rich. But the political life of the country was stifled by a powerful and determined military government which, with a war to be won, could not be bothered with immature nationalism. What had been intended to be a request for volunteer help ended as confiscation and enforced labor. Thus, the Egyptians came out of the war, as did many new nations, embittered and determined to achieve independence.

So it was that a former protégé of Lord Cromer, Saad Zaghlul, approached the British Residency, the seat of power, on November 13, 1918, at the head of a delegation (Arabic: *wafd*) to demand the right to petition for freedom in London and Paris. When he was refused, Zaghlul organized committees throughout Egypt, circulating petitions calling for an end to British rule. These committees grew into the Wafd party. This was in violation of martial law, and the British authorities, who always held a low opinion of Egyptian will and daring, warned Zaghlul to stop his activities. When he refused, he was deported to Malta on April 7, 1919.

Few then realized the strength of the nationalist movement or the bitterness which years of wartime suppression and social contempt had engendered in the Egyptians. On the day after Zaghlul's arrest Egyptian students, in the first of their forays into the streets of violence, began what was to become a full-scale national rebellion.

In Syria the war had ended on strident notes of national liberation but muted voices of national organization. Everyone was restive with new aspirations, but among the Arabs there were few with the sophistication to move to the grand stage of Europe where the future was being decided.

Amir Faisal, who had led the Arab Revolt, was then thirty-five years old but quite inexperienced in international politics. He knew his limitations but thought he had some hope, as he put it himself, with Zionist money, connections, and *savoir-faire*. It was immediately evident that the Zionists had these. The Zionist Organization had secured the appointment of a pro-Zionist as the chief political officer in the Arab area, had the support of Lord Balfour and other senior British officials, and had a powerful American delegation, close to President Wilson, led by Justice Louis Brandeis. During Faisal's visit the British officer closest to him, Colonel Cornwallis, reported, "I understand that Dr. Weizmann, in return for the Emir's help in Palestine towards realization of Zionist aspirations, proposes to give money and advisers, if required, to the Arab Government and claims that the Zionists can persuade the French Government to waive their claims of influence in the interior." At a dinner given by Lord Rothschild, Faisal himself was reported to have said,

> Dr. Weizmann's ideals are ours, and we will expect you, without our asking to help us in return. No state can be built up in the Near East without the goodwill of the Great Powers, but it requires more than that. It requires the borrowing from Europe of ideals and materials and knowledge and experience. To make these fit for us, we must translate them from European shape to Arab shape—and what intermediary could we find in the world more suitable than you? For you have all the knowledge of Europe and are cousins by blood.

It is clear that at this period Faisal was far more worried about French intervention in the Levant than he was about any possible future clash with Zionism. France had laid claim to most of the Levant coast. Faisal realized before he left the Middle East, that even if the French chose not to push into the interior their geographical position would give them a strangle hold on the Arab state. The British Foreign Office seemed to want to set aside the Sykes-Picot Agreement, on which France's claims rested, but seemed equally firm on insisting that the Balfour Declaration must stand. Faisal realized, as few Arabs have since, that in these circumstances politics is indeed the science of the possible. So he came to a provisional agreement with Dr. Weizmann. The agreement was written up as a formal document in eleven articles. In brief, the two recognized the need to work together to achieve mutual aims, to give effect to the Balfour Declaration, to facilitate Jewish immigration provided the rights of the Arab peasant and tenant farmers be protected, to ensure freedom of worship and protection of the Holy Places, to provide Jewish economic help to the Arabs, and to constitute the British government as their arbiter. To this agreement Faisal appended in Arabic, above his signature, the following condition: "Provided the Arabs obtained their independence as demanded in my Memorandum dated the 4th of January, 1919, to the Foreign Office of the Government of Great Britain, I shall concur in the above article. But if the slightest modification or departure were to be made I shall not then be bound by a single word of the present Agreement which shall be deemed void and of no account or validity, and I shall not be answerable in any way whatsoever."

Faisal realized that the local population of Palestine strongly opposed the creation of a Jewish state, but he thought he could act on his own, compromising as necessary in order to save his state from the French. Like other figures at the Peace Conference, Faisal lost touch with the mood of his countrymen. In Palestine itself, the visit of the first Zionist commission had roused the strongest antagonism and fears in the population. The British political officer in Jerusalem warned in August 1919 that "if we mean to carry out any sort of Zionist policy we must do so with military force."

Faisal was not alone in being confused as to the desires of the population. The Middle East was far away from Western Europe and America, unknown save as the Bible Land to all but a few, and even that small band violently disagreed. The American and British delegations were in favor of an international commission to ascertain the wishes of the natives, in the spirit of the various wartime statements on self-determination issued in the names of all the Allied governments. The French were opposed to a commission unless it were understood, as the senior French representative in the Levant put it, that its purpose was "to keep Faisal in the dark while partition of Syria is being arranged." British forces then held the north of Iraq and Palestine, large parts of which areas had been promised to the French under the wartime Sykes-Picot Agreement. At the Paris Peace Conference, France demanded that the commitment be honored, but the British, aware of the need to control the north of Iraq to make the Iraqi state viable and of the need for more territory than the area around the port of Acre-Haifa to honor the Balfour Declaration, refused to go by the letter of the Sykes-Picot Agreement. After a serious diplomatic crisis between the two countries, the issue was resolved in September 1919 by Prime Minister Lloyd George and Premier Clemenceau. It was agreed that Mosul should be given to Iraq, Palestine should come under British control, the British should withdraw from Syria, which would come under French control, and France should share in the exploitation of Middle Eastern oil.

French accusations that the British were trying to make it impossible for the French to enter Syria embarrassed the British and caused them to give up urging the appointment of an investigating commission. But President Wilson unilaterally appointed his own, the King-Crane Commission. It visited the Middle East in the summer of 1919 but its report was probably never read by President Wilson and was not published for nearly four years. The report was, however, reproduced in British diplomatic reports. Essentially, the King-Crane Commission found that the population of Syria was strongly opposed to a French mandate, wanted, above all, independence and unity, but would settle for an American or British mandate. Its methods of gathering impressions have often been criticized (mainly by those who were unhappy at the results) but its findings are borne out by the investigations of all the experienced British political officers then resident in the Middle East.

Meanwhile, Faisal's popularity was slipping badly in Syria. He had made no progress in keeping out the French, who were gathering forces on the Levant coast, and he had been reported

to have virtually given away Palestine to the Zionists. His understanding with the Zionists was in the words of the political officer
in Jerusalem, "a noose about Faisal's neck . . . he is in favour
with [the Arabs only] so long as he embodies Arab nationalism
and represents their views." Indeed, the Arab congress at Damascus did repudiate the substance of his agreement with Weizmann.

When he returned to London in September, Faisal informed
the Zionists that he could agree only to limited immigration and
that he had intended that the Jewish homeland be thought of as
a province of the larger Arab state. "I quite understand," he said,
"the desire of Jews to acquire a country, a homeland. But so far
as Palestine is concerned . . . it must be subject to the right and
aspirations of the sentiments of the present possessors of the
land." Jewish rights he brushed aside as the sort which would
give the Arabs a right to take over Spain, which they had ruled
for as long as the Jews had Palestine.

Another trip to Europe was equally fruitless. The French were
determined to extract their pound of Syrian flesh and the British
bluntly informed Faisal that he must go to Paris and make his
terms. As Lord Balfour later told the chief political officer, "We
had not been honest with either French or Arab, but it was now
preferable to quarrel with the Arab rather than the French, if
there was to be a quarrel at all." British troops gradually pulled
out of Syria and Lebanon, turning over their positions to the
French on the coast and to the Arabs in the interior; the British
monthly subsidy of £150,000 (upon which Faisal's state depended) was cut in half with the understanding that the French
would then begin to contribute £75,000. Faisal, meanwhile, was
not allowed to build up his army or police force and received no
new equipment; his own position was by then so compromised
that in the north of Syria a strong movement was begun to re-
create the Ottoman Empire and the army passed into the control
of Arab officers whose sympathies and service had been on the
Ottoman side during the war.

At the eleventh hour Faisal recognized that there was no future
in his course of moderation. Since he could expect nothing but
sympathy from the British and obviously nothing from the

Americans who, due to the illness of President Wilson, had virtually dropped out of the Peace Conference, Faisal threw himself into the ranks of the nationalists. He completely repudiated his understanding with the Zionists—which had always been conditional upon the granting of Syrian independence — and in March 1920 had himself proclaimed King of Syria and Palestine by the Arab congress at Damascus; he was not recognized as such either by the French or the British. The San Remo Conference in April awarded a mandate over Syria to France. The French army at this time had concentrated some 90,000 troops on the coast. A minor incident in July led to a French ultimatum that the mandate be accepted, the outbreak of hostilities, an invasion of Syria by the French, and the overthrow of the Arab government. The seeds were sown for a harvest of hatred of the French which was to be reaped yearly for a quarter of a century.

PART FOUR DEVELOPMENT OF THE ARAB STATES

IX. The Mandates: Iraq, Syria, Lebanon, and Transjordan

Neither in Lebanon, which benefited from French protection and favor, nor in Transjordan, where the population was primarily nomadic, was there, at least initially, much opposition to the mandates. Both in Iraq and Syria the mandate period began badly. In both, significant portions of the population regarded the mandates, as did many European statesmen, as "a substitute for old imperialism."

In Syria the tone of the whole mandate period was set in the initial contacts between the French and the Arabs. As we have seen, Sharif Faisal, as head of a state, had participated in some phases of the Paris Peace Conference, had negotiated with the British and French governments, had accepted the title of king from the General Syrian Congress on March 7, 1920, and was in control of the government in Damascus. The French, at the same time, were in control in Lebanon and had gradually built up strong military forces there. After their long, frustrating, and bitter contest with the British at the Paris Peace Conference, at Sèvres, and at San Remo over the division of spoils in the middle East, the French were not prepared to be stopped by a motley crowd of semi-savages, as they regarded the Arabs, and on July 14, 1920, issued an ultimatum to Faisal. Among the demands listed were reduction of the Syrian army, acceptance of the French mandate, punishment of those who had opposed France, acceptance of the French-controlled currency, permission to station French garrisons in most Syrian cities and important towns, and prior acceptance of other, then undisclosed, demands which the French might make later. Three days were allowed for compliance.

Recognizing his inability to resist, Faisal tried to temporize but finally on July 20 agreed to submit. At this point Arab mobs attacked the government and demanded that it fight for national independence. Whether for this reason or others, the telegram of capitulation from the Syrian government to the French high commissioner General Gouraud took seven hours to reach Lebanon. When it arrived the French troops had already marched. To the Arab negotiator who tried to get the invasion stopped, the French set forth a new schedule of demands. Clearly, the French were intent upon a definitive assumption of power, unhampered by any conditions or restraints. On July 24, after a skirmish at Maisalun, the French moved toward Damascus whose occupation they completed on July 25. Faisal tried to compromise, even at that point, but was rebuffed and on July 29 went into exile in the British zone of what is now Jordan.

Meeting much hostility in the interior of Syria, primarily from the Muslim Syrians, the French acted to create for themselves a more pro-French and more powerful Lebanon. On August 31 General Gouraud issued a proclamation which recast the frontiers of "Greater Lebanon" so that it became about four times as large as the Lebanon which had existed prior to World War I. Though this move made some of the Lebanese more pro-French, it accentuated the divisions both between the religious groups in Lebanon and between Christian Lebanon and Muslim Syria, divisions which underlay the 1958 Lebanese civil war and which even today are the source of bitterness. In the short run the French policy appeared successful, but, ironically, the inclusion of large areas wherein the population was predominantly Muslim has made Lebanon less secure as a Christian state.

The rest of Syria was dismembered also. The coastal area north of Lebanon, centering on the port of Latakia, was split off and put under a separate administration and even, in 1922, temporarily made a separate state. Alexandretta, on October 20, 1921, was separated and put under a special administration which eventually resulted in its incorporation in Turkey. Jabal ad-Druze, south of Damascus, was made autonomous under the mandate. Finally, Aleppo and Damascus were separated with each as capital of an autonomous area. From an administrative point of view these were such expensive attempts to divide and control local opposition that within a year the French rejoined three of the areas in a federation.

Throughout the French mandate period, although one administrative division after another was tried, the threat of violence was never far behind the outward face of events. Damascus, invaded in 1920, was bombarded in 1925, 1926, and 1945, and martial law was enforced periodically until the very end of the mandate. Constitutions were tried and suspended and independence was proclaimed or promised time after time until finally gained in 1945. Divisions between religious groups and districts were certainly not created by French policy, but were as certainly magnified by it. It would, perhaps, be fair to categorize the mandate period as less a school in government than one in administration wherein tendencies toward unrest, rather than being corrected by political means, were temporarily restrained but ultimately increased in violence.

In Iraq the situation was quite different. As we have seen, between November 22, 1914, and October 30, 1918, the British were in the process of capturing Iraq from the Turks. During this period they were forced to lay the base for what became the state they helped to create. Efficient military government was necessary to the conduct of war: lack of sufficient shipping space required the maximum amount of local production, especially of cereals, and the maintenance of forces required the construction and management of such facilities as ports and railroads. Above all, public security had to be established and maintained. Half a government was clearly impossible. Moreover, the British, unlike the French in their subsequent efforts in Syria, had a workable model in the Indian empire. Cadres of men familiar with problems of public security on the Northwest Frontier and in the Persian

Gulf were imported into Iraq to handle analogous problems. In the caliber of these men is one of the most striking contrasts to the French in Syria. Included in the British forces were many of the Englishmen who, for a generation, dominated Western writings on the Arabs and who became legends in their own rights. But having said this, one must also say that their overt paternal system could not and did not work.

Sir Arnold Wilson was the very personification of the government of Iraq. Highly intelligent, well educated—his two-volume memories of his difficult years in Iraq is a model of its kind—strongly principled, inspiring, and personally liberal, he was an authority on the Persian Gulf area. Under his control the government was honest, efficient, and paternal. His aim was order and economy. He tended to divide the country into three groups: the bedouin and the Kurds, who composed the first, were the noble savages; the second, the peasantry, were pitiful and in desperate need of succor; but the third, the urban literati—the "town Arabs"—were deceitful, dangerous, pompous, inept, and best kept out of all affairs. If let into government, the town Arabs would only strip the bedouin of his nobility and would complete the ruin of the peasant. Neither the peasant nor the bedouin could rule; so the British must. Any other view was simply naïve and irresponsible.

Naïve and dangerous was Sir Arnold's description of the "romantic" policies which had flowed from President Wilson's declarations on self-determination and from the British promises to the Arabs. Without these Britain and France could rationally have carved out spheres of interest, and Britain's share would have been of great value to its empire in India. Wilson's bête noire was Colonel T. E. Lawrence, a flamboyant newcomer to the area who had captured the public imagination and the ear of senior British officials in London. But it was not Lawrence so much as a tired and nearly bankrupt England on which the plan for a greater Indian empire went aground.

Lacking the force to garrison the whole of Iraq while they also fought the determined and brave Turks, the British tried to create order in the countryside by "promoting" the shaikhs of clans or sections of tribes, the largest *effective* units of tribal life, to paramount status, making them responsible to the government for public order. To keep an eye on the shaikhs and their tribesmen, political officers with small detachments of locally levied police forces were stationed throughout the country. Since communications were often unreliable and always slow, the political officer relied largely upon his personal daring and bluff to maintain his authority.

Announcement in Iraq, at the end of the war, that Britain intended to assume the mandate for Iraq led to widespread popular discontent. Pro-Ottoman sentiment was not dead, and the Syrian government had dispatched a small group of nationalists who, calling themselves the Northern Iraq Army, had tried to capture Mosul in May 1920. Agitation against the government, particularly because of its measures of taxation and its friends among the new tribal paramount chiefs, increased during the summer. Finally, on June 30, a minor incident set off the great tribal rising which spread all over southern Iraq. As railroads were cut and trains derailed, the scattered and partly immobile British force was unable to act promptly to relieve the outlying detachments. For a while, indeed, only the area immediately surrounding Baghdad was secure. Not until mid-October, after the loss of 1654 British men, the expenditure of £40 million—or more than six times the total given to the Arab Revolt in the First World War —and the infuriation of the war-weary and impoverished English government, was order restored.

In a letter to the London Sunday *Times* in August 1920, T. E. Lawrence stung Wilson's imperial policies where the hurt was worst, the purse: "Our government is worse than the old Turkish system. They kept fourteen thousand local conscripts embodied, and killed a yearly average of two hundred Arabs in maintaining peace. We keep ninety thousand men, with aeroplanes, armoured cars, gunboats and armoured trains. We killed about ten thousand Arabs in this rising this summer. We cannot hope to maintain such an average: it is a poor country, sparsely peopled. But Abd el Hamid would applaud his masters, if he saw us working . . . How long will we permit millions of pounds, thousands of imperial troops, and tens of thousands of Arabs to be sacrificed on behalf of a form of colonial administration which can benefit nobody but its administrators?"

It was the power of the purse that moved Iraq toward freedom. To the great credit of the British, they recognized, after a severe shock of tribal war, that they could not afford to govern Iraq directly as a colony, and they found a less overt system, with English advisers behind an Arab façade, which was more economical. In recognition of this fact, Sir Arnold Wilson was withdrawn from Iraq.

On October 21, 1920, the newly arrived civil commissioner, Sir Percy Cox, announced the formation of a provisional government under Arab ministers with British advisers. Meanwhile, the British sought a head of state. As provisional president of the Council of Ministers, they chose an old and venerated religious leader under the umbrella of whose prestige they set about organizing a government and administration. As the tribes submitted they were amnestied. At this time about 250 of Amir Faisal's supporters, many of whom had served in the Turkish forces, but who were born in the area which had become Iraq, petitioned to return. Wisely, the British decided to make them into an asset. In the first group, which returned early the following year, was Nuri Said, who was to serve as prime minister many times until his death in 1958.

At Cairo, in March 1921, Winston Churchill met with senior British advisers and worked out, essentially, the administrative arrangements that were to endure for the next forty years. Recognizing the need to cut expenditures and the fact that the mandate was unpopular in Iraq, Churchill decided to negotiate a treaty with Iraq, parallel to that between Britain and Egypt, which would, bilaterally and in name at least, end the mandate (although in the eyes of the League Iraq remained a mandate) and give Iraq that degree of nominal independence which would lessen the danger of hostilities or civil war. Recognizing also that Britain's position in Iraq would, in large part, depend upon the selection of a ruler, Churchill decided to move vigorously for the selection of Sharif Faisal, so lately king of Syria. To this end, a program was worked out to ensure his election in the forthcoming referendum. "Popular" support was mobilized and Faisal's only serious opponent was arrested and deported on vague charges of sedition. Faisal arrived in Iraq in June 1921, met with a disappointingly cool reception, but was declared king on July 11, 1921.

Thus the British imported into Iraq, to make possible their indirect rule, the very man whom the French had at the cost of an invasion expelled to make possible their direct rule. Herein lay an essential contrast in methods. Throughout their period in the Arab East, the British sought the cheap ways of rule, making virtues of necessities and assets of rivals, while the French plunged on, often into unnecessary and costly clashes with nationalism. Whereas the French never consolidated their position, the British success is striking: reductions in British personnel in the Iraq government reached such proportions that by 1927 they controlled the country with only a handful of civil servants and small detachments of the Royal Air Force.

Like Lebanon, Transjordan was created as a separate unit without serious opposition by the local population. Transjordan was the product of Churchill's Cairo Conference. Its territory had been originally a part of the mandate of Palestine, as approved by the League of Nations, but was always administered under a separate regime and on May 26, 1923, was formally separated. Since April 1, 1921, it had been controlled by the Amir Abdullah, brother of King Faisal, who agreed to give up his plan to attack the French in Syria, to avenge his brother, if he were given control over Transjordan. The British, whose relations with France were still strained, agreed. They also had another reason. The British declared that Transjordan as constituted, was not subject to the Balfour Declaration and that Jews were forbidden to buy land there; thus the British could feel that in Transjordan they had honored their wartime promises to the Sharif Husain.

It is not important for our present purposes to follow in detail most of the developments of the mandates in the four countries. Major trends in the control of the hinterland, in the development of national markets, in the development of organizational cadres of the new states, and in the rise of education are, however, of such a formative influence on the area and the people of today as to require close attention.

Possibly the most significant aspect of the mandate period in Jordan, Iraq, and Syria was the spread of urban control over rural and desert areas. From time to time, under powerful and able governors, public security had been secured, but normally, as one left the Mediterranean coast it steadily declined. As we have seen, the nomadic tribes were autonomous "nation-states" which lived beyond the reach of urban government. As long as they were mobile, the tribes constituted a danger to public security; only when they had invested in immovable objects, particularly land, could they be brought to heel.

The great tribal rebellion of 1920 was the rock on which the British dream of empire had broken: it simply was far too costly to retain Iraq as the imperialists within the British government wanted. To cope with the tribes, the British relied upon two methods. On the one hand, they made clear that they had the power and the will to enforce public security in those areas of importance to them; and on the other, they appointed responsible chiefs to whom they gave incentives to control the tribes. Since all of the other clan chiefs would conspire against the government-appointed paramount chief, the British high commissioner, in a report to the League of Nations, reckoned that "as the authority of the central government increases, the problem [of security] should be logically solved by the gradual dissolution of the tribal bond." The first job, however, was to cope with the tribes militarily.

The British at the end of the First World War, like Egyptians in Lebanon in 1832, profited from a revolution in arms technology. Between 1840 and 1918 the Turks lacked a clear superiority in arms. The rifles they used were about the same as those used by the tribes. Their position was not dissimilar from that of the American army when the American Indians began acquiring repeating rifles. The First World War introduced several new sorts of weapons. The first was the armored riverboat which enabled the British to bombard fortified towns in the Tigris-Euphrates delta. The stunned Arabs whose mud forts crumbled had to surrender, lamenting that, in the words of one old warrior, "but this is not war." A second weapon and perhaps the most striking of all was the airplane. The rapid development of the airplane came just at the end of the war in Europe and air power got its first major test in the Middle East.

To control the vast expanses of steppe and desert, both the British and the French came speedily to rely on air power. For example, in 1924 occurred the last of the great tribal raids out of Arabia. In this raid, which was not unlike the original Arab invasion after the rise of Islam, some 26,000 sheep were seized and taken from southern Iraq and Syria to Arabia. The devastating effects on the tribes within Iraq and Syria, which had been more or less brought under government control by that time, was immediately recognized by officials. The Royal Air Force in Iraq was then called upon to police the vast frontier land of the great Syrian desert. Thereafter, the RAF patrolled the frontiers so that a bedouin tribe would be spotted as it got anywhere near the frontier area. If an "invader" were seen, the plane would radio to alert ground troops who rushed to the area in "armed Fords." The armed Ford was simply a truck with a machine gun mounted on the top, but between it and the camel was a gulf as wide as that between a Jenny and a jet. This combination of air power and mobile ground units gave the government the ability to reach out into the desert as no government ever had in the past.

In a report from the high commissioner of Iraq in 1923 the effect of this new power is vividly described: "a main factor in the pacification of the country has been the Royal Air Force. By prompt demonstrations on the first sign of trouble carried out over any area affected, however distant, tribal insubordination has been calmed before it could grow dangerous . . . In earlier times punitive columns would have to struggle towards their objectives across deserts or through difficult defiles, compelled by the necessities of their preparations and marching to give time for their opponents to gain strength. But now, almost before the would-be rebel has formulated his plans, the droning of the aeroplanes is heard overhead, and in the majority of cases their mere appearance is enough. By its means (air power), it has been possible to achieve a highly centralized yet widely understanding intelligence which is the essence of wise and economical control."

The building of roads and the rapid rise of public transport made it unnecessary for notables to retain expensive bands of retainers. The local political officer in Kurdistan remarked in a report to the League in 1928 that in the town of Sulaimaniya one could see a good example of the pacifying influence of the motorcar. "Formerly, a tribal chief from the vicinity of the Persian border having business at administrative headquarters would make the two days' journey accompanied by a large escort of armed horsemen. Following the construction of a pioneer motor road, with police posts, from Sulaimaniya to [one of the administrative posts], a regular taxi service has sprung up. The tribal chief, finding that he can take a seat for three rupees and perform the journey without fatigue in two hours, ceases to entertain large bodies of expensive armed retainers. The practice of carrying arms thus tends to grow less." Thus, not only was it possible for the central government to move more rapidly and dramatically against rebellious people, but the people gave up a part of their means of rebelling.

The opening of roads tended to bring about the creation of national markets. This trend had been stimulated by the wartime conditions. Since shipping was everywhere at a premium and supply of large numbers of troops was difficult, the military administrations tried to organize sufficient production to meet local needs. The demands of war forced the administration to create a cash crop economy to replace the honeycomb cells of largely autarkic groups of villages and to encourage production of cereals needed by the army. This was a trend which the settlement of tribes, the building of roads, and the creation of an export market in the following decade was greatly to extend.

Moreover, British troops brought with them the desire for, and small supplies of, the accouterments of Western civilization: kerosine lamps, flashlights, pocket knives, cheap cotton cloth, automobiles, and trucks. These became objects of intense desire for the wealthier civilians not only for their utility but, no doubt, as status sumbols of a civilization that was so obviously powerful and successful. The British army was not, however, able or willing to supply such things to the local inhabitants. So it was natural that a new commercial class should spring up on the foundation of large-scale purchases by the army and casual spending by troopers which had pumped money into the economy. New styles were introduced as influenced by the army: sandals to headdress, the Iraqi shed his Arab dress for Western. His Syrian cousin was not far behind.

As roads were built across the desert from Damascus to Baghdad along the Euphrates route and connecting the various Iraqi cities, the areas which had been largely autarkic, which had supported themselves and had a considerable degree of economic autonomy, came to sell their goods one to the other and to buy from central points those things which they could not produce as economically. The Kurds in the northern area of Iraq, for example, who had prior to this time bought very little from the outside world, began to buy cotton goods from England or India, chinaware from Japan, cigarettes from Baghdad. As they acquired new tastes, locally produced goods were no longer satisfying to them, and they were anxious to move in and out of the places like Baghdad and to acquire the accouterments of European life. Markets grew in strategic locations throughout the country and more and more people were drawn into the system which the state itself represented. Thus, more and more people came to have a stake in supporting the political existence of the state. It is interesting that Basra and Beirut, where this commerce developed earlier and most rapidly, saw almost none of the armed unrest that some of the northern areas of Iraq and Syria witnessed.

As the city governments extended their control over the countryside, townsmen extended the limits of their cultivation far beyond what had been considered relatively safe in Ottoman times. Of course, this meant that townsmen took over many of the watering places and extensively used farming lands of the semi-nomadic and nomadic tribes. Particularly in Iraq, something comparable to the "enclosures" of eighteenth century England or the changes brought about on the American range by the advent of cheap barb wire happened during the first decade of the mandate.

In all of the mandates, but particularly in Iraq, the development of the economy was dependent upon security in the rural areas. Not only physical security, of the sort that could be supplied by military means, but also security of investment was essential to get money out of strong boxes and into the land.

As early as the enactment of the new land code in 1858 the Ottoman government had recognized the utility of the security of tenure. In 1869, during his short stay in Iraq, Midhat Pasha, the greatest of the Ottoman governors of the nineteenth century, tried to bring order into the system of land tenure. Similar efforts were made in Lebanon in the decade of the 1850's and in Palestine somewhat later. The details of the Ottoman system are complex, but the general purpose was twofold: to give sufficient title to those who would invest in the land and hire others to farm it, and to give the nomadic tribes lands on which to settle.

Before this time the Ottoman governments had concentrated their efforts in the towns and left the countryside to itself until the harvest, when tax collectors, accompanied by military escorts, collected what they could from the unwilling peasants. The effective law of the countryside, except when taxes were collected, was local custom. Peasants cared little what the records in the distant cities might say; they knew who owned the land. Even when encouraged to register their lands, they feared to do so since they suspected that land registration might be a government ruse to raise their taxes or to conscript their sons into the army.

Profiting from this disaffection from government of the peasant and the tribesman, the larger merchants and officials obtained formal rights to vast tracts of tribal and village lands. Later, when the Iraqi land system was studied by Sir Ernest Dowson, he found that "with the introduction of tapu tenure many village areas appear to have been wholly or partially registered as the personal possessions of local notables, without any consideration of the immemorial rights of those who had regularly occupied and tilled the land or pastured the flocks thereon. The pinch in these cases seems to have been mainly felt when the lands were pledged, and forfeited, to town-dwelling merchants for debt."*

As to tribal lands themselves, the Turks regarded them as government-owned, merely being used by the tribes with no rights of ownership. Taking up the Turkish definitions of ownership and the Turkish records, the Iraqi courts according to the high commissoner's report to the League for 1925, reached the momentous decision that "all lands excluding urban mulk (freehold) properties belong primarily to the State and that good title to such lands can only be obtained in consequence of alienation by Government . . . acquisition of title to lands by long and undisturbed possession, is a legal impossibility in Iraq." This one blow placed the tribes on the danger list. Their lands could be encroached upon at will by city dwellers who could arrange with the government to buy or lease land. The tribesmen involved were forced to emigrate or to settle. Whereas in Turkish times they had been able to keep their lands by making it impossible for others to take possession, in 1925, under the droning of the airplane, they were powerless.

During the period 1920 to 1932 great tracts of land along the rivers which had in the past been lightly used by semi-nomadic and nomadic tribes as grazing, water, and winter-wheat areas became regularly cultivated private property. In 1921 along the Iraqi rivers were 140 water pumps, irrigating a total of 72 square miles; by 1929 the number of pumps had risen to over 2000 and the area irrigated to over 2670 square miles. In the three years from 1927 to 1930 some 1057 new pumps were installed with a substantial increase in the size of the area cultivated. The pumps were mostly owned by city men who expected to get from the government rights to the land. And, in fact, according to the land sales of the period, they did. In the year 1927, for example, the government sold 7917 pieces of government land and 448 pieces of mortgaged land. As the report to the League of that year described the development, a gradual transition to an enclosure of arable land was being promoted. "The prospective pump-

---

* Sir Ernest Dowson, *An Inquiry into Land Tenure and Related Questions* (printed for the Iraqi government by the Garden City Press, Ltd., Letchworth, Eng., [1932]), p. 20.

owner is usually an enterprising capitalist townsman, lacking land and anxious to develop a portion of the Domains already subject to tribal occupation."

The policy of the government was to grant a limited term tenure to the shaikh as the representative of the tribe, but in practice title to the land often passed to the shaikh, so that what had been in fact tribal land became in law his land. This, and the large investment necessary for irrigation, tended to produce a heavy concentration of land. Ultimately nearly 70 percent of the arable land of Iraq was held in blocks of over 250 acres. In southern Iraq the concentration was even more impressive. In one province 75 percent of the land was in units in excess of 2500 acres and only 6 percent in units less than 125 acres.

Shortly after achieving independence in 1933 the new national government passed a law which virtually converted the formerly free tribesmen into serfs. The key to the relationship between the owner and the tenant in the new land was debt. So widely was it defined that it is almost inconceivable that any peasant could ever be out of debt. The peasant incurred a debt for any work done by the owner, any seed advanced, any work *not* done by the peasant. If the peasant tried to leave the land, the owner was entitled to call out the armed forces of the government to have him brought back. Then he was blacklisted so that he could get no other job.

The shaikh who in the time of the peasant's father or grandfather had been the honored elder, the generous host who dared not inflict the most trifling punishment on the poorest man in the tribe, had become an absolute master, perhaps a member of Parliament, who lived far away in the city and who had all of the power of the government behind his word. This was nothing less than a social revolution, one whose legacy was to have profound —and violent—influence in the midst of the Iraqi revolution of 1958–59 and, perhaps, will again. At the least, it has been largely responsible for the creation of those vast concentric rings of slums which lean on Arab cities.

In all four mandates the governments were pressed to organize relatively cheap means of control. In general they sought to recruit local people to work for the government so that the more expensive Europeans would be required only for senior positions. This was particularly evident in the area of public security. Britain, as we have seen, was strongly opposed to the continued outlay of large amounts of money on public security and demanded a cut in the size of the British garrison in Iraq. Transjordan never had more than a handful of British officers and no sizable force.

The French, to the contrary, throughout their tenure in Syria and Lebanon were compelled to retain very large military establishments. In 1921 the French had over 50,000 troops in Syria and shortly after the two-year rebellion of 1925–27 sent in even more. Additionally, from 1921 the French began recruiting Syrian and Lebanese auxiliaries and by 1925 had over 7000 of these under arms. Ten years later, at the high point, these *troupes spéciales* totaled 14,000. Until the bitter end of French rule in Syria in 1945, when they formed the basis of the incipient Lebanese and Syrian armies, the French were to retain control of these troops. To patrol the steppe and desert, they also formed in 1921 camel companies under French officers. But French efforts were always expensive since they could not entrust any significant role to the Arabs of Syria.

The British position was quite different. After the 1920 Iraqi revolt, the more settled areas of Iraq were relatively peaceful. Only in Kurdistan and in the desert areas was public security seriously threatened. Security in these areas, after the inauguration of the government of King Faisal, was the concern of the government of Iraq, with which the British had treaty relations (although under the terms of League they formally exercised a mandate). This government had primary responsibility and was assisted to create and sustain its own military force under British guidance.

In 1926 the mandate government organized an "armed Ford police unit" to control the great bedouin tribe of the Shammar, and in 1928 a similar group was created in the south of Iraq. So successful was it that it became the model for changes in all the frontier guard forces organized in the area. In Transjordan the former commander of the Egyptian camel corps had formed a desert patrol in 1920 to fend off tribal raids from across the border and to bring a degree of security to the desert. The force, however, was not entirely successful as it could not gain the cooperation of the bedouin and had to meet raiders on their own ground with their own weapons. It was the scheme of enlisting bedouin into a special highly mobile desert force that made John B. Glubb (Glubb Pasha) famous and brought order and security never before imagined into the desert.

In Iraq the British had formed units of Assyrian and Kurdish levies to assist in the garrisoning of the country during the war. These forces proved loyal to the British during the 1920 revolt and by 1925 reached a strength of 7500. Since they were under British officers, paid by the British, and drawn from the non-Arab minorities, it was decided that they could not be a proper nucleus for an Iraqi army. However, throughout the mandate period they matched or overshadowed the young Iraq army. The Iraqi army, itself, was formed in 1921 under the command of former officers of the Ottoman army of whom the chief was Nuri Said, later to be prime minister. A military college was also opened. By 1925 this force had reached 7500 (just matched by the levies 7500) and was able to replace departing British ground units.

The young Iraqi army was impelled into politics sooner than any of the other forces of the mandates since it had early "tasted blood" in the Kurdish revolt and then in 1933 had attacked and massacred large numbers of Assyrians whom the British had used as the base of their power in Iraq. In the 1930's, as later, the Iraqi army was always close to or involved in political power. Seven times between 1936 and 1941, it made or supported coups d'etat. The reason is not difficult to find. The army was by all odds the most efficient organization in the country. Its dedication and discipline contrasted as sharply with the often self-seeking politicians and their merchant allies as did its ability to communicate and move with the rest of the population. Moreover, it was used and permitted itself to be used by the government as "a valuable means of fostering a true National Spirit." From this position in the mid-twenties was no great step to the military coups of the mid-thirties.

One can argue that what happened in Iraq in the mid-1930's occurred twenty years later in Syria, delayed by the nature of the French-controlled military structure there. In the late 1950's the Syrian army began to intervene decisively in politics. This is a phenomenon which came to distinguish virtually all of the Arab countries by 1960.

With the exception of Syria, which had existed as an independent kingdom, though with uncertain frontiers and a rudimentary administration for two years until the French invasion, and to a lesser extent Lebanon, whose nucleus of Mount Lebanon had enjoyed autonomy for several centuries, the new mandate states did not exist even in the minds of the leaders of Arab nationalism in 1920. Tribal groups were divided—often bitterly —amongst themselves and held both their urban cousins and members of the minority groups in contempt. In Iraq the Shii community was politically attached to Iran, dependent upon its charities and culturally Persian. In northern Syria pro-Turkish sentiment was sufficiently strong to allow Turkish guerrilla bands a free hand. In Lebanon the several groups whose religions divided them still thought of their churches as their "nations." And in Transjordan statehood was a mockery, opposed by the Palestinians, both Arab and Jewish, scorned by the bedouin, and referred to by the British as "Churchill's inspiration."

It was long before any of these governments was to achieve a sense of identity. Even today the issue of nationality—whether a man of Damascus is a Syrian or an Arab or, if both, which is the object of his deepest loyalty—is unresolved. Even King Faisal, the hero of the Arab Revolt and the popular victim of French tyranny in Damascus, was far from accepted. A British report to the League of Nations for the year 1922–23 admitted that "Faisal and his government could not be maintained without British support and friendship." The real job of the mandate period, then, was the schooling of the Arabs in the requirements of statehood.

The creation of states, each distinct from its neighbors, was in large part a mechanical process. The growth of administration created jobs and careers; to travel a man had to have a passport which bore the name of his country; the forms and procedures of daily life developed in different patterns. Linguistic differences resulted from the fact that technical vocabularies, created to give instruction in fixing trucks or filling out government papers, were patterned on different models. The Iraqi army manual was unintelligible to the Syrian gendarme. Even the goods available from Europe differed as each copied the European metropole— the French radio using 110-volt electrical current would not work in Baghdad where the British installed 220. And, at least as important, each area developed its own enemy: The Syrians carried an abiding hatred of the French but remembered Britain with some favor, while the Iraqis who had never seen the French but who were captivated by stories of Paris felt no anger toward the French but were resentful of the British. Transjordanians, on the contrary, rather liked the British and, at least in the early days, admired the gallant band of Englishmen who knew the desert and the bedouin like the best of Arabs. The Lebanese, profiting from French benevolence and attracted by French culture while fearing Syrian nationalism, threw themselves almost wholeheartedly to the French. So, on the "new politics" the Arabs of Beirut, Damascus, Amman, and Baghdad literally had no common language.

From this to statehood, however, is a long jump.

Many small impulses contributed to that jump but none was more important than education. As an American educational consultant informed the Iraqi government some years later, "Without a public school system it is obvious to everyone that an independent nationality could not be maintained even if established."

Education in the Turkish era had been directed toward government service. Special schools were established to enroll the sons of tribal shaikhs—with the double purpose of impressing the young men with the power of the empire and holding them hostage for their fathers' conduct. Those of the city men who did not go abroad and wanted more than the religious schools could offer were obliged to learn Turkish. With little developed native industry or commerce, moreover, the roads of advancement led through government civil or military service. Most of those who achieved prominence in government service in the generation after the First World War had been Ottoman army officers. It was a principle of the British administration, but not of the French administration, to bring these young men right into responsible posts as early as possible.

Since the Ottoman craft of state aimed at creating essential public security, raising tax revenues, and maintaining territorial integrity at minimum cost, it is not surprising to find that little was done in the field of education. The few schools which Iraq had were mostly on the primary level and all, after the Young Turk revolt, offered courses in Turkish. In 1913 about 6000 students were registered but probably most of these were only part-time and very few got beyond the first two or three years of classes. Religious schools taught recitation of the Koran and literary Arabic; weak and unimpressive as they were, they did preserve in Iraq some unity of form in Islam and, for a very small part of the population, a standard of the written language.

When the British surveyed the educational system, they found little other than the buildings to be of any use. Most of the relatively modern teachers were not qualified to teach in Arabic while those who could teach in Arabic did not know the subjects needed by the class of clerks and administrators the British wanted to staff the mandate government and business enterprises. In 1920 less than one half of one percent of the population was registered and in attendance in the schools. In that year the government opened two secondary schools—one with seven and the other with twenty-seven students. The British viewed education in highly specific and utilitarian terms. In its 1923–24 report to the League of Nations the mandate government stated its view that "in this country, it is neither desirable nor practicable to provide Secondary education except for the select few."

In that same year some 15,000 students were in Iraq's 300 religious schools and about 5000 adults were enrolled in anti-illiteracy classes. But pressure of necessity forced the government gradually to increase its outlay from 3 percent to 8 percent of the budget in the field of education. However, even as late as 1932, when the mandate ended, the average rural school child got only two years of schooling, and of the 154 existing government schools only 14 had as many as six grades. Whole districts of Iraq had no schools with six grades.

In Syria the situation was similar but for different reasons. The French defined their mandate as an obligation to bring European, that is, French, culture to the benighted natives; it made little difference that the natives were Arabs, with a vast literary heritage. That heritage was eschewed to the extent possible. Students were encouraged to study French and the best among them found their ways to French universities and institutes. But caution was the keynote. Since the French attempted to retain for themselves a far larger share of administrative and political power than did the British, they regarded education as a dangerous fuel for the fires of nationalism.

It is significant that the number of students in school rapidly increased when Iraq obtained its independence. By the end of the British mandate Iraq had 19 secondary schools with 129 teachers and 2082 students; within three years the number of students doubled, and by the eve of World War II it had reached nearly 14000. But even more significant was the change in the materials of instruction: school books became increasingly directed at fostering nationalist feeling. The function of these schools, as seen by the Iraqi government, was to "select and train leaders for all the essential phases of life of [the] nation."

The British educational adviser was not rehired and the example of Germany came increasingly to attract Iraqi educators. Education, always considered as a means to the end of national betterment in the larger sense, became so in all points of detail. For example, the aim of teaching history was to "strengthen the 'national and patriotic feeling' in the hearts of the pupils." This was to be accomplished in Iraq, as in the Palestine school system of the same period, by means of study of Arabic literature and with "stories about famous Arabs and their qualities . . . taught in such a way [as] would lead to the growth of national feelings."* This was a difficult task, for far from burning with a sense of national mission, the students were apathetic. An American consultant wrote that "there is evident among teachers and pupils no great patriotic fervor for their new nationalism . . . Somehow the youth of the secondary school and their teachers must get a vision of what the nation demands of them and an inspiration from these new possibilities of national culture and political achievement. These things they do not seem to have, nor does the school experience contribute in any extent to them."†

This lack of purposefulness in what they were doing and disappointment with their much advertised new "democracy" were to be of great significance in the troubled days of the 1930's. As in Europe so in Iraq, the failure of democracy to put the meat of practice on the bone of its theory left the educated elite with little more than whetted appetites and sore teeth.

Consciousness of the apathy of the Iraqi people and shame at the weakness of the nation before Europe was a potent political mixture in the 1930's in Iraq. Despairing of adults, the government encouraged the rise of paramilitary youth groups. Even the Boy Scouts were involved and grew by 1930 to 12,000 members. But the most significant was the *Futuwah*—the name evoked the memory of the efforts of the last Abbasid caliph to restore his regime to its former glory on the eve of the Mongol conquest, but the spirit was more akin to the fascist youth movements of Europe—whose director urged Iraqi youth to "get tough for ease spoils virtue." "That nation," he admonished Iraqi high school students in 1933, the first year of independence, "which does not master the art of death with steel and fire will be trampled to death [shamefully] under the hooves of cavalry and the boots of foreign soldiers." Essentially, this "art of death" was an attempt to state in a modern and national form the famous pre-Islamic verse

* Matta Akrawi (later director general of education of Iraq), *Curriculum Construction in Economic, Social, Hygienic and Educational Conditions and Problems of the Country* (New York, 1942), pp. 186-187.

† Paul Monroe, *et al.*, *Report of the Educational Inquiry Commission* (Government Press, Baghdad, 1932), p. 37.

memorized by generation after generation of school children: "Who holds not his foe away from his cistern with sword and spear, it is broken and spoiled: who uses not roughness, him shall men wrong." This inculcation of pre-Islamic values, which ultimately made up the whole syllabus of the humanities in the public school system of all the mandates, was in part an attempt to find a national image which could transcend the bitter and divisive religious problems of the Sunnis and the Shiis, of the Christians, Jews, and Muslims.

Education was the road to advancement through government service, but few wanted to get their hands dirty in the process of building the nation. The law college, the high road to government, prospered, but in the agricultural state of Iraq in 1930 an agricultural college was closed for lack of students. The glittering lure in the educational system was a tour abroad. To imbibe Western learning at its source was to be on the road to success in Iraq.

In a broad sense the entire mandate system was conceived as a sort of giant school in self-government. In no sense had the Turkish government aimed at such tutelage. And, as in any school, the "students" eagerly pressed for graduation.

In its report to the League of Nations in 1928 the mandate government noted that "From the beginning, the idea of a mandate has been abhorrent to nearly all educated elements in the country, and it was this fact which, in 1922, caused the British Government to negotiate with the 'Iraq Government a Treaty of Alliance to define Great Britain's relations with 'Iraq. It was not long, however, before the view became prevalent in 'Iraq that the Treaty of Alliance was in effect only the mandate in another form and it was approved by the Constituent Assembly in 1924 on condition that negotiations should be opened with a view to amending it."

Iraq achieved its formal independence in 1932 when it joined the League of Nations. The Syrians, remembering with pride their prior independence, pressed for their freedom, and it was only with great difficulty, at considerable cost in lives and property, that the French were able to hang on. Ironically, Syria was economically a losing proposition for them since it was British trade which always predominated in the Syrian market and French administration was always expensive. A full-scale civil war raged in and around Damascus in 1924–25. Damascus and other Syrian towns were bombarded three times during the mandate. Finally, after another outbreak in 1944, Syria and Lebanon achieved their independence.

Many of the problems which the mandate system was designed to solve were merely deferred and still form a part of the Middle Eastern scene.

X. Arabia and Egypt: Isolation or Humiliation

Egypt and the Arabian Peninsula present a sharp contrast in their development in the twentieth century. In their experience with the West, this contrast is particularly instructive and illustrates another aspect of "the impact of the West." Egypt profited in its relations with the West by gaining the most advanced Arab economy and by passing rapidly into the modern era, but has paid a heavy price in the psychological scars so evident in its political life. Arabia, unscarred, was also unassisted and unorganized by imperialism. While enjoying what has been termed "the ancient and comfortable right to be let alone," the states of Arabia have paid for their seclusion. None of the infrastructure associated with the mandate system or Western tutelage was created and, especially in those areas of the peninsula where oil was not found—in Yemen, for example—the people suffer from material and cultural backwardness.

The geography of Egypt is an invitation to invasion; and the regulation of the Nile irrigation system requires strong, centralized authority. These two facts have dominated Egyptian history. After suffering a series of invasions by the so-called Hyksos in the midst of its classical period, Egypt was invaded by the Persians in 525 B.C. and then conquered by Alexander the Great in 332 B.C. Never again, until after the First World War, when Egypt attained formal independence, or, as many Egyptians aver, after the Second World War, when the British troops were evacuated, did Egypt live under Egyptian rule. Its rulers were Greeks, Romans, Arabs, Armenians, Abyssinians, Turks, Circassians, French, and British. So deeply ingrained was the notion that it was not the métier of Egyptians to rule that, as we have seen, Napoleon's attempt to get native Egyptians to accept official responsibility was violently rejected. Forty years later, in the midst of the rule of Mehmet Ali Pasha, Egyptians told visitors that they were unsuited to rule themselves, that rule was the profession of others while they, the Egyptians, excelled in the law of Islam and in arts, crafts, and agriculture.

Egypt to Mehmet Ali Pasha and his successors was a base of power, not a homeland. Thus, though Mehmet Ali's dynasty rid themselves of the Albanian, Circassian, and other foreign slave or mercenary troops, they did so because these men refused to modernize, were expensive and unreliable; though they recruited native Egyptians, they did so because the Sudanese did not perform well and the Egyptians were available. Yet, Mehmet Ali Pasha and his more vigorous successors were personally if not nationally vitally interested in the growth of Egyptian power and in the achievement of Egyptian independence.

Twice during his long rule, Mehmet Ali had the Ottoman Empire in his grasp but both times the European powers forced him to withdraw. European statesmen realized, during most of the nineteenth century, that the sudden and dramatic breakup of the Ottoman Empire would endanger European peace and stability in a way unacceptable to them all. Thus, as has been said, British policy aimed at keeping the Ottoman Empire strong enough to withstand Russian pressure in the north but not so strong in the south as to constitute a barrier to the thrust of British commerce or imperialism. Russia wanted either no Ottoman Empire or one amenable to Russian policy; therefore, it alternated a policy of aggression with one of support against the aggression of others. France lacked such a clear conception of its national interests. Napoleon III sent an expedition to Lebanon in 1860 but withdrew, and in 1882 the French sent ships to Alexandria with the Royal Navy but took no part in the bombardment or the invasion of Egypt which established British power there. In general France tried to maintain friendship with the empire and its rivals, suffusing both with French culture and assisting in the development of both through commercial loans and entrepreneurial activity.

Mehmet Ali realized that his only security of tenure rested on his military power. Other rebels before his time in Egypt and elsewhere throughout the Ottoman Empire had gained a measure of autonomy only to lose their heads on the executioner's block. Safety lay in the acquisition of such power as to rival or replace that of the empire itself. Therefore, Mehmet Ali undertook his program of modernization of the army and the economy. To gain foreign exchange, he introduced cotton, encouraged agriculture, built and manned factories, sent missions of students and technicians abroad for training, and hired foreign specialists. Recognizing the geographic facts of Egypt, he instituted a strong, centralized regime, becoming himself the "landlord" of Egypt to get the most out of the country, and invaded surrounding areas to protect the open, defenseless Nile Valley. At the peak of his power, he ruled much of the Middle East and had armed forces totaling nearly 10 percent of the population of Egypt.

After the British-led invasion of Syria and the retreat of the Egyptian army in 1841, Mehmet Ali was forced to cut his army to 18,000 men, to give up a large part of his fiscal policy, particularly the monopoly system which sustained his industry and prevented the influx of cheap European manufactured goods, and to forgo the attempt to rival the Ottoman Empire. With his road to independence blocked and in declining health, Mehmet Ali lost interest in his reforms. In his last years and under his successors Egypt, in the words of an Egyptian historian, "was going slowly to sleep again."

But if this was true of the government, it was not true of the country as a whole. The growth of export agriculture, particularly in cotton, had tied the Egyptian to the world market. Even more significant was the intellectual ferment, at first affecting very few people, occasioned by the creation of a group of men who had been exposed to European culture and who, upon their return, infused their fellow countrymen with information and curiosity concerning Europe. In the shock of discovery of Europe, Egypt came, gradually, painfully, and partially, to recognize itself. Avant-guarde Egyptian writers began to speak of the nation, love of the homeland, and nationalism as something Egyptian. It was long, however, before the seeds thus planted were to take hold and grow in the soil of Egypt.

Meanwhile, Egypt had much to learn of the power and influence of Europe. The lesson began in earnest in 1854 when the ruler of Egypt granted to Ferdinand de Lesseps a concession to dig the Suez Canal. The sorry story of this episode, in which the Suez Canal Company, backed by a powerful consortium of Europeans and uncontrolled by inexperienced or venal Egyptians, committed grand larceny, has been told above. Oriental delight in pomp and circumstance and the genuine need to develop the Egyptian economy led the ruler of Egypt deeper and deeper into the trap of the great European banks. And the refusal of the European powers to allow Egypt to break loose from the Ottoman Empire saddled it with additional expenses. Prime Minister Disraeli announced to the House of Commons on March 23, 1876, that the khedive had requested that the report of an inquiry into Egyptian finances be suppressed. This was the coup de grace to the unsound finances of the country. Ultimately, Egypt was literally placed in receivership with its government under the control of a debt commission. This sparked native resentment against the weak Egyptian government and its European masters. A coup against the Egyptian government by a group of Egyptian army officers was put down by a British invasion and Egypt became in fact though not yet in name a British protectorate.

Immediately after their assumption of power over Egypt, the British announced that "although a British force remains in Egypt for the preservation of public tranquility, Her Majesty's Government are desirous of withdrawing it as soon as the state of the country and the organization of proper means for the maintenance of the Khedive's authority will admit of it." As the years went by the British government, according to a British historian, promised some 66 times to evacuate the country. Britain finally withdrew its last base in 1956 only to attempt later in that year to invade the country again.

British administration of Egypt was always a curious arrangement. The British did not claim possession or even protection over Egypt for three decades, the senior British official was the "consul-general," and Egypt remained a part of the Ottoman Empire. Essentially, British rule over Egypt was the quintessence of enlightened imperialism: It was the international version of government by a city manager. Under Consul-General Lord Cromer, who ruled Egypt from 1883 until 1907, improvements in irrigation, notably the completion of the first Aswan Dam in 1902, made possible an increase in the cropped area from 4.7 million to 7.7 million acres, debts were repaid to the full face value, and many substantial improvements were made in the government. Following the reconquest of the Sudan in 1898, Egypt was made a nominal partner in the Anglo-Egyptian Condominium established to rule it. Egyptians have complained, and rightly, that little was done in the field of education and that they were excluded from participation in social as well as administrative affairs.

But Egyptians, having acquired a better educated minority, stirred by a native religious revival which at the least encouraged a belief that in the Arabic-Islamic past there was much of which to be proud, and watching the national assertiveness of Japan and Turkey, aspired to a larger control over their own destiny. Political parties espoused the slogan, common in sentiment to others in many parts of the world, "Egypt to the Egyptians." To some degree the British found this political agitation useful to keep the ruler, the khedive, more dependent upon them. In any case the nationalists posed no serious threat as they were merely a small group of urban professional and trades people without much popular backing. It was not until the Denshawai incident of 1906 that hatred of foreign rule stirred the average Egyptian.

Successors to Lord Cromer were somewhat more willing than he to allow Egyptian participation in government or, at least, expression on political affairs. In 1907 the first national congress was held, and more encouragement was given to education. Again, however, the government tightened down on public demonstrations, enacting a press censorship law in 1909 and instituting exile as a punishment for undesirable politics. Thwarted resentment found an outlet in the assassination of the Coptic prime minister Butros Ghali, whom many regarded as a puppet of the British.

Egypt had become more prosperous. The government had been extremely frugal and had managed to cut most taxes and duties to the bone. Yet income increased as more lands were brought under cultivation as a result of the Aswan Dam, and the population increased by nearly 30 percent. By the First World War exports had increased 30 percent over Lord Cromer's best year.

When the First World War broke out, both the khedive and the British agent were out of the country—the khedive in Constantinople and Lord Kitchner in London. In November, when Britain declared war on Turkey, Kitchner joined the British war cabinet. The cabinet voted to annex Egypt, but British officials resident in Cairo were opposed. In December Egypt was declared a protectorate, with all ties to the Ottoman Empire severed, and its pro-Ottoman khedive deposed.

Ironically, it was to be Lord Cromer's protégé, Saad Zaghlul, who was to lead the charge against the British. Zaghlul, picked to be minister of education in 1906, was commended to the Egyptian people by Cromer as one who "possesses all the qualities necessary to serve his country."

We have noted above Zaghlul's petition to the British, and how, when he was refused, Zaghlul set about organizing committees throughout Egypt and circulating petitions for an end to British rule. The arrest and deportation of Zaghlul led in March 1919 to nearly a month of violence in which the British won all the battles, but the Egyptians won the war. Caught, as in Iraq, between expensive civil strife and frugal war-weariness, the British invited the Egyptians to submit proposals for reform and announced in April that Zaghlul was to be released. A state of tension continued with one prime minister after another resigning, so the British government appointed a commission of inquiry to investigate the causes of the disturbance and to plan for a more peaceful future.

On its arrival in Cairo in December 1919 the commission met with a silent boycott from all Egyptians outside the palace since its terms of reference had restricted it to modification of arrangements *within* the protectorate rather than allowing it to consider independence. Again the pace of violence was stepped up, with a steady procession of terrorist attacks on British soldiers and on those Egyptians who cooperated with the British.

Zaghlul, who had failed to achieve anything in Paris, then approached the commission of inquiry in London and attempted to negotiate with the British for what he had failed to get in Paris. A memorandum was drawn up to show what the British were prepared to accept, but Zaghlul, impelled by now by the very public emotion he had helped to create, found consideration of any proposal short of outright British evacuation impossible.

The main items in the British proposal called for Egyptian independence, a mutual defense treaty between Great Britain and Egypt, British right to maintain military forces in Egypt, Egyptian assumption of control over financial affairs, centralization of the capitulations under British control, and Egyptian right to discharge foreigners employed by the Egyptian government at a future date. These points are important both in that they indicate how far Egypt was from true independence and in that they form the base line for all future Anglo-Egyptian negotiations. The very fact that Britain was willing to negotiate thus with a man who had no official standing in Egypt—Zaghlul was not then even a member of the government—was itself tantamount to a British admission that the government of Egypt was a sham. This served to strengthen the nationalist movement and to concentrate still further the leadership in Zaghlul's hands.

Failing to work out an acceptable pact with the nationalists, the British government agreed in December 1921 to negotiate Egyptian independence. To ensure that events went smoothly, the British again arrested and deported Zaghlul. But at this point the British government, despite the urgent pleas and even threats to resign by its able high commissioner, Lord Allenby, again delayed. Again Egypt was torn by violence. Finally, on February 28, 1922, London unilaterally announced the independence of Egypt, leaving "absolutely reserved" four areas: British imperial communications, Egyptian defense, protection of the minorities and foreign interests, and the Sudan, over which, in theory, Britain and Egypt exercised a condominium.

It is a part of the tragedy of the contrast between the ruler and the ruled, the powerful and the powerless, the donor and the recipient, that events which appear to the one in one guise do not so appear to the other. As the British saw it, after frustrating and often infuriating negotiations, undertaken in good faith by the British but punctuated by violence in Egypt, the Egyptians, acting with the encouragement if not under the direct leadership of the very men carrying out the negotiations, refused a reasonable and logical solution in which Britain agreed to independence, reserving for itself only those matters of vital national interest or international moral concern.

From the perspective of the Egyptians, the events appeared quite the contrary: In the midst of a great war, ostensibly and vocally proclaimed to be for freedom—so ringingly announced by President Wilson—the great powers showed, under their thin new masks, the old faces of greed, oppression, and cunning. At the Peace Conference in Paris when it suited their purposes they dealt with half-savages or phony representatives, but would not meet the legitimate demands of representatives of such advanced and civilized peoples as the Egyptians for self-determination. After so constituting all of the "legitimate" avenues to power as to exclude the true representatives of the people, they accused these of breaking the law when they resorted to the course of true patriotism in the face of tyranny. Finally, when violence became too costly, they gave in, but did so with such cunning as to produce a stillborn state with matters of integral national concern like self-defense, maintenance of public security, and control over the headwaters of the Nile withheld. If any lesson had been learned, it was that Britain respected only force. Such was the Egyptian view.

Zaghlul was allowed to return to Egypt in September 1923. In the elections for the new parliament, the first conducted on a mass basis, he won an overwhelming victory with 190 out of 214 seats. Zaghlul was asked to form the cabinet and was invited by the British to negotiate a new treaty; he agreed to form a cabinet but refused to enter negotiations with the British unless there were no "absolutely reserved" points. On this, negotiations again broke down, and Zaghlul, flushed with what he thought was the proximity of victory, threw his Wafd into demonstrations in Egypt and the Sudan. In the atmosphere of hostility and passion the British officer who was commander of the Egyptian army and governor-general of the Sudan, Sir Lee Stack, was assassinated in Cairo on November 19.

The British reacted in a white fury, presenting an ultimatum to the Egyptian government which, after stating that "this murder, which holds up Egypt as at present governed to the contempt of civilized peoples, is the natural outcome of a campaign of hostility to British rights and British subjects in Egypt and the Sudan, founded upon a heedless ingratitude for benefits conferred by Great Britain," demanded "ample apology," "condign punishment" for the criminals, suppression of all "popular political demonstrations," payment of a fine of £500,000, withdrawal of all Egyptian officers from the Sudan within twenty-four hours, and notification of the Sudanese (that is, British) government that it could draw unlimited water from the Nile—thus appearing to strike at the jugular vein of Egypt. Moreover, Egypt was to "withdraw all opposition in the respects hereafter specified to the wishes of His Majesty's Government concerning the protection of foreign interests in Egypt."

The Egyptian government immediately agreed to apologize amply, to punish the criminals, and to pay the fine, but refused the other demands. In reply the British instructed the Sudan government forcibly to eject the Egyptians there and to renounce restrictions on its use of Nile waters. The British seized a part of the Alexandria customs to ensure Egyptian fulfillment of conditions. Further, the high commissioner suggested that hostages should be taken to be shot in the event of further assassinations.

Powerless to react but too proud to remain, Zaghlul resigned as prime minister and was replaced by a government that was little more than a British puppet. In December Parliament was dissolved and new, carefully rigged, elections were staged, but even in these the Wafd won almost half the seats. So Parliament was again dissolved. In yet another election the Wafd won 144 out of 201 seats but a British show of force, fear of palace intrigue, and, probably, weariness caused the 67-year-old Zaghlul to take a moderate position until the end of his life in 1927.

Once again, the Wafd took power in 1928 but was dismissed on charges of corruption and scandal—often more potent political weapons than gunboats—and in confusion, the Egyptian nationalist movement seemed itself in danger of being as discredited as were the very institutions of popular participation in government, the Parliament and the ministries. It appeared that long before it had reached its goals, the Wafd "sold out." Indeed, the man who followed Zaghlul as leader of the nationalists, Nahhas Pasha, was deeply involved in the scandals and corruption which so divided his party.

So Egypt faltered through the early 1930's, having lost all the élan of its nationalist period, led by men with an increasing stake in the status quo, dissatisfied but apparently, even in seeming victory, unable to achieve real independence. By 1936 the government was ready to sign a treaty with Great Britain which gave Britain essentially what she had asked for in 1922, military control, joint participation in British control over the Sudan, and British endeavors to end the privileged position of other foreign powers in Egypt. In 1937 on this basis Egypt was able to join the League of Nations.

Egyptian frustration and anguish is perhaps best documented in the rise of such extremists as fascist youth groups and the Muslim Brotherhood. The Egyptians, now really leaderless and with uncertain or complex goals, were unable to find a path to their future. Although formally independent they did not find themselves to be free.

Egypt broke diplomatic relations with Germany when World War II began and with Italy when Italy entered the war in the summer of 1940, but did not declare war. The country be-

came a huge armed camp for the British Eighth Army as the
western desert became a major theater of operations, and in the
exigencies of the situation such freedom of action as was possessed by Egypt was quickly subordinated to the demands of
the British military. Egyptian reticence or sympathy for the Axis,
widely shared in the Arab world, was overcome by a coup de
main in which British forces surrounded the palace of King
Farouk in February 1942 and threatened to depose the king unless he named a prime minister of their choosing. Ironically, the
government so installed was of the Wafd, long since tamed and
friendly to the British.

Even those who have criticized the British admit that they
acted under the most extreme conditions, with the war apparently being lost in most theaters and the beginnings of a German
drive in North Africa which would bring Field Marshal Rom-
mel's tanks to a point within 70 miles of Alexandria. But British
actions in Egypt as in Iraq and elsewhere did lend reality to the
contention of nationalists that so long as British forces remained
on Egyptian soil, Egypt was a good deal less than fully independent.

Perhaps as potent a factor in Egyptian thought as any that
could be adduced in economics or politics was the scar tissue
caused by the blatantly evident and utter scorn felt by many
Europeans for the Egyptians. "Wog"—Wily Oriental Gentleman—and "Gypo" became soldiers' taunts; the words of the
Egyptian national anthem were redrafted as a smutty joke on the
Egyptian king and queen. The typical English-Arabic phrase
book always prominently featured the words "Get out," *imshee,*
and "Beat it," *yalla,* and were largely restricted to those words
used by an impolite patron to a waiter. But perhaps most of all,
the central and most inviting piece of real estate of Cairo, the
island in the middle of the Nile, was largely taken up by a sporting club which was restricted to Englishmen and, toward the
end, to acceptable Europeans and Americans. Even the king of
the country was unwelcome. Later there was to be no prouder
victory of nationalism, even the Egyptianization of the Suez
Canal or the National Bank of Egypt, than the capturing of the
board of directors of the Gazira Sporting Club.

As the tides of war changed, after the battles of El Alamein and Stalingrad, the British position eased considerably. Britain not only was prepared to allow more autonomy within Egypt itself but encouraged Egypt and other Arab states to move toward the realization of at least a part of their aspirations for some form of federation. It was in Alexandria in October 1944 that the Arab Unity Conference was assembled under the chairmanship of Egypt. And, in order to be allowed to join the United Nations, Egypt in February 1945 finally declared war on Japan and Germany.

Once again, Egypt emerged from a war with appetite whetted for real independence. Students and members of the Muslim Brotherhood and other groups dominated the streets of Cairo for some months. The Egyptians were able to begin negotiations with the new Labour government on a revision of the 1936 treaty, but the Wafd, attempting to recapture its faded youthful vigor and purity, refused to be bound by the negotiations or to take part in them. In beginning the negotiations Great Britain agreed to evacuate all of Egypt except for the Suez Canal Zone, which became the major British base in the Middle East, but the future of the Sudan, which the Egyptians regarded as a part of Egypt since, at least, the 1899 convention establishing the condominium, led to a break in the talks. Egypt then took to the United Nations her case against the 1936 treaty, which she held was negotiated under duress, and against British moves to alienate the Sudan, but the Security Council was unwilling to do more than urge continued discussions between the two parties.

Almost immediately upon the heels of the defeat at the United Nations came the Palestine War in which Egyptian forces, after glowing speeches by leaders of the Egyptian government, were defeated. The bitter consequences of this humiliation were not long delayed for a government by now almost devoid of the respect of its people.

The Arabian Peninsula, where Islam was born, ceased to be the major stage of Islam in the time of the fourth caliph, Ali, when the capital of the empire was shifted to Kufa in what is now Iraq. But Arabia, with Mecca as the target of prayer and goal of pilgrimage and Medina, the birthplace of the Islamic state, never lost its sentimental and religious hold on Muslims. Particularly after the bedouin "defected" from the caliphate, returning to their pre-Islamic ways, in the second century of Islam, Arabia remained the "blood bank" of Arab civilization. From it all but Arabs were excluded and to it the faithful sent their pious donations to support religious and cultural institutions. Indeed, as the routes of commerce and the centers of industry were concentrated elsewhere, religion became the major "business" of Arabia. Little scope existed for agriculture, for few areas other than Yemen and the southeastern coast had sufficient rainfall or springs—Arabia has no rivers—to support more than occasional farming, and until this century no other significant resources were exploited.

Periodically in Islamic history, a reform movement has come from Arabia, paralleling the rise of Islam. The last, and greatest, of these is the Wahhabi revival of fundamentalism.

A successor in spirit if not in fact to other attempts to return to the bases of the faith, Wahhabism was begun in Arabia in the eighteenth century when a religious reformer, Muhammad Abdu'l-Wahhab, made common cause with the shaikh of the princely tribal family of Saud. The classic Islamic combination of the "Book and the Sword" which thus resulted led to a wave of conquest and tribal raids into Syria, Iraq, and all parts of Arabia in the early nineteenth century. Temporarily suppressed in the second decade of the nineteenth century by the Egyptian armies of Mehmet Ali, Wahhabism survived in the highlands of Nejd and on the eastern shores of Arabia. Its influence was, however, contained by the rise of a rival Arabian dynasty, the Rashidis of Hail, and by the Ottoman protection and support given to the office of the sharif of Mecca. In 1890 the Rashidis forced the Sauds to flee from the Nejd, to seek safety under the protection of the shaikh of Kuwait. In 1902 the late Abdu'l-Aziz ibn Saud, with a small band of Kuwaiti and Nejdi retainers, in a predawn coup de main, recaptured Riyadh. The Rashidis, weakened by internal disputes, were unable to cope with the revival of Wahhabi power not only in the Nejd but also in the Ottoman province of al-Hasa which the Saudi forces captured in 1913.

In December 1915 the British government signed a treaty in which it agreed to recognize Ibn Saud as sultan of the Nejd and to grant him a subsidy of £5000 monthly. Essentially, the British were interested in keeping Arabia quiet internally so that the Arabs under the influence of the sharif of Mecca, the British chosen instrument, could carry the war to the Turks in the Hejaz and in what is now Jordan and Syria.

The British were at the same time negotiating with Sharif Husain on the terms under which *his* Arabs would enter the war. In the Husain-McMahon Correspondence the British had specifically undertaken to restrict his activities from interference with other Arab rulers with whom they had treaties. Consequently, the British refused to recognize Husain's claim to be "King of the Arabs." Meanwhile, an Arabian force under Husain's son Faisal captured Damascus and took over Syria.

However, in Arabia supporters of Husain and Ibn Saud clashed in 1918, and Ibn Saud decisively defeated the Hejazis in 1919. Preoccupied with his Rashidi rivals until 1921 when he overcame their last resistence, Ibn Saud made no move against the Hejaz until 1924. In that year, after the abdication of Husain in favor of his eldest son Ali, the Hejazi forces were defeated again and both Taif and Mecca taken. A year later, in December 1925, Ibn Saud completed the conquest of the Hejaz, taking Jiddah, and King Ali went into exile. In 1927, in the Treaty of Jiddah, Great Britain recognized Ibn Saud as King of the Hejaz in return for his recognition of Faisal as King of Iraq, Abdullah as Amir of Transjordan, and the special status of the British-protected shaikhdoms on the Persian Gulf. Except for a brief Saudi war with Yemen in 1936 the Arabian Peninsula was at peace from 1927 to 1961 when a coup d'etat in Yemen developed first into a civil war and then a "civil war with outside intervention" as Egyptian troops landed in Yemen and the Saudis assisted the Yemeni royalists.

The British and the Ottoman Turks were almost the only foreigners in Arabia until the end of World War I, when interest in the possibility of oil brought in Americans. The major British interest in Arabia, until the discovery of oil in this century, has been the route to India. The Persian Gulf was a link in the

Euphrates-Mediterranean route and so involved vital communications. We have seen that one effect of Napoleon's invasion of Egypt was to accentuate the importance of securing the northern Persian Gulf gate of the route, Kuwait, just as an earlier rivalry with the Portugese and then the Dutch had brought the British to the lower end of the gulf and the Island of Hormuz in 1622. By 1639 the British had secured rights to open a trading post at Basra, and by 1764 had a consul there. By the end of the century the British placed a resident in Baghdad to superintend the post route to Europe. By 1820 they had established complete control over the Gulf, suppressed piracy, and entered into treaty arrangements with the shaikhs of the "Pirate" (renamed "Trucial") Coast.

From the time of Napoleon the British were deeply worried about the use by other powers of the Euphrates–Persian Gulf route to attack India. At first Russia was thought to pose such a danger and then Germany. One after another the petty shaikhdoms came under increasing British influence and protection. In 1869 the Trucial shaikhdoms agreed not to deal with foreign governments except through Great Britain; this was extended to Bahrein in 1880, Muscat in 1891, and Qatar in 1916. Kuwait, from the middle of the nineteenth century the key port on the gulf, was originally planned as the Persian Gulf terminus of the Berlin-Baghdad–Persian Gulf railway; but in 1898 it was effectively removed from the Ottoman Empire when, finding that the Russians intended to establish a logistics base there, the British entered into treaty arrangements similar to the others concluded with the gulf shaikhdoms in previous years.

The shaikh of Kuwait was recognized by Great Britain to be independent under British protection on November 3, 1914. On April 30, 1915, the Idrisi Sayyid of Sabya in Asir was recognized similarly. These areas were backwaters in the general war effort, which was concentrated in western Arabia, in the Hejaz, where Sharif Husain instituted the Arab Revolt. But they were areas of immediate concern to the government of India and consequently their special status was reserved in the British commitment to Husain.

Aden, on the southwest tip of Arabia, was also affected by the thrust of Napoleon toward the East. In 1799 a British force occupied the island of Perim, which forms a sort of stopper in the mouth of the Red Sea, and then moved to Aden. In 1802 the British concluded a commercial treaty with the sultan. Relations later were strained and an incident involving the passengers and crew of a wrecked British ship gave the British a pretext in 1839 to bombard and seize the town of Aden. In an ensuing peace treaty a stipend was allotted to the sultan, but five times before 1857 the town came under attack. Aden became a crown colony in 1937. As a part of the South Arabian Federation, which was formed in 1959, even today Aden is the object of a three-way tug of war between the British, the Arabic-speaking natives, and the large Yemeni community resident there.

Yemen, "Arabia Felix" of the classical writers, is the second largest of the states of the Arabian Peninsula. With a climate quite different from the rest of the peninsula and cut off by vast deserts from the north, Yemen has been strongly influenced by its nearer neighbors in Africa. But it has also been ruled by Ethiopia and Persia. The legendary seat of the Queen of Sheba, Yemen has the longest settled and recorded history of any part of Arabia. Its relatively heavy rainfall has made settled agriculture possible, and this has caused men to invest in the land in a way quite different from the use of nomadic areas to the north. Both Judaism and Christianity have, at periods, dominated the religious life of the country. Following the advent of Islam, Yemen became Muslim but most of the people espoused a non-Orthodox branch of Islam, the Zaidi Shii sect, which has had its "patriarch" the ruling imam of Yemen from the ninth century to the present time.

In 1517 Yemen was nominally conquered by the Ottoman Empire, but more effective threats to the autonomy of the area came from the Europeans, mainly the Portuguese, who alternated trade with piracy and imperialism. Invaded in the nineteenth century by the Egyptians, who drove out the Wahhabi tribes of Arabia, restored the imamate, and re-established Ottoman suzerainty, Yemen served in World War I as the base for Turkish operations against the British in Aden. In the Armistice of Mudros, Yemen achieved its independence. Although Yemen had a treaty with the Soviet Union in 1928, it was not recognized by the United States until 1946.

Internally, the history of Yemen is a sordid and bloody tale, but the country has been so isolated from the outside world and so poor in resources or strategic value as to preserve not only a large measure of autonomy but also a culture and a way of life. Well might a commentator say, when civil war broke out after the death of the old imam in 1962, "Yemen is rushing headlong into the fourteenth century."

When the "impact of the West" came in Arabia, it came not in the uniform of the soldier, in the ledger of the European banker, or with the humiliating attitude of the imperialist, but with the magic wand of the oil drilling rig. Far from refusing to let the Arab into its posh clubs, the oil industry was delighted to sit as a guest in the bedouin tent or to build for the Arab Western, air-conditioned cities, railroads, schools, and hospitals in return for the privilege of being allowed to drill in the desert wastes for oil. Undreamed of wealth poured into the peninsula—by 1964 almost one billion dollars yearly. The sudden infusion of wealth was almost too much. None of the petty states had the institutions or the people to handle such sums, and they cannot be said to have been efficiently used. Much was wasted or used on nonproductive luxury items. But while the Arabian Peninsula has not had the profit of foreign tutelage in the creation of a trained people, in the development of the infrastructure of a modern state, and in the imposition of the institutions of constitutional government, it has also avoided the trauma of the deep wounds of national humiliation. The pride that the poorest of bedouin has retained is only now being regained, at great cost and effort, by the richest of the Egyptians.

XI. Palestine: The Promised Land

On February 18, 1947, the British government announced to the world what had been evident to many long before, that "there is no prospect of resolving this conflict [in the Palestine mandate] by any settlement negotiated between the parties . . . We have . . . reached the conclusion that the only course now open to us is to submit the problem to the judgment of the United Nations."

As with so many simple and straightforward statements in international relations, behind the words lies a complex, emotion-fraught, and bitter story, many of whose ramifications lie far outside the scope of this book, yet one whose influence permeates the whole history of the modern Middle East—and the world—and which, therefore, commands out greatest and most sensitive attention. It is not incumbent upon the author or the reader to join the emotional fray—quite enough authors and readers have already done this—but it is essential for anyone who aspires to understand the Middle East today to know the sources, the extent, and the depth of those emotions in order to be the better able to cope with the events and men they have so profoundly affected.

The history of the Palestine problem is a long and spotty one; for the present purposes, only a few things need to be said about it: (1) though Palestine remained the emotional center of Zion, the Jewish population was almost totally expelled or drawn away from Palestine under the Roman Empire; (2) the Arab invasion in A.D. 636 brought relatively few new people to Palestine, so that the ancestors of most of the "Arabs" were actually converted (either to Islam or to use of the Arabic language) over the centuries of Arab and Turkish rule; and (3) the immigration of Jews, other than the small number who came for religious reasons over the centuries, began in the late nineteenth century and was the result of persecution in Europe.

During the First World War, as we have seen, much or all of what subsequently became the Palestine mandate, entrusted to Great Britain under the League of Nations by the Paris Peace Conference in April 1920, was promised to France under the May 1916 Sykes-Picot agreement, to the Jews for "the establishment in Palestine of a National Home for the Jewish people" in the November 1917 Balfour Declaration, and, at least under one reasonable reading, to the Arabs by the Husain-McMahon Correspondence of 1915–16. The war ended with Great Britain in control of the area and the other three contenders attempting to secure their rights. A serious diplomatic clash with France over what the French regarded as British bad faith on the issues of Palestine, Syria, and Mosul was settled in Paris. This left two contenders, the Zionists and the Arabs, with the British holding an uneasy and unstable balance for nearly thirty years.

Initially, as we have seen, the Arabs were less concerned with opposition to the Zionists than to the French. The Arab leader Amir Faisal thought that if he came to terms with the Zionists, they could persuade the French government to waive their claims of influence in Syria. In a formal understanding with Dr. Weizmann, Faisal agreed, on behalf of the Arabs, to work together with the Zionists to achieve their mutual aims, to give effect to the Balfour Declaration, to facilitate Jewish immigration provided the rights of the Arab peasants and tenant farmers be protected, to insure freedom of worship and protection of the Holy Places, and to constitute the British government as their arbiter, provided the Arabs achieved their independence. Also a part of this agreement was Jewish economic aid to the Arabs. But the Arab Congress at Damascus repudiated the essence of Faisal's agreement with Weizmann, saying: "We regard their claims as a grave menace to our national, political and economic life. Our Jewish fellow-citizens shall continue to enjoy the rights and bear the responsibilities which are ours in common."

Faisal, himself, had little more time on the world stage as spokesman for the Arabs of the Levant. On July 14, 1920, French troops invaded Syria and, after routing the small Arab forces sent to oppose them, seized Damascus and overthrew the Arab government. Never again were the Arabs of Palestine to find a spokesman of international stature, and not for years were they to be represented by an Arab state with even the shadowy authority enjoyed by Faisal's Syrian kingdom.

Meanwhile, events in the occupied territory of Palestine had begun to assume, as they had in Iraq, a shape of their own. As in Iraq, so in Palestine, it was discovered that the administration was in a state of chaos. This was particularly evident in Palestine in questions of land ownership. Not only had the retreating Turks taken with them most of the administrative personnel but also had either taken or destroyed official registers of land holdings. Confusion was compounded. In Palestine, due to the Turkish ban on foreign ownership of property, dual sets of land ownership records had been maintained since the middle part of the nineteenth century. The many foreigners who had bought land registered it in the name of a subject of the empire. Over the years the land might have been sold or inherited several times. Moreover, since the Ottoman land tenure system was superimposed on local usage, rights of various sorts were often exercised by different parties in any given piece of land. In some instances land cases begun in the immediate postwar years were hardly settled by the end of the Palestine mandate.

The first chief administrator of Palestine urged that the Zionist program be dropped as inimical to public security in Palestine. The King-Crane Commission, which President Wilson sent to the Middle East to ascertain the wishes of the population, of which about 10 percent was Jewish, reported an overwhelming rejection by the population of Zionist aspirations. But before the end of the military administration and the inauguration of the mandate, upwards of 5000 Jewish immigrants were allowed to enter the country, and Hebrew was adopted as one of the official languages.

Meanwhile on July 1, 1920, authority in Palestine was handed to Sir Herbert Samuel as the first high commissioner of the mandatory government. But it was not until 1923 that Palestine legally ceased to be a part of the Ottoman Empire and became a mandate of the League of Nations. A little over a month after taking power the new civil government issued the land transfer ordinance which reopened the registry office so that lands once more could be bought and sold. The first major purchase of land, by the Jewish National Fund and the Palestine Land Development Company, Ltd., encompassed seven Arab villages in Galilee.

At the same time Sir Herbert Samuel, who had been a principal supporter of Zionism in England during the war, set the quota for the first year's immigration of Jews at 16,500. Just before the publication of the quota on immigration, occurred the second of what was to become a series of Arab-Jewish clashes. In the following year, in May 1921, immigration was suspended after another series of Arab attacks on Jews and Jewish settlements. Everyone, even among the Arab moderates, feared that sooner or later a Zionist state would be created if a sufficiently large number of Jews had moved to Palestine. This was the finding of an investigation commission. However, immigration was allowed to continue the following month with fewer restrictions than prior to the outbreak.

Thus, in 1921 two precedents were set by the government which were to be followed for the next quarter century. In the first place, the government in the face of acts of violence, *did* temporarily accede to the aims of those committing the acts of violence: it did temporarily suspend immigration. In the second place, after the situation had been brought under control and an investigating commission had studied the underlying causes of the trouble, the government *did not* address the identified causes in its subsequent policy.

In 1922, after further Arab outbursts against Zionism, the high commissioner requested that the Colonial Office define exactly the meaning of the phrase "a National Home." The then Colonial

Secretary, Winston Churchill, published a statement of policy. After affirming that the Balfour Declaration was to remain the bedrock of British policy, he restricted, more narrowly than any senior British official had to that date, what was meant in the Balfour Declaration: "Unauthorized statements have been made to the effect that the purpose in view is to create a wholly Jewish Palestine. Phrases have been used such as that Palestine is to become 'as Jewish as England is English'. His Majesty's Government regard any such expectation as impracticable and have no such aim in view . . . They would draw attention to the fact that the terms of the Declaration referred to do not contemplate that Palestine as a whole should be converted into a Jewish National Home, but that such a Home should be founded in Palestine."

In 1922 the British government decided to separate Transjordan legally from the mandate of Palestine. Transjordan, said the British government, was not included in the Balfour Declaration and Jews were forbidden to buy land there. This move satisfied no one. The Zionists felt that if their historic claim was justified in principle, it was justified in its particulars; so they argued at that time, as they had previously argued at the Peace Conference, that Transjordan was necessary for the development of their National Home. The Arabs, in their turn, argued that Britain's act tended to weaken the position of those who lived in the Palestine mandate by appearing to settle the Arab claim to the dubious benefit of the small number of nomadic tribesmen moving about in the Jordan desert. Further, they pointed out, this action gave a larger degree of independence and self-government to Arabs far less advanced than they, and so sapped the idea of tutelage in statecraft inherent in mandate conception.

In Palestine itself the high commissioner tried in 1922 to establish a government agency in which Arabs would have a voice— at least in lesser issues of policy. The plan called for a council of twenty-three members, including the high commissioner. Ten of the other twenty-two would be official appointees; of the remaining twelve elected positions, two would be Christian, two Jews, and eight Muslims. The Arabs opposed the plan since they would have only ten votes—a minority—on such fundamental matters as land policy, immigration, and Zionism. In the face of Arab hostility the high commissioner dropped the whole project. The following year he suggested that the Arabs form "an Arab Agency" analogous to the Jewish Agency, so that the Palestine Arab community would have voice in the affairs of government. This also the Arabs refused.

There can be no doubt that the Arabs were mistaken in not accepting this proposal, for their refusal deprived them of all effective concentration of their activities in the Palestine mandate. Again and again in the following years the Arabs refused to be involved responsibly in political affairs. They argued to themselves that if they accepted responsibility for any part of the affairs of the mandate they would thereby acquiesce in the basic policy of creating a Jewish National Home and would become actually, as the mandate suggested they were politically, but a single part of the population of Palestine.

In Palestine, as in the other mandate states, noteworthy developments in education, public works, health, and other "social overhead" facilities took place. In the excitement of the developmental activity so evident within the mandate, the political questions appeared briefly in the 1920's to have been shelved.

This is true to a certain extent because the worst fears of the Arabs had not been realized. The country had not been "swamped" by Jews, a Jewish state seemed no nearer to establishment than in 1922, and as long as times were good, everyone was prepared to deal in the present and leave the future worries for bad times. Then, somewhat curiously, the arrival of a sharp economic depression, which resulted partly from a collapse of the Polish currency, instead of increasing Arab discontent tended to lessen Arab fears. From 1925 to 1928 no meetings of the Palestine Arab Congress were held, and no protests were voiced over Jewish immigration. The immigration figures themselves provide an index.

The year 1925, when a series of Arab protests were made to the mandate authority, was the largest immigration year to that date, with a net Jewish immigration increase of 31,650. In the next year, however, only about one sixth as large a net immigration was recorded. The Arabs reached the conclusion that with their high birth rate they were not in danger of losing their majority of the population. In 1927 the Jewish community had 2358 more emigrants than immigrants. By the Arabs this was taken as a sign that the National Home had failed, the Jews were leaving, and the Arabs could relax in victory. In the following year, however, the trend was reversed; a very slight net gain was made. And in 1929 the net gain was 3503. The optimism of the Arabs was shattered. They also observed that the Zionist crisis had tended to heal the breach between the Zionist and non-Zionist Jews and even led to an enlarging of the Jewish Agency.

The relative calm of the middle years of the 1920's was ended by a riot in 1929, begun when a number of Zionists organized a demonstration at the Wailing Wall in Jerusalem in the course of which the Zionist flag was raised and the Zionist anthem sung. Within two weeks of violence 472 Jews and 268 Arabs were among the casualties. The commission which investigated the disturbances noted: "The Arabs have come to see in the Jewish immigrant not only a menace to their livelihood but a possible overlord of the future . . . and the result of Jewish enterprise and penetration have been such as to confirm that they will be excluded from this soil."

After questions were raised in the League of Nations Permanent Mandate Commission, the British government decided in May 1930 to appoint a special commission under Sir John Hope-Simpson of the League of Nations Refugee Settlement Commission for Greece, and formerly of the Indian Civil Service, to investigate the underlying causes of the recent disturbances. The Hope-Simpson report recommended an immediate halt to immigration, but suggested that it might become possible again on a limited scale in future years.

The British government accepted the report and on the basis of it issued the Passfield White Paper which went even further toward granting Arab desires than did John Hope-Simpson's report. Jewish reaction was both immediate and effective. Zionist leaders protested to the Colonial Office, and the president of the

Jewish Agency, Chaim Weizmann, resigned in protest. From a wide variety of public figures, including the leadership of the opposition Conservative party, protests flowed in. In hasty retreat, the British government took the unusual step of redefining its action in a letter published in *The Times* in which the prime minister denied that the government intended to stop the development of the National Home. Subsequent speeches in Parliament and statements to the press further modified the intent of Passfield White Paper. In February 1931 the British prime minister, in a letter to Weizmann which was published in *The Times*, proclaimed that immigration "can be fulfilled without prejudices to the rights and positions of other sections of the population of Palestine," and so repudiated the Passfield White Paper.

Coming as this letter did, only as the result of protests by one group in Palestine and their supporters, without benefit of another government study or commission, it was naturally taken by the Arabs as concession to political pressures. They called it, in bitter jest, the "Black Letter" which canceled the White Paper. For the first time Arab hostility began to be directed at the government rather than toward the incoming Jews.

The immediate result was an Arab boycott and a refusal to work together with the Jewish community on civic affairs. But on a positive program, the Arabs spoke with many voices when they spoke at all. Lacking a constituted representative, as the Jews possessed in the Jewish Agency, the Arabs divided into a number of mutually hostile groups which were ineffective in expressing their desires to the government. Moreover, the minimum Arab program was independence, end of immigration, and restriction of land sales. On these terms the government had shown itself unwilling, if not unable, to negotiate. As a result, moderate Arabs could have no concrete and positive program to urge upon the government.

Meanwhile, with the rise to power in Germany of the Nazis in 1932, a new sense of urgency and, eventually, desperation was felt by the Zionist organization, and its ability to act was stiffened by the increasing scale of immigration from Germany. Between

1932 and 1933 the number of immigrants tripled. As the subsequent royal commission pointed out: "As the National Home expanded from 1933 onwards, so the Arab hate and fear have increased." The attitude of the Arab leaders became more hostile toward the government, and the tone of the Arab press more bitter. In the autumn of 1934 the Arab executive submitted to the high commissioner a formal expression of its view that the safeguards for Arab interests embodied in the mandate had broken down. In the single year of 1935, 61,854 Jewish immigrants arrived. This figure was as large as the total immigration of the first five years of the mandate, and in the four years from 1932 to 1936 the Jewish population of Palestine quadrupled.

Meanwhile, in other Arab countries, notably Egypt and Syria, the British and French governments appeared to give way before violence and nationalist demonstrations. So once again, the Palestine Arab community resorted to direct and violent action. On April 13, 1936, a series of terrorists attacks began throughout the country. Violence bred further violence between the Jewish and Arab communities. Throughout Palestine committees were formed in the Arab towns to demand the establishment of a representative government, prohibition of sales of land to Jews, and end of Jewish immigration. The normally mutually hostile Arab political leaders were forced by their rank-and-file supporters to form a united front and call for a general strike. This time, the government refused to submit to pressure and on May 18 issued an immigration schedule which was somewhat higher than in any previous year. The general strike quickly developed into a civil war. Two trains were derailed, a bridge blown up, and guerrilla bands which included soldiers from Syria and Iraq began to operate in the hill country. On May 23 mass arrests of Arab leaders were made, and in June members of the Arab Higher Committee were interned in a concentration camp.

In June 1936, 137 Arab senior officials and judges in the Palestine government presented a memorandum in which they set out their contention that the disturbances were caused by the fact that the Arab population of all classes, creeds and occupations is animated by a profound sense of injustice done to them. They feel that insufficient regard has been paid in the past to their legitimate grievances, even though those grievances had been inquired into by qualified and impartial official investigators, and to a large extent vindicated by those inquiries. As a result, the Arabs have been driven into a state verging on despair; and the present unrest is no more than an expression of that despair.

The fact must be faced that that feeling of despair is largely to be traced to loss of faith on the part of the Arabs in the value of official pledges and assurances for the future, and to the fact that they are genuinely alarmed at the extent to which His Majesty's Government have from time to time given way to Zionist pressure. Their confidence was severely shaken as far back as 1931, when the Prime Minister's letter to Dr. Weizmann was issued as an interpretation of the White Paper of 1930. But more recently, when the projects regarding the Legislative Council and the restriction on sales of land were hotly challenged in Parliament, their loss of confidence turned to despair.

Coming as this did from the most moderate, committed, and responsible members of the Arab community, the memorandum made a considerable impression both on the government and on the royal commission which was subsequently sent to investigate the cause of the disturbance.

By September 1936 some 20,000 regular troops had been sent to Palestine to try to re-establish public security. Severe punishment, including the destruction of villages and the quartering of troops, was meted out to those accused of harboring rebels. Arab casualties amounted to over 1000. Both Amir Abdulla of Transjordan and the prime minister of Iraq offered to mediate, but the British government could not allow mediation to include the issues of any of the terms of the mandate or the goal of the establishment of a National Home. Their offer of mediation having been refused, the rulers of the other Arab states advised the Arabs of Palestine "to rely on the good intentions of our friend Great Britain who has declared that she will do justice." By mid-October the strike had ended and the Arab bands had dispersed.

A royal commission, appointed to investigate the underlying causes of the disturbance, arrived in Palestine in November 1936.

After careful study of the situation the commission decided that the mandate was unworkable in its existing form. Their conclusions, published in 1937, are still worthy of attention.

An irrepressible conflict has arisen between two national communities within the narrow bounds of one small country. About 1,000,000 Arabs are in strife, open or latent, with some 400,000 Jews. There is no common ground between them. The Arab community is predominantly Asiatic in character, the Jewish community predominantly European. They differ in religion and in language. Their cultural and social life, their ways of thought and conduct, are as incompatible as their national aspirations. These last are the greatest bar to peace . . . The War and its sequel have inspired all Arabs with the hope of reviving in a free and united Arab world the traditions of the Arab golden age. The Jews similarly are inspired by their historic past . . . In the Arab picture the Jews could only occupy the place they occupied in Arab Egypt or Arab Spain. The Arabs would be as much outside the Jewish picture as the Canaanites in the old land of Israel. The National Home . . . cannot be half-national . . . This conflict was inherent in the situation from the outset. The terms of the Mandate tended to confirm it [and] the conflict has grown steadily more bitter . . . In the earlier period hostility to the Jews was not widespread among the fellaheen. It is now general . . . The intensification of the conflict will continue . . . it seems probable that the situation, bad as it now is, will grow worse. The conflict will go on, the gulf between Arabs and Jews will widen."

The recommendation of the royal commission was that Palestine be partitioned between the two communities since the only alternative appeared to be a rule of repression which would lead nowhere. The British government accepted the royal commission's report and issued a White Paper announcing that partition would be the basis of British policy. In the debate in the House of Lords, however, Lord Samuel, the first high commissioner, pointed out that the Jewish state, as small as it necessarily would be, would contain a population of Arabs almost equal to that of the Jews. Later he wrote that "the Commission seems to have picked out all the most awkward provisions of the Peace Treaty of Versailles, and to have put a Saar, a Polish corridor, and a half a dozen Dansigs and Mamels into a country the size of Wales." Such a monstrosity, he warned, would be impossible either to administer or to defend. After an initial cool reaction, the hostility of all parties to the conflict hardened against the plan. The Zionist Congress refused it outright. The League of Nations was not in favor but, in the final analysis, could do little but accept the advice of the British government. Those Arabs whose districts would be lost to the Arab state brought pressure on their leaders to oppose the plan. To see if a better redrawing of the map of Palestine might not be possible, a partition commission was appointed and sent to Palestine.

Meanwhile, in September 1937 the acting district commissioner of Galilee, which under the royal commission proposal would have been given to the Jewish state, was murdered by Arab terrorists. On October 1, a week after the assassination, the government outlawed the Arab Higher Committee and all national committees, ordered the arrest and deportation of six leading Arab figures, and froze the funds of the Pious Foundation which had supported Arab political activity. Almost 1000 people were interned. During the year, 438 attacks with bombs or fire arms were made on police posts, Jewish settlements, and Arab houses.

When the partition commission arrived in Palestine in April 1938, the leaders of the Arab community were for the most part under detention, but the community itself was united as never before and not one Arab collaborated with the commission. To counter Arab hostility, the government armed nearly 5000 Jews as active and reserve police, but the period of Zionist cooperation with the government was short-lived. Following the June 1938 hanging of a Jewish revisionist terrorist convicted of firing on an Arab bus, the Jews attacked government buildings and bombed Arab markets. In one such attack in Haifa 74 Arabs were killed and 129 others wounded.

During 1938 the government reported 5708 "incidents of violence" including over 1000 attacks on troops or government facilities. Some 2500 people, almost all Arab, were interned, and it was estimated that at least 1000 rebels had been killed by the police and army.

The partition commission published its recommendations in November 1938. After admitting that "the Arabs remain inflexibly hardened to partition" and that "it is impossible to divide a country of its size and configuration into areas the frontiers of which, having regard to the conditions of modern warfare, will have any real military significance," the commission presented three plans for partition. The unsolved dilemma was simply the need to create a Jewish state of sufficient size as to be economically viable and yet one which would not have an Arab majority.

The ensuing government White Paper admitted that "the political, administrative and financial difficulties involved in the proposal . . . are so great that this solution to the problem is impracticable."

The next British move was to summon yet another conference —this time only of the more moderate Arab leaders and those of the Jewish community—to London in February 1939. There, the government decided to review the basis of the Arab case including the Husain-McMahon Correspondence which, for the first time, was made public. A committee was established to evaluate the correspondence as it related to Palestine. Though this committee was not able to agree, the British government representative admitted that the Arab condition was found to be stronger than was thought before. The conference adjourned without having reached any agreement, and with both Jews and Arabs resolved to resist any limitation on their rights. The Arab rebellion continued in the hills of Palestine with covert and overt support from Arabs in surrounding countries. At the same time Jewish legal and illegal immigration was greatly accelerated.

To cope with the dilemma in which it found itself, the British government decided to issue a new statement of policy in which it proposed to adhere to *its* original contention that Palestine was not included in the area promised to the Arabs, but that neither was it the intent of the Balfour Declaration to convert Palestine into a Jewish state against the will of the Arab population. Therefore, the British government offered a plan whereby Palestine would, if possible, within ten years, be given representative institutions and a constitution. After five years Jewish immigration would cease, and Arab land sales would be permitted only within selected areas. The White Paper ended with a plea that both Jews and Arabs take note of the reverence "of many millions of Muslims, Jews and Christians throughout the world who pray for peace in Palestine and for the happiness of her people."

In Palestine the Jewish community was outraged. The transmission lines of the broadcasting station were cut so that announcement of the White Paper was delayed. Government offices were burned or sacked, police were stoned, and shops looted. The government thus found itself under attack from both the Arab and Jewish communities at once.

Meanwhile, in Europe the lights were dimming, and on September 1 the Second World War began with the march of the German army into Poland.

In Palestine reactions to the war were mixed as members of both communities rallied to support the British government against the Germans. Altogether some 21,000 Jews and 8000 Arabs served in branches of the British armed forces. However, both Jews and Arabs did maintain their opposition to the local government, and demonstrations and terrorist attacks never ceased throughout the war. Shortly after the immediate German threat to the Middle East was ended with the British victory at El Alamein in 1942, public manifestations of hostility increased. Members of the Stern Gang clashed with the police in a number of instances. On August 8, 1944, a Jewish attempt was made to assassinate the high commissioner, government installations were raided and looted, and the commander-in-chief of the British forces in the Middle East was moved to issue a communiqué pointing out that the "active and passive sympathizers of the terrorists are directly impeding the war effort of Great Britain and assisting the enemy." On November 6, 1944, the British minister of state resident in Cairo, Lord Moyne, was murdered by two members of the Stern Gang. In the late spring of 1945 the incidence of attacks on the government and on British army units greatly increased. Raids were made with great precision on arms dumps, banks, and communication facilities. As Europe emerged from the war, Palestine took up war in earnest.

As the full horror of the war in Europe and Nazi massive murder of Jews came to the public attention, the already critical situation was inevitably further inflamed in Palestine. The British government was blamed, because of the restrictions on immigration which followed the 1939 White Paper, for the death of hundreds of thousands of Jews who failed to escape from Europe.

With an unbroken record of failures in its attempts to settle the Palestine problem the British government asked the United States to participate in one further inquiry. The resulting Anglo-American committee of inquiry had as a key part of its terms of reference instructions to inquire into the *European* Jewish community's needs. So it was at the assembly points for the survivors of Nazi bestiality that the Anglo-American committee began its short life. The heart-rending tour was an emotional gauntlet for the committee members who eloquently described in the report "the depths of human suffering there endured."

In Palestine the committee found the observations of the royal commission to be valid, as valid in 1946 as in 1936. Hostility of the Arabs to Zionism was unanimous. The major difference between the two dates was the new and increasing power of the Jewish Agency with its unofficial army, the Haganah, then estimated at 60,000. The committee's description of Palestine will be recognized by all who saw it in these violent days. "Army tents, tanks, a grim fort and barracks overlook the waters of the Sea of Galilee. Blockhouses, road barriers manned by soldiers, barbed wire entanglements, tanks in the streets, pre-emptory searches, seizures and arrests on suspicion, bombings by gangsters and shots in the night are now characteristic."

While awaiting the report of the Anglo-American committee the government of Palestine had set the immigration quota at 1500 monthly and tightened up on penalties for armed attack, possession of firearms, and membership in terrorist groups. These police measures did little to calm the situation.

On the night of June 16 the paramilitary activity in Palestine became more concentrated as the commando group of the Haganah, the Palmach, destroyed nine bridges in different parts of the country. The next night the Stern Gang attacked railway installations in Haifa, and on the eighteenth the Irgun kidnapped six British army officers and held them as hostages. The government published a series of intercepted telegrams which showed that the Jewish Agency was involved in the activities of the terrorist groups as well as of its own army, the Haganah. On June 29 the government arrested a number of key figures in the Jewish Agency and occupied its headquarters long enough to seize a part of its files. Twenty-seven hundred people were arrested, of whom about seven hundred were detained after questioning. Most of the personnel of Palmach was included among those arrested, and large supplies of arms were discovered and seized by the British troops. In reprisal the Irgun blew up the King David Hotel, where the senior staff of the government of Palestine was housed, on July 22.

Meanwhile, in London, American and British officials discussed the possibility of solving the problem of Palestine in a way which went far beyond the cunning of Solomon. The proposal was to divide the Jews and Arabs into separate zones or provinces but to leave these provinces as autonomous members of one state. This was actually a contingency plan worked out some years before by the Colonial Office as a last resort. The plan was considered in London by representatives of the Arab states, who rejected it. Neither Palestine Jews nor Arabs even accepted the British government invitation to discuss the plan. The Arab position remained that Palestine should become an independent state ruled by its native majority with due protection for the rights of the minority. The Zionist position likewise was familiar: Palestine should be a Jewish commonwealth, open to Jewish immigration as controlled by the Jewish Agency.

As yet another attempt at compromise, the British government suggested in February 1947 that Palestine be administered for five years as a trusteeship with substantial local autonomy in areas with Jewish or Arab majorities, the protection of the minority being the responsibility of the British high commissioner, with provision for nearly 100,000 refugees to enter the country in the first two years. This proposal was rejected by both the Arabs (including the Arab Higher Committee) and the Jewish Agency. In these circumstances, failure, heavy expenditure of men and money, and what the British regarded as American irresponsibility—in 1946 both the Democratic and Republican parties attempted to win Jewish electoral support by declarations favoring mass immigration into Palestine—Britain decided to turn the problem over to the United Nations. Speaking in the House of Commons on February 18, 1947, Ernest Bevin said the government had "been faced with an irreconcilable conflict of principles. There are in Palestine about 1,200,000 Arabs and 600,000 Jews. For the Jews, the essential point of principle is the creation of a sovereign Jewish State. For the Arabs, the essential point of principle is to resist to the last the establishment of Jewish sovereignty in any part of Palestine. The discussions of the last month have quite clearly shown that there is no prospect of resolving this conflict by any settlement negotiated between the parties . . . We have, therefore, reached the conclusion that the only course now open to us is to submit the problem to the judgment of the United Nations . . . We shall then ask the United Nations . . . to recommend a settlement of the problem. We do not intend ourselves to recommend any particular solution."

The United Nations had previously taken official recognition of the problem of Palestine, in the Security Council and General Assembly, but it had not itself investigated the situation. On May 15, 1947, the General Assembly voted to create a Special Committee on Palestine (UNSCOP), to submit not later than September 1, 1947, "such proposals as it may consider appropriate for the solution of the problem of Palestine."

UNSCOP members arrived in Jerusalem on June 14. Once again the Arab Higher Committee showed itself inflexible by refusing to participate in the meetings of the special committee. The Arab states, however, did make their views known by repeating arguments they had previously advanced.

The Jewish Agency, to the contrary, cooperated in full with UNSCOP and provided its members with extensive documentation and appeals. Even the Irgun, then engaged in a game of hide-and-seek with the whole of the British forces in Palestine and not always on friendly terms with the Haganah, managed to hold a lengthy meeting with the chairman of the committee.

The committee found little that was different from what its predecessors had reported. It pointed out that Palestine was a small country and of its limited extent of somewhat over 10,000 square miles, only about half was inhabitable by settled people. although the country was principally agricultural—65 percent of the population gained a living directly from agriculture—some 50 percent of the cereals used by the population had to be imported. Palestine, it noted, "is exceedingly poor" in all of the resources needed for modern industry. The population was then 1,203,000 Arabs to 608,000 Jews or about 2 to 1. Since the Arab birth rate was much higher than the Jewish, by 1960 these figures would probably become by natural increase, if immigration were stopped, 1,533,000 to 664,000—or almost 5 to 2. Lastly, to complicate the problem of any sort of partition, UNSCOP found that there "is no clear territorial separation of Jews and Arabs by large contiguous areas." "Jews are more than 40 percent of the total population in the districts of Jaffa (which includes Tel-Aviv), Haifa and Jerusalem. In the northern inland areas of Tiberias and Beisan, they are between 25 and 34 percent of the total population. In the inland northern districts of Safad and Nazareth and the coastal districts of Tulkarm and Ramle, Jews form between 10 and 25 percent of the total population, while in the central districts and the districts south of Jerusalem they constitute not more than 5 percent of the total."

Unquestionably the problems involved in partition were great, yet the urgency of the problem was even greater than in the previous year. Some 17,873 illegal immigrants were under detention and 820 Palestinians were under arrest for security reasons; if anything the situation reported by the Anglo-American committee had worsened. "The atmosphere in Palestine today is one of profound tension . . . In the streets of Jerusalem and other key areas barbed wire defenses, road blocks, machine gun posts and constant armoured car patrols are routine measures. In areas of doubtful security, Administration officials and the military forces live within strictly policed security zones and work within fortified and closely-guarded buildings."

The British administration found that virtually its whole energies had to be devoted to public security and eventually, in all truth, to self-defense. "The right of any community to use force as a means of gaining its political ends is not admitted in the British Commonwealth. Since the beginning of 1945 the Jews have implicitly claimed this right and have supported by an organized campaign of lawlessness, murder and sabotage their contention that, whatever other interests might be concerned, nothing should be allowed to stand in the way of a Jewish State and free Jewish immigration into Palestine."

This being the situation, UNSCOP recommended that the mandate be terminated "at the earliest practicable date," that independence be granted, and that until independence the United Nations assume responsibility. It further recommended that the international community assume *its* responsibilities in assisting the 250,000 Jewish refugees assembled in Europe so as to relieve the pressure on Palestine. Finally the committee urged that whatever other divisions be made in Palestine, it be preserved as an economic unit. The majority of UNSCOP voted to approve a plan of partition with economic union. The states thus created would have the following populations: Arab state, 10,000 Jews and 725,000 Arabs and others; Jewish state, 498,000 Jews and 407,000 Arabs and others; internationalized district of Jerusalem, 100,000 Jews and 105,000 Arabs and others.

This was about the best UNSCOP felt it could do. The Arab state would contain a 1½ percent Jewish minority but the Jewish state would contain a 45 percent minority of Arabs (not including an estimated 90,000 bedouin). In the international zone there would be an almost 1 to 1 equality. The United Nations Secretariat estimated on the basis of past returns for the various districts of Palestine that the Jewish state would have a revenue three times larger than the Arab.

A minority of the committee—India, Iran, Yugoslavia—proposed that a federal state be created. The major motive behind this solution was to "avoid an acceleration of the separatism which now characterizes the relations of Arabs and Jews in the Near East, and to avoid laying the foundations of a dangerous irredentism there, which would be inevitable consequences of partition in whatever form." Moreover, the UNSCOP minority pointed out that the vast majority of both Jews and Arabs opposed partition. The Arab and Jewish states within the federal state should have full powers of self-government under the federal constitution. The boundaries suggested differed slightly from those proposed by the majority.

At the United Nations, before the proposals of UNSCOP were published, Soviet delegate Andrei Gromyko expressed the Russian position on the Palestine issue. He stressed the "bankruptcy of the mandatory system of administration of Palestine." In this he agreed (except, perhaps, in choice of words) with almost every observer of the problem from the royal commission onward. He then went on to support the "aspirations of the Jews to establish their own State." However, he agreed with the Arabs that the responsibility for this state of affairs was European, was due to the "fact that no western European State has been able to ensure the defense of the elementary rights of the Jewish people." Finally he supported the sort of dual state proposed in the minority UNSCOP report. The British and American delegates wanted to avoid discussing the possible solutions until the UNSCOP report was available and clearly wanted to avoid any approach to solution that might involve Russian entry into the Middle Eastern sphere.

When the UNSCOP proposals were published, the British government announced its intention to remove its military installations from the Palestine–Suez Canal area deep into central Africa, to an area which then seemed relatively quiet, Kenya. In effect, Britain was getting ready to wash its hands of Palestine. As desperately as everyone had wished this in the past, there was an immediate realization that such action would precipitate a grim and bloody struggle, that as violently condemned as the British had been, they had exercised the only existing restraint.

The Jewish Agency could be satisfied in having gained recognition of its early claim to independence and a much larger slice of territory than ever before offered, except in the limited "National Home" sense suggested in the Balfour Declaration. The Arabs felt that they had lost everything, and they publicly announced that they intended to resist the implementation of UNSCOP's proposals by force. The Egyptian newspaper *al-Ahram* predicted in September 1947 that "the Palestine Arabs will launch a relentless war to repel this attack on their country, especially as they know that all the Arab countries will back and assist them, supplying them with men, money, and ammunition."

The rival communities prepared for war, the Arabs in two—rival—paramilitary organizations neither of which proved to amount to much when tested. The Jews of course had large cadres of men who had served in the British army or the American army and air force during the war, and they already had standing, if concealed, armies in the Haganah, its Palmach elite corps, the Irgun, and the smaller Stern Gang. Quantities of equipment and ammunition were being seized from British stores and soon the Jewish purchasing agents were able to send into Palestine considerable amounts of American and Czech equipment.

At the United Nations both the United States and the Soviet Union supported partition, and by agreement, arrived at on November 10, decided that the British mandate should end May 1, 1948, and that the two states would be established by July 1. The British delegate announced that the British army would have evacuated the country by August 1, and that Britain would thereafter not participate in whatever efforts were made to police partition. When the General Assembly met on November 26, Sir Alexander Cadogan announced that Britain wanted to make quite certain that the General Assembly realized it could not count upon British forces to impose its decisions on either Jews or Arabs.

In the Middle East outside of Palestine itself, the growth of anti-Zionism among the Arabs had reached a fever pitch. Ugly demonstrations broke out in many points all over the Middle East. In points as widely scattered as Aden, Libya, and Baghdad a growing feeling of anger over Palestine which could not be expressed against the distant Palestine Jewish community was vented locally upon Jews who in most cases had little or no contact with Zionism. The Jewish communities in their turn recoiled in fear from the nations in which many of them had participated, often at the highest levels of government. This ugly situation in the ensuing months led to a large-scale migration from Iraq and Yemen which further increased the immigration pressure upon Palestine.

After study by various subcommittees and lengthy debates on the floor at the United Nations, a proposal was made to partition Palestine, in general according to UNSCOP's recommendations with minor frontier changes (the main feature being to include Jaffa within the Arab state). Finally on November 29 the partition proposal was passed by a vote of 33 to 13 with 10 abstentions. The end of the mandate was in sight.

In Palestine the Arabs managed to gain a semblance of unity by reverting to their 1936 model of local national committees. The first of these was established in Jaffa just before the United Nations voted partition. Arab attacks on Jews and Jewish settlements and Jewish reprisals and attacks on Arabs began at the end of November and rapidly gained in intensity. In January 1948 Arab volunteers from other states began to enter Palestine. The Arab leader of the 1936 revolt was again in Palestine with about 5000 volunteers in scattered and uncoordinated bands. The streets of all towns and many villages were already forests of barbed wire, and only the foolhardy and the combatants moved about at night.

As the British troops exposed themselves less and less and began to withdraw from remote positions, Arab bands raided settlements and even managed to cut the road from Tel Aviv to Jerusalem, but they soon showed they were no match for the Jewish military units. Both Jews and Arabs set up shadow governments by drawing on the personnel of the mandate government and their respective organizations. In the Jewish Agency, of course, the Jewish community had a ready-made government. The Arabs were more restricted in their experience. They never had an organization comparable to the Jewish Agency, and even their few leaders had been absent for a decade.

The day-to-day events in Palestine from December 1947 to May 1948 belie the arbitrary classifications of peace and war. There were 5000 casualties—one in every 350 people in the country—in this five-month period, and the damage to property may be estimated in the millions of dollars. In some days as many as fifty "incidents" were reported all over Palestine. Trains were blown up, banks robbed, government offices attacked, convoys ambushed, and mobs and gangs looted, burned, and clashed with troops or rival mobs.

The surrounding Arab states prepared for war, and their presses proclaimed in lurid and strident tones that they would resist to the death the UN decision. However, on March 21, the political committee of the Arab League unexpectedly made a bid for a compromise peace. It decided to insist that the original British proposal, which the American government was also considering, be enforced. This would have put Palestine under a temporary trusteeship. The committee further urged that the Jews then on Cyprus be accepted into the several Arab states as immigrants and that those in Palestine be assured of their rights as a minority in an Arab state. If the proposal was in earnest, it was certainly too little and too late. Psychologically no one could retreat, least of all the Arab governments.

On the surface the Arabs appeared infinitely stronger. After all, the whole Arab world was publicly pledged to intervene in the war. Egypt, Iraq, Syria, Lebanon, and Transjordan all had standing armies and were receiving surplus British or French equipment. Public enthusiasm, especially among students and the middle class, was high. Yet, it was already evident how weak the Arab governments were. None of the governments was "popular" in its own home, and subsequent events proved that corruption was not only prevalent but existed to such an extent as to all but incapacitate most of the Arab forces. The army commands proved inefficient particularly in logistics but lacked initiative in tactics as well. The troops were poorly trained and often poorly led. And finally, even in dire need, the Arab governments proved that their jealousies and personal quarrels were of much more importance to them than their declared interest in Palestine. None of the Arabs, Palestinian or other, except the Arab Legion of Transjordan, could begin to match the level of technical competence of the Jewish forces. Moreover, among the Arabs of Palestine they found little support. These had been virtually leader-less since 1938 and had never really recovered from their rebellion of 1936–38. By the end of the mandate, they had become terror-ized, psychologically defeated mobs, fleeing in all directions.

Early in April the pattern of events began to assume some shape. British forces had been steadily pulling out of the country. The March 20 statement by the Secretary General of the Arab League, that the Arabs would accept a truce and limited trustee-ship for Palestine if the Jewish Agency would agree, was rejected out of hand by David Ben-Gurion "for even the shortest time." Fighting raged over most of Palestine. On March 27 Jewish air-craft had begun to participate in the fighting for the first time. Then on April 8 the most active and popular Arab leader, Abd el-Qadir Huseini (who was then chief of the Arab national guard) was killed. On April 10 the Irgun with the help of the Haganah attacked and took the village of Deir Yasin. After the Haganah left, the Irgun, in a deliberate attempt to promote terror among the general Arab population, massacred all the village in-habitants and widely publicized its action. Arab attacks on settle-ments and Jewish areas began to be beaten off and on April 15 the Haganah launched a major counterattack against the main Arab army under Fawzi el-Qawaqchi. From then on the Arab forces began to fail in their attempts and to assume the defensive. On April 19 the Haganah took Tiberias as the British evacuated its Arab population. April 21 saw the Irgun and Haganah offen-sive on Haifa, which surrendered and was evacuated by the Arab population. Early in May Jaffa was declared an open city under Haganah control, and on May 14 the Haganah captured Acre. Staggering from these defeats, Arabs were pouring out of the country by every road. On May 14 in the afternoon at Tel Aviv, David Ben-Gurion proclaimed the establishment of the State of Israel.

The mandate had ended.

XII. Formal Independence: A Short Flight on Fledgling Wings

The end of World War II marked the close of a period of overt and covert guidance and restraint by the West and the emergence of the Arab states into the community of nations. On the surface this statement is simple enough. However, the precise definition of the time framework and the realities of power which lie behind it pose the key issues of Arab politics of the last generation.

Though no part of the Arabian Peninsula was under Western domination or tutelage, the entire economic life of that area was financed, managed, and developed according to the decisions of the international petroleum industry, and rightly or wrongly—in scorn or envy—Arabs then as now ascribe to that area something less than full independence. More significant and more measurable, however, was the Western impact on the political history of the other, more advanced, and more populated Arab states.

Egypt, which had been declared a protectorate at the outbreak of World War I, entered into a treaty with Great Britain in 1922 which gave it formal independence with four "absolutely reserved" areas of British control. In 1936 this treaty was revised so that Egypt got more independence of action, and in 1937 she joined the League of Nations. However, British troops remained in Egypt, and from the perspective of Egyptians they were the trump card which made the British the final arbiters of Egyptian affairs. In 1942 the British did, *in extremis*, use their military power to impose upon the Egyptians a prime minister of their choosing. At the end of World War II Egypt finally declared war on the Axis, joined the United Nations, and got the British to agree to withdraw their troops from Cairo and to restrict their military presence to the Suez Canal Zone. It was not until 1954 that the bulk of the British troops withdrew from the Suez Canal, and in 1956 the British and French made an effort forcibly to re-enter Egyptian affairs.

In Iraq the story was similar with a few changes in dates and names. After a costly attempt to rule Iraq as a province, loosely attached to the Indian empire, the British organized a national government in 1921, installed a more or less popular monarch of their choosing, and accepted a mandate from the League of Nations. The mandate was, however, so unpopular in Iraq that while maintaining it vis-á-vis the League Great Britain negotiated a treaty in 1922 in which Iraq's special status was recognized. In 1930 a new treaty was negotiated which gave to Iraq sufficient independence for it to join the League of Nations in 1932. The British continued to maintain garrisons there. These made no attempt to intervene in the political unrest of the mid-1930's, but when in 1941 a pro-Axis government came to power, the British and their Arab allies invaded the country to replace the government with one composed of Britain's friends. Iraq declared war on the Axis in 1943 and joined the United Nations. An attempt to negotiate a new treaty in 1946 (the Portsmouth Treaty) led to an outbreak of riots in Baghdad. The treaty was dropped, but behind the shield of the monarchy and the astute political leadership of Nuri Said, British interests remained safe. As Iraq joined the Baghdad Pact in 1955, the British relinquished more of the form of their special position.

Transjordan, which had been separated from the Palestine mandate in 1922 and placed under the rule of Amir Abdullah, remained a client state of Britain. In 1946 it was declared independent but was in fact dependent upon Britain for financial support and for the leadership of its army. Growing resentment at the recognition of this dependence led to the ousting of Glubb Pasha, the British general who commanded the Arab Legion from

1939 to 1956 and to attempts to find other sources of revenue, including Egypt and Saudi Arabia and, after the failure of these, the United States.

Lebanon, which had benefited from French favor in 1920, when its area was multiplied in size, became in that year a French mandate. In 1926 it was given a constitution, but this was amended twice and suspended in 1932. After a period of direct French rule the Lebanese government was restored but with strictly limited powers. The constitution was reestablished in 1937. The period before and immediately after the outbreak of war saw French power retained but operating behind a façade of Lebanese political activity. Then, following the Franco-German armistice in June 1940, Lebanon and Syria went under the Vichy government, and a year later both were invaded by a British–Free French military force. At that time Lebanese independence was promised, and this promise was repeated and reaffirmed in various forms until in 1945 when the British ordered the French to evacuate their military forces. At that point Lebanon joined the United Nations.

In Syria the story parallels that of Lebanon, but the actions were at each stage considerably more bitter. Syria was not augmented by the French in 1920 but rather was invaded and then divided into a collection of petty states. In 1924–25 the Druze and others revolted against French rule, and the French retaliated by bombing villages and shelling Damascus on two separate occasions, in October 1925 and May 1926. In 1928 a constituent assembly was convened in Damascus, and the constitution was put into effect in 1930 but suspended in 1932. In 1936 Syria was rent by a general strike, attended by considerable violence and national agitation, which the French met with an attempt to negotiate a treaty, patterned on those the British had made in Iraq and Egypt. If concluded, this would have made Syria a member of the League of Nations with certain military facilities left in French hands. But the French government refused to ratify the treaty.

Syria, like Lebanon, was invaded by the British and Free French forces in 1941 and received the same assurances of inde-

pendence. Continued delays in the implementation of these assurances created an atmosphere of smoldering resentment which
burst into flame in May 1945 when, after a general strike and
sporadic outbursts of violence, the French shelled and bombed
Damascus and other Syrian cities. On June 1, 1945, the British
ordered the French to cease all military actions and to withdraw
all their forces. Syria at last achieved de facto independence
which was symbolized by participation in the San Francisco
Conference of the United Nations.

As a move toward the realization of the generally held aspira-
tion of Arab unity, the Arab states, with the encouragement of
Great Britain, in 1945 formed the Arab League. Actually, as
early as May 29, 1941, alarmed by the pro-German activities of
the Iraqi government, Anthony Eden, in a widely publicized
speech at Mansion House, encouraged the Arabs to look to
Britain as a friend of Arab unity aspirations. "This country has
a long tradition of friendship with the Arabs . . . It seems to me
both natural and right the cultural and economic ties between
the Arab countries, and the political ties too, should be strengthened. His Majesty's Government for their part will give their
full support to any scheme that commands general approval."
Taking up this encouragement, Nahhas Pasha as leader of the
Wafd and Prime minister of Egypt spoke of "the bonds which
bind us to the Arab and Eastern peoples [as] many beyond
numbering and strong beyond sundering . . . with Egypt in the
forefront [they will build] a powerful and cohesive bloc." Somewhat later, in January 1943, in announcing the Iraqi declaration
of war on the Axis, toward which, as the enemy of Britain, many
Iraqis were still sympathetic, Prime Minister Nuri Said proposed
the formation of a new state, composed of Syria, Lebanon, Transjordan, and Palestine—"Greater Syria"—with which Iraq would
join to form an Arab League. Finally, after consultations and
negotiations among all of the Arab leaders, delegates of the several Arab states and the Palestine Arab community met in September 1944 at Alexandria and agreed to form a League of Arab
States.

Thus, it may be said that the end of World War II marked a real beginning of independence and self-assertion in the Arab countries. With the departure or the formal "nationalization" of the military and paramilitary forces which had been created in the mandate states, national governments had more real power but also accepted more real responsibility than ever before.

At this point the old objects of national struggle became irrelevant: little merit attached to anti-French activity in Syria when the French had departed. A single new issue of nationalism took the center of the Arab stage, an issue for which all of the Arab governments eagerly sought responsibility and to which they turned all of their suppressed energy and ardor of nationalism. That issue was Palestine.

Not only through the Arab League, whose attentions were largely devoted to the Palestine problem during the immediate postwar period, but singly each Arab government became deeply involved in the issue in consultation with the British government, at the United Nations forums, and in virtually every public media in the Arab countries. Even the religious leaders of the Mosque-University of al-Azhar declared a Holy War. An irregular "Arab Liberation Army," financed and condoned by the Arab governments, of some six or seven thousand men, infiltrated into the Palestine mandate. As the mandate drew to a violent close, the Arab radio and press publicized the plight of the Palestine Arab community, particularly the massacre at Dair Yassin in which almost the entire village population was killed, and thereby stimulated Arabs everywhere to demand action by their governments.

On May 14, 1948, when the mandate ended, the Arab governments had to try to implement their decision to intervene. However, no government was really prepared to act. The most effective force, that of Transjordan, consisted of only four battalions with very little ammunition or other supplies and was under the command of British officers. It had virtually no logistical base or transport. The other Arab armies were ill-equipped and ill-trained. Their commands, moreover, were timid and mutually antagonistic. The governments behind them were suspicious of one another. The Egyptians, fearing King Abdullah's ambition to take over Palestine, deliberately took action to undercut Transjordanian effectiveness by seizing military supplies destined for Transjordan.

Military forces of Egypt, Transjordan, Syria, Lebanon, and Iraq were sent to Palestine. After a month of fighting the Arab states agreed to a truce which the United Nations undertook to monitor. This period, which lasted just a month, was used to bolster the fighting capacities of both forces, but truly herculean efforts on the part of the Israelis enabled them to emerge at the end of the truce far stronger than they were before. However, the public announcements by the Arab governments led their peoples to expect an early victory and the Arab governments refused to extend the truce.

Fighting broke out again on July 8 but the Arab armies were hopelessly disorganized and had no common plan of action. Israeli forces used the next ten days before the second truce greatly to enlarge their area of occupation. During the truce itself, an "Arab Government of All Palestine" was proclaimed in September, recognized by all the Arab governments except Transjordan, which organized a rival "National Congress." The open split between the governments of Kings Farouk and Abdullah encouraged the Israeli military command to concentrate all their strength against the Egyptian forces, and after winning air superiority the Israelis captured the southern area of the former mandate in October. Yet another cease-fire was proclaimed on October 22 in the south, but on that day fighting which spilled over into Lebanese territory broke out in the north. Meanwhile Abdullah had been declared by his supporters to be King of Palestine, and this led to violent reactions in the other Arab countries. Again the Israelis hit the Egyptians on December 22 and penetrated Egyptian territory.

In Cairo public outcries, at first directed against foreigners, quickly turned against the government whose ineffectiveness, despite propaganda and censorship efforts, had become clear. On

December 28 a member of the militant Muslim Brotherhood assassinated the prime minister. At this point, seeing that hostilities threatened its interests, Great Britain announced that it would invoke the 1936 treaty to intervene unless Israel withdrew her forces from Egyptian territory and some stability were achieved in Egypt. The Egyptian government wished to avoid British intervention above all, and notified the United Nations that it was prepared to discuss an armistice.

Armistice agreements were negotiated bilaterally between the Israelis and the *separate* Arab countries in the early months of 1949. In the midst of the negotiations the Iraqi government withdrew its forces and so exposed the Transjordanian forces' flank; consequently the Transjordanian government, under threat of a resumption of the war, was forced to cede to Israel additional territory. The Syrian government was unable seriously to undertake armistice negotiations until April, when the others had been concluded, due first to violent public demonstrations leading to a fall of the government and then to a military coup. The latter almost caused Iraqi and Jordanian military intervention in Syria and further split the Arab governments.

The fact, however dressed up or explained, was simply that the Arab states were beaten in the Palestine War.

Fairly uniformly, there was the realization that below the façade of government and authority little real power existed. "But how could this be" was the implicit question behind the outpourings of the critics. The governments of the Arabs who created Islam, who conquered half the world, whose caliphate shone with the bright glow of civilization while Europe slept in the ignorance of the Dark Ages, and whose vast corpus of literature and rich language were admired all over the world, were spotlighted as impotent, backward, corrupt bombasts. The shock of this discovery created a trauma from which Arabic society suffered for a decade. Many sought excuses—the governments, mere puppets left behind in the wake of imperialism were rotten; the arms furnished the Arab armies were worthless; Israel was a front for a combine of the great powers and of course the Arabs were not able to defeat this combine. Radio propaganda warfare, with each state blaming the "other" Arabs for the defeat in Palestine, started in late 1948 and was increased in violence in 1949. Since then it has been a regular feature of the Middle Eastern scene. Many Arabs blamed the West: Israel was the "last stage" of imperialism, was the stepchild of the West, was the way Westerners, shamed by the horrors of the Nazi "final solution," sought to repay the Jews (at the expense of the Arabs), and so forth.

Other Arabs sought the causes in more complex problems of Arab society and politics. A bitter critic of the failure of the Arabs, the former ambassador of Syria to the United States and president of the National University in Damascus, Constantine Zurayq, wrote immediately after the events in 1949, in *The Meaning of the Disaster,* "Seven Arab states declare war on Zionism in Palestine, stop impotent before it, and then turn on their heels. The representatives of the Arabs deliver fiery speeches in the highest international forums, warning what the Arab states and peoples will do if this or that decision be enacted. Declarations fall like bombs from the mouths of officials at the meetings of the Arab League, but when action becomes necessary, the fire is still and quiet, the steel and iron are rusted and twisted, quick to bend and disintegrate. The bombs are hallow and empty. They cause no damage and kill no one." Equally bitter was the statement by the Palestinian Musa Alami, who had helped to found the Arab League, "In the face of the enemy the Arabs were not a state, but petty states; groups, not a nation; each fearing and anxiously watching the other and intriguing against it. What concerned them most and guided their policy was not to win the war and save Palestine from the enemy, but what would happen after the struggle, who would be predominant in Palestine, or annex it to themselves, and how they could achieve their own ambitions. Their announced aim was the salvation of Palestine, and they said that afterward its destiny should be left to its people. This was said with the tongue only. In their hearts all wished it for themselves; and most of them were hurrying to prevent their neighbors from being predominant, even though nothing remained except the offal and bones."*

* *Middle East Journal,* 3(1949):385.

Most Arabs found it hard to disagree and the press was filled with bitter reproach against the Arab governments. In an oft-quoted passage, from his *Philosophy of the Revolution*, Gamal Abdul Nasser later wrote: "In Palestine I met only friends that shared the work for Egypt, but there I also discovered the thoughts that shed their light on the road ahead. I remember the days I spent in trenches pondering over our problems. Falougha was then beseiged and the enemy had concentrated his guns and aircraft heavily and terribly upon it. Often have I said to myself, 'here we are in these underground holes besieged. How we were cheated into a war unprepared and how our destinies have been the plaything of passions, plots and greed. Here we lay under fire unarmed.' As I reached that stage in my thinking my feelings would suddenly jump across the battlefront, across frontiers to Egypt. I found myself saying, 'What is happening in Palestine is but a miniature picture of what was happening in Egypt. Our Mother-Country has been likewise besieged by difficulties as well as ravaged by an enemy. She was cheated and pushed to fight unprepared. Greed, intrigue and passion have toyed with it and left it under fire.' "

The events of the period from the winter of 1948, when it was obvious that the war was lost, onward make clear how widespread was the feeling of malaise in the Arab world. To take Egypt as an example: On November 9 an attempt was made to kill former prime minister Nahhas; on November 13 the printing plant of the major European-language Egyptian newspapers was blown up; on November 28 the leaders of the Muslim Brotherhood were arrested; and on the same day police opened fire on a demonstration in a provincial city; on December 4 the Cairo chief of police was killed by a hand grenade; on December 28 the prime minister was assassinated; and on February 12 the leader of the Muslim Brotherhood was killed. Riots, attempted bombings, and threats were almost daily occurrences. Minor episodes were the divorce by the unloved King Farouk of his popular wife and the bitter, degrading, but revealing fight in the Egyptian parliament over passage of Egypt's first progressive income tax in February 1949.

The first government to collapse, however, was not in Egypt but in Syria where on March 30, 1949, a Kurdish colonel seized power in a bloodless and rapid coup. In all likelihood the coup was "popular" since the public was sick of the failures and ashamed of the weakness of the old regime. But the Syrian parliament refused to legalize the new government and was dismissed. Dismissal of a discredited parliament was not enough and the new government could not build a base of popular support; on August 14, in his turn, the colonel was arrested, tried, and shot by another military clique. The ensuing government was greeted with less warmth than apathy by the Syrian public. This government, in turn, was overthrown by an army lieutenant colonel on December 19, 1950.

Egypt in January 1950 held general elections, won by the Wafd party, which had been out of office during the Palestine War and which now promised a program of basic reforms. Education in particular was to be brought to the whole people as never before, but the government also promised to modernize the army and industrialize the country. These were bold programs and deeply stirred the Egyptian public, for the Wafd, despite many tales of corruption, still had a powerful organization and, comparatively, some luster of its nationalist days in the 1920's.

Recognition that more was wrong with Arab society than a government, or a collection of governments, was made manifest in the United Nations–sponsored conference on social welfare in Cairo in November 1950. Explicit was the notion that poverty and backwardness were direct results of structural defects in Arab society, and implicit was the notion that governments could act to remedy these if they had the will and the intelligence. Titles of many of the papers given at the conference centered on "How should a . . . project" be undertaken or "The practical steps which can be undertaken."

In concluding the conference its chairman, the Egyptian minister of social affairs, said: "This [giving of needed social services and raising the standard of living of the mass of the population] is their right from the State. The time is passed in which social services were rendered as a form of charity. The responsibility of the States has developed; it is no longer confined to matters of order, security, defence and the like, but its prime duty is to secure the welfare of its people, by providing possibilities of employment and adequate wages for a decent living, together with social services including education, medical care, suitable housing, and so forth . . . This is the prime responsibility of the States." This admission, not particularly important in itself, was typical of many which all of the Arab governments made either explicitly as here or implicitly in beginning programs of development as Iraq did in 1950.

Once made, the admission of responsibility, and possibility, raised further questions: If development is, in fact, possible and if the well-being of the citizenry is the "prime responsibility of the States," then does not the blame for past weakness, misery, lack of development, and humiliation fall upon those same states? If development is possible now, was it not possible before? And if it is now possible, is it not possible faster and more fundamentally? Is the development going to be real or merely the subject of wordy conferences? Can it be carried out by parliaments which represent those groups in society—landlords and tribal shaikhs—most firmly and obviously opposed to change? These were the questions of political discussion in the press, where it was free, in the army officers' messes, the coffee houses, and in every gathering of students.

As if in partial answer to the feelings behind such questions, the Wafd government had passed in July 1950 a law making journalists liable to a year in prison and a fine for publishing even innocent information on the biggest Egyptian landlord, the royal family, without government consent. Censorship, fear of confiscation or retaliatory action, caused the press to moderate its attacks, except on the "fair game"—governments in neighboring states. But throughout the area discontent was seething. No one who visited Egypt could miss it. As Sir Malcolm Darling wrote in the Manchester *Guardian* on December 7, 1950, "In the village ignorance may not be bliss, but it is some protection against discontent. Now, however, a new wind blows. With the greatly increased facilities of communication and the steady if very gradual spread of education the seed of new ideas, of new hopes, is carried from town to village. Ignorance of the outer world is no longer universal, but almost universal poverty remains. Herein lies the danger. Poverty and ignorance can lie down more or less happily together, but not poverty and education. That nowadays is likely to be an explosive mixture."

The peasants, themselves, did nothing to overturn the regime, but in the ruling class a split rapidly became manifest. The students, as they often had, led the revolt. Street demonstrations were common during this period, and the government retaliated by cracking down on the students. The Wafd government, originally a product and benefactor of student violence, imposed fines and jail sentences on anyone who incited students to demonstrate. Even professional men had to be banned from striking. By suppression of legitimate protest and itself stimulating the desires of the people for reform, the government contributed to the rise of violence. By December 1950 the press reported agitation in the army of a group known as "The Free Officers."

Meanwhile, the Egyptian government proved unable to win any concessions from the British government on a revision of the 1936 treaty, but encouraged the activity of paramilitary groups against the British army in the Suez Canal Zone. When the British refused Egyptian demands, however, the government turned on those who had supported its anti-British program.

Caught between its own nationalist propaganda, its weakness in dealing with the British forces, and the militancy of its own people, the Egyptian government faltered and fumbled from one mistake to another. While continuing its violent verbal attacks on the British, it ordered the police to fire on demonstrators who repeated its slogans and closed schools and universities where the agitation was carried on. Encouraging a belief that reform was possible and publicly condemning senior officers of the army and even members of the royal family for corruption in supplying faulty arms to the Egyptian forces in the Palestine War, it failed to produce any tangible results of reform or progress.

In July 1951 King Abdullah of Jordan was assassinated by a Palestinian Arab in Jerusalem. This was an act of violence which ripped away the already thin and tattered veil of kingship which had held at least some of the rulers aloof from the sorry plight of their peoples and what an increasing number of army officers and students regarded as the sordid gluttony of the politicians. Revealed were weak men with tarnished scepters. At once they were pulled knee-deep into the muck of corruption and intrigue.

Finally, on January 26, 1952, "Black Friday," anti-Western and anti-privileged-class mobs raced through Cairo, burning, pillaging, and killing. Among the casualties was the world-famous Shepheard's Hotel in Cairo. The Wafd government fell, only to be replaced by a series of weak and less popular teams of ministers. Just hours after the last of these was announced, the army led by the "Free Officers" seized power on July 23, arrested many senior officials, and forced King Farouk to abdicate and leave the country.

XIII. Coups, Conflicts, and Conferences

The coup of July 23, 1952, in Egypt was an event of the greatest significance in the Arab countries. Even at its inception, it was viewed by other Arabs as qualitatively different from the coups which had punctuated Iraqi politics in the 1930's or Syrian politics in 1948–50. To many it seemed, from its beginnings, the most needed reform—total abolition of the old regime—before real progress could be made.

In a mood of jubilation other Arabs demanded revolution *à l'Egyptienne*. Even in Lebanon, where cooler heads have created a tradition of commercial shrewdness since the time of the Phoenicians, editorials called for a "complete revolution" which would sweep away the past and all its memories, to bring immediately power, progress, and above all dignity. Plagued by scandals of truly epic proportions, threatened by general strikes, and not supported by the army, the president of Lebanon resigned on September 19, 1952. The chief of staff of the army became prime minister *ad interim*, and a new president was elected by the Chamber of Deputies on September 23. In Lebanon, however, the army refused to stay in politics; in fact, so quickly was power turned back to civilian politicians that the new president had to come to terms with the very forces and vested interests, as represented in the parliament, he presumably had come to office to supplant. The poisonous plant of discontent, so vigorous in the

Lebanon of 1952, was pruned but not extirpated; it was to grow again and to bear the bitter fruit of civil war in 1958.

In Iraq, meanwhile, the process of development had begun under the development board formed in 1950. The rather sudden infusion into the economy of massive oil royalties, as both production and profits soared in the early 1950's, produced a shock to the whole society. The vista of a real and proximate new world seemed to open ahead. Everything appeared ready to sail forward on a wave of change. Yet, the current was neither uniform nor rapid enough to suit many.

Young women, held apart from society more strictly than their cousins in the Levant or Egypt, suddenly emerged into educated society. They, like their brothers, began to win government fellowships for study abroad, and they were "liberated" from the long black gown, the *abba*, which had symbolized their confinement and social disability. But the end of confinement, in some spheres, led to great emotional stress, to the accentuation of a sense of doubt, loneliness, frustration, and fear which haunted and distorted Iraqi intellectual life in the 1950's. In the spring of 1952 a young Iraqi woman was expelled from her college for writing a short story depicting a young woman's hunger for meaning in a time of "tasteless emptiness" in which an "ignorant, leaderless people" still clung to "crippling and immoral social mores."

Similarly, the Iraqi young men returning from long periods of education abroad ran head-on into the roadblocks of Iraqi society and bureaucracy. The backward Iraq to which they returned both embarrassed them and spurned them. They were prevented from putting into effect their new learning and felt themselves to be aliens in their own homes. A best seller in those years was an Arabic translation of Turgenev's *Father and Sons*, which was set in a Russia of comparable anguish and dislocation. But, in the early 1950's the number of able, energetic, and uncommitted people in Iraq was very small; by the end of the decade it had become powerful. In 1951–52, for example, Iraq had only five native mechanical engineers, but so many of Iraq's more able people were abroad studying that by 1958 it had over a hundred mechanical engineers. Changes of proportional magnitude were in train in all the professions and in other parts of the society as well.

Movement and change were "in the air" in Baghdad. At first each individual rushed headlong toward a better future. There was no focus to the obvious discontent. Times were clearly better. But the "new men" of Iraq were cramped by the contrast of a potential future and an actual present. It was only as the government got more efficient and devoted more resources to the development program that its end was hastened. The irony of Iraq lies precisely in this fact: Iraq had the resources and the capital and was developing the people for the inevitable over-throw of the government. If it had none of these, the old regime might still exist.

The government, however, was led by a wise and experienced stalwart, trained in the Ottoman army, who had fought in the Arab Revolt, who had weathered many a storm and three times fled for his life from (and returned to vanquish) more powerful enemies than what he regarded as mere children of some educa-tion. This was Nuri Said who ruled Iraq with a sure hand. Even his enemies respected him, and so popular—or so accepted—was he that his most bitter opponents admitted that he would have won even a free election. He knew what he wanted and how to get it. But Nuri's government was creating a new Iraq in which he and men of the old school would have no place. Great eco-nomic and social change was unmatched in political life, which, like a dam, held back the forces of protest. Pressures built steadily until 1958.

The military officers who had engineered the coup in Egypt in July 23, 1952, were clearly unsure what to do with their power. They *were* sure they had to destroy the power of the monarchy and so forced King Farouk to abdicate and leave the country within a few days. It was eleven months, however, before the monarchy was formally abolished. The relationship of the older politicians to the new order was more open-ended. First the government was entrusted to a "clean" politician of the old regime, but the officers also moved to destroy both public recognition of the old elite, by abolishing titles connected with the monarchy, and the base of its power, the ownership of huge tracts of fertile, irrigated lands along the Nile. On September 7 the army took over formal power as General Nagib, the figurehead of the "Free Officers," became prime minister. Most of the ministers, however, were civilian, and as late as March 1954 the officers were still flirting with a return to civilian rule.

It appears clear, in retrospect, that the Free Officers really did not have any precise notion of the structure of the new Egypt they sought. They wanted to abolish much of the old structure, but just how much was determined more by the events of the first two years after they seized power than by any preconceived ideas. For example, it appears that the land distribution program was suggested to the Free Officers *after* the coup as a popular move, one needed for any real progress in the country and the sure way to sap the foundations of their potential opponents, the men of the old order. They did not seize power to carry out land reform, but having seized power set about learning what they could do to improve their chances of staying in power and of uplifting the country. Similar was their attitude toward civilian politicians. It was not until the Muslim Brotherhood militants had tried to assassinate Gamal Abdul Nasser on October 26, 1954, that rival political groups began to be suppressed. And in pressing to get the Sudan recognized as a part of Egypt and to get the British to evacuate Egypt, the new government was carrying forward, more vigorously perhaps, policies espoused by Egyptian governments for over half a century and in other forms for time out of mind of man.

Nasser has suggested that he never thought his group would have to build a new regime, but that he conceived of his job as one of destroying the old. In his *Philosophy of the Revolution* he speaks bluntly of his "shock," "sorrow," and "bitterness" at the lack of support for the coup. "Prior to that date I imagined that the whole nation was on tip-toes and prepared for action, that it awaited the advance of the vanguard and the storming of the outside walls for it to pour down in a solid phalanx marching faithfully to the great goal . . . After July 23rd I was shocked by the reality. The vanguard performed its task; it stormed the walls of the fort of tyranny; it forced Farouk to abdicate and stood by expecting the mass formations to arrive at their ultimate object. It waited and waited. Endless crowds showed up, but how different is the reality from the vision! The multitudes that arrived were dispersed followers . . . We needed discipline but found chaos behind our lines. We needed unity but found dissensions. We needed action but found nothing but surrender and idleness . . . Personal and persistent selfishness was the rule of the day. The word 'I' was on every tongue."

It is not really necessary to question whether or not the military had always intended to retain power: even if they wished to turn it back to another group, the Free officers could hardly have done so safely, for having seized the tiger by the tail they had to hang on or be eaten themselves. The question was not whether to retain power but who would exercise it and for what ends. This brought to the surface a power struggle between General Nagib and Lieutenant Colonel Nasser which involved the army, the Muslim Brotherhood, and civilian politicians. Ultimately, after much covert and some overt struggle and maneuver, Nagib was ousted from power and placed under house arrest on November 1, 1954. But the regime was still very far from having an established and agreed policy on domestic issues. Up to that time its energies had largely been absorbed in consolidating power.

The most emotion-laden and popularly watched if not important issue with which the new regime had dealt grew out of its relations with Great Britain. When the British evacuated Cairo in 1945–6, the bulk of their forces, at times as large as 80,000 men, moved to bases in the area of the Suez Canal. Successive Egyptian governments tried to get them to leave Egypt but to no avail. Appeals to the United Nations were unsuccessful. As we have seen, the inability of the last series of precoup governments to satisfy nationalist goals, in large part stimulated by the same governments, was a major factor in their being discredited. After lengthy negotiations the new government achieved this aim in the October 1954 Anglo-Egyptian treaty. By April 14, 1956, the British had evacuated the last of their Suez installations.

The regime was less successful in its attempt to reunite the Sudan and Egypt. The importance of the Sudan to Egypt had long been recognized: it was the conduit through which the Nile River passed and from which Egypt historically derived cheap labor. The Sudan was conquered by the forces of Mehmet Ali Pasha in 1821 and indifferently ruled until it revolted in 1881. When the British came to Egypt, they and the Egyptians reconquered the Sudan in the battle of Omdurman in 1898. After 1899, when it was administratively separated from Egypt, the Sudan was ruled as an Anglo-Egyptian Condominium. Reacting to the nationalist agitation following World War I, when Sir Lee Stack was assassinated in Cairo, the British almost totally excluded the Egyptians from participation in the Sudanese government.

Thus, while Egyptian cultural contacts, particularly through the spread of Islamic teaching from Cairo's Azhar Mosque-University, remained strong, the Sudan began to develop a separate system of administration, to deal directly with Great Britain, and to achieve some sense of separate national identity. Economic activity was sparked by the creation of a rich cotton-growing agricultural area at the confluence of the Blue and White Niles. This brought a degree of prosperity to the Sudan but raised two problems in Sudanese-Egyptian relations: was the amount of water taken from the Nile for use in the Sudan harmful to Egyptian agriculture and was the amount of cotton grown in the Sudan a threat to Egyptian exports. These issues were debated regularly in the press and in various intergovernmental conferences up to 1952 when Britain decided to allow the Sudanese self-determination.

At that time the Egyptians made a determined effort to woo the Sudanese into a union with Egypt. The British and the Egyptians agreed to allow the Sudanese to elect a provisional government which would, after a three-year period, decide whether or not to join Egypt. It is easy to see why this was a serious tactical mistake for the Egyptians: once the Sudanese had tasted the sweet fruit of self-government, they were unwilling to give it up.

Syria also was unable to achieve a sense of identity or national cohesion. The sequence of coups of 1959 was followed by an interlude in which a civilian government served as a façade for military power. Then Lieutenant Colonel Adib Shashakli openly took power in December 1951, became president in July 1953, only to be ousted from power in February 1954. A civilian government returned to office but the real nature of its power was probably only the relative exhaustion of the many rivals.

Whether Syria was to be an independent state, a part of "Greater Syria," in union with Iraq and/or Jordan, or ultimately a part of the United Arab Republic was a question for which Syrians found no answer in the 1950's and which is still under debate.

The issue which pointed this up most clearly was the Western attempt, particularly from 1953 to 1955, to get the Arab World into an area defense pact. Following the Korean War the United States sought to forge a "shield" of interlocking alliances from Europe to the Far East. It was United States policy to encourage its allies to take the leadership wherever possible in forging these alliances. Since the Middle East was an area of British influence and expertise, Britain's advice and leadership were sought. In British thinking Egypt was the center of military power. Britain's base at Suez contained the major military facilities for the whole area. Therefore, Britain sought, as early as 1951, to bring Egypt into an alliance. But London was unwilling to meet Egyptian demands on the Sudan and the weak and corrupt government of Nahhas Pasha could not compromise on this issue.

American thinking on Middle Eastern defense turned increasingly to what came to be called "the Northern tier," Greece, Turkey, and Iran. This resulted in United States military assistance programs and bilateral military pacts between Turkey and Pakistan in the spring of 1954. At that time the United States began giving military aid to Iraq, but the suggestion that Iraq might join such a pact was strongly attacked by Egypt. Throughout the summer of 1954 it appeared that Egypt might, itself, be receptive to some sort of alliance with Turkey, but her incentive was sharply reduced when Britain, unilaterally, agreed to withdraw from Suez. By December it was clear that Egypt was opposed to other members of the Arab League joining any Western-oriented military pact.

In Iraq, however, the motivations of the government were quite different. Nuri Said, whether in the government or working behind the scenes, was firmly committed to a pro-Western orientation. Iraq, moreover, had begun to benefit by United States military assistance and was on the eve of its great "leap forward" through the development plan, with which it needed Western help. Iraq had its "Suez" also. It sought to get the British to terminate the 1930 Anglo-Iraqi treaty. Great Britain agreed to do this if Iraq joined in an open-ended collective security pact with Turkey. So in February 1955 the Baghdad Pact was born, and in April Britain terminated the 1930 treaty. This led to a violent outburst from Egypt, which accused Iraq of having betrayed the quest for Arab unity. In riposte Egypt sought compensatory stronger ties with Syria and Saudi Arabia and, for a time with Jordan.

The whole relationship of Arabs one to another remains the key unresolved issue in Arab politics. The ideological basis of this problem is discussed below but here it should be pointed out that moves toward some degree of Arab federation or unity had been made or talked about since 1919 when Sharif Husain of Mecca proclaimed himself "King of the Arabs." During the latter phases of World War II, as described above, the Arab states had founded an Arab League. But the Arab League was always as much a cockpit as a coordinating committee. It had effect on the policies of its members only on key issues and then only sporadically. It tried to achieve a coordinated approach to the Palestine War, but it failed. Its attempts to establish what sort of entity "Arab Palestine" should be only high-lighted the profound differences between Kings Farouk and Abdullah. Subsequently, as King Farouk was ousted and Egypt acquired a militant, reforming government of young men while Iraq and Saudi Arabia remained under the control of what the Egyptians regarded as old regimes, the lack of accord became painfully obvious.

As the *Economist* Middle Eastern correspondent Tom Little wrote of the October 1955 meeting of the Arab League in Cairo "The Arab League met in Cairo in October in 'an atmosphere of cordiality.' To judge by reports of every meeting it has held in the eleven years in its existence, it has never done otherwise . . . the simple fact that the League met at all, after the violent polemics between Egypt and Iraq during the first nine months of 1955, was enough to warrant satisfaction of the Arab statesmen . . . Arab unity does not exist. I question whether it has ever existed . . . The Arab League revealed from the outset this historical condition of the Arabs: their persistent inability to unite politically but their abiding belief that union is a natural condition of their peoples which only required political formulation. In the Arab League, the Arabs trod a little too heavily upon their own dreams."

Meanwhile, the Palestine problem continued to occupy the attentions of the Arabs and others. When Secretary of State John Foster Dulles visited the Middle East in 1953, he found that whenever he attempted to discuss the Communist menace, his Arab counterparts rejoined with what they considered the more immediate danger of Israel.

Peace, indeed, had never really come to the Middle East. Despite the armistice of the Spring of 1949, the borders of Israel were fronts rather than frontiers. Raids and counterraids, intelligence probes, commando attacks, or foraging expeditions were the order of the day, almost every day. Shootings back and forth across the Syrian-Israeli, Jordanian-Israeli, and Egyptian-Israeli frontiers were normal operating procedure. The United Nations Mixed Armistice Commissions were kept busy sorting out conflicting claims and charges and passing judgment, or recommending censure by the Security Council, for acts of aggression. Between 1949 and 1955 thousands of incidents occurred.

Armistice lines, drawn to fit a haphazard pattern of military events rather than to meet economic, social, or even strategic criteria, make notoriously bad frontiers. In this case they cut off from their normal means of earning a living, either their places of employment or their fields, an estimated 150,000 Arabs. These people, technically not refugees since they still retained their dwellings, were the most grievously hurt of all of those who lost in the Palestine War. As such, they constituted an angry, hungry, and desperate element in the political life of Jordan where most lived.

The others, the legally certified refugees, almost a million strong, were scattered in the surrounding Arab countries. The bulk were in refugee camps maintained by an agency of the United Nations at a cost per person—including everything they got—of less than $2 monthly. That gave them medical attention and food measured at 1600 calories daily. But they were idle, miserable, and sustained by intoxicating memories of an idealized past and enervating dreams of an unlikely future. Idleness became the dry rot of character. As more "refugees" were born each year and the older refugees died off, the number who had ever known a life outside the confines of the camps declined. Able to do little for themselves—few had any skills to sell while most fell into that already saturated economic category of landless agricultural laborers—they bitterly reproached their Arab hosts for their plight. It was a refugee who killed the Arab statesman regarded by non-Arabs as the "most sensible" and realistic on the Palestine issue, King Abdullah. This lesson was not lost on the public figures in the other countries. Everywhere, even if inarticulate, passive, and humbled, the refugee was a reminder of the Arab humiliation and shame in the war and a living indictment of those who had promised to protect him.

Israel had embarked upon a policy of "massive retaliation" for Arab border violations. Demonstrations of this policy came in Israeli raids with regular army units against Nahhalin, Jordan, in March 1954 and Gaza in February 1955. In the latter case the Gaza headquarters of the Egyptian army was the target, and there were sixty-nine Egyptian casualties. Apparently that raid alarmed the Egyptians as no previous raid had and made obvious to them their need for better equipment. When this was not forthcoming from the Western powers on the schedule, on the terms and in the amounts desired, Egypt decided to explore other sources. In September 1955 Nasser announced that Czechoslovakia would supply large quantities of late-model military equipment to Egypt on terms not then known.

It speedily became apparent that the United States viewed this development with alarm, for it appeared that the "northern tier" had been hurdled. But the Arabs, still conscious of a long and often unhappy history of relations with the West, were gleeful. Nasser had done what no other Arab had thought possible. He had used the Cold War to internationalize Arab affairs and so, apparently, gained a lever to extract better terms from both the West and the East.

Meanwhile border friction grew rather than lessened. Israeli forces attacked Syrian positions on October 22, Egyptian positions on November 2, and Syrian outposts on December 11. For these attacks Israel was censured by the Security Council. For its impartiality in voting for censure, the United States got less credit than an outsider would have thought due. The Arabs regarded Israel as a Western state, and Arab, particularly Egyptian, propaganda grew more bitterly anti-Western. In Jordan demonstrations were held in December against the pro-Western government and the Baghdad Pact. The government fell and violence continued well into 1956 until finally, on March 2, the British officer who commanded the Jordanian military forces, Glubb Pasha, was discharged by King Husain in what was perhaps the most popular move made by a Jordanian government. In his place the king named a young Jordanian Arab nationalist. Putting aside the colorful bedouin headgear of the Legionnaires, he dressed them in the drab but "modern" caps of Western armies.

In Iraq, in a bid to win more popularity, the government decided in April 1956 that it would shift its development emphasis from massive but remote and unseen projects, such as it had undertaken, to "impact" projects in the populated areas. But the Iraqi government remained politically and emotionally isolated from the currents of change in the Arab world—for example, in June 1956 it banned a visit by a popular Arab hero, the young Algerian nationalist leader Ahmad ben Bella.

Worsening relations between Egypt and the West induced Secretary of State Dulles to announce on July 20, 1956, that the United States would withdraw an offer to lend Egypt $200 million toward the construction of the Aswan "High Dam." In riposte Nasser nationalized the Suez Canal on July 26.

Western reaction was swift and sharp. The foreign ministers of Britain and France and the American secretary of state met in London on August 2 and organized the first conference of "user states" for August 16. This group sent a mission to Cairo in the first week of September to attempt to work out a compromise solution. None proved possible. Egypt continued to run the canal despite the removal of most of the pilots. Threats and the freezing of Egyptian assets abroad failed to move Nasser. Egypt offered to pay compensation to shareholders in the company but insisted that the canal had been and would continue to be Egyptian. After various moves and pronouncements by all the parties, Israel attacked Egypt on October 29, despite warnings from the United States not to do so. Great Britain and France issued an ultimatum ostensibly to both sides and then on October 31 bombed Egypt and on November 2 invaded the canal zone. On November 5 the Anglo-French force captured Port Said but agreed to a United Nations–ordered cease-fire on November 7.

Insofar as there had been careful Allied planning, it presumably had as an immediate object the fall of Nasser. That did not happen. The Egyptians—particularly the guerrilla and paramilitary forces—fought better than had been expected, and there was no attempt at a palace coup.

As the dust settled it was clear that major changes had taken place in the Middle Eastern scene. Suez was going to remain Egyptian; Egypt was going to pay any price to get what it regarded as adequate arms to prevent another defeat; the Jewish, English, and French communities of Egypt, as minority communities always do in such circumstances, paid the price for the acts of those associated with them, had their property sequestered, and for the most part left Egypt; and Israel gained one objective, the right of passage through the Straits of Tiran to her port in the Gulf of Aqaba, Elath. The United Nations was brought into even closer contact with the Palestine problem as a United Nations Emergency Force (UNEF) was established to monitor the withdrawal of Israeli troops. For Egypt the withdrawal of British and French forces symbolized the end of a century of foreign interference—one of the first things Egyptian troops did upon entering Suez was to blow up the statue of Ferdinand de Lesseps.

The Suez crisis had made Nasser an Arab hero. Before his nationalization of the Suez Canal Company and his purchase of arms from the Soviet Bloc, Nasser had been regarded by many Arabs as a strong but colorless modernizer, but weighed in Arab scales, Suez was Stalingrad, El Alamein, and the Battle of Britain rolled into one. In the Arab view Egypt had stopped Britain, France, and Israel and Nasser had defied the world and won. In expression of support for the Egyptians, the Lebanese cut the oil pipeline at Tripoli and the Syrians blew up the Iraq Petroleum Company pipelines. ARAMCO, as an American company, was unharmed. So strongly, in fact, did this emotional wave of pro-Nasser feeling carry the Arabs that young King Husain of Jordan, believing he was about to lose his throne to it, himself struck against the more extreme nationalists in April 1957, dismissing his prime minister and the chief of his army and installing a government in the style of his grandfather, King Abdullah.

Continued Syrian instability led, in February 1958, to a merger of Syria with Egypt to form the United Arab Republic. Moves toward some sort of closer association between the two countries were begun in 1956. In January of that year the new Egyptian constitution proclaimed that the Egyptians were "a part of the Arab nation," and the Syrian parliament, in July, voted to set up a negotiating committee to explore plans for a federal union with Egypt. After an interval of some months, November 1957, a joint parliamentary session was held in Damascus. This group urged further steps toward a federal union. Finally in February, when the Syrians grew alarmed at the rise of Communist power in Syria, the formation of the United Arab Republic was announced. Other Arab states were invited to join in a larger union called the United Arab States. Rather curiously,

Yemen, alone among the other Arab states, decided to adhere to this new, and largely theoretical, entity.

Stung by the challenge the formation of the UAR seemed to offer to their security, integrity, and pride, the governments of Iraq and Jordan speedily, on February 14, formed the Arab Union, taking as their flag the banner of the Arab Revolt. Little that had made them separate states was actually affected. It was clear that the initiative and the leadership were in the hands of President Nasser of the United Arab Republic, and the Arab Union aroused few patriotic sentiments.

In Saudi Arabia, where the sudden and vast inflow of riches had produced something like an Arabian nights dream come true, mounting criticism of extravagance, corruption, and decadence led, in April 1958, to a gentle, intrafamily palace coup in which King Saud, the son of King Abdul Aziz, who had died in 1953, handed over power to his brother Crown Prince Faisal.

Just a month later the political and religious factions of Lebanon, which had been at one another's throats since the 1830's, broke into open warfare again. The issue this time was the extent to which Lebanon should be overtly committed to the West, through the Eisenhower Doctrine, or be attached to the major powers of the Arab World, particularly Egypt and Syria. These and other issues tended to divide the country along religious lines with the Christians, in general, favoring closer ties with the West, and the Muslims, with the Arab countries. In these troubled waters the Egyptians and others were fishing. The president of Lebanon, himself a product of the coup of 1952, sought to retain office beyond the constitutional limit and invited the help of the United Nations and ultimately of the United States to this end. All eyes were upon Lebanon when, suddenly and with no apparent warning, the Iraqi army overthrew the government of Nuri Said.

The American reaction was quick and powerful: within hours the first contingents of American marines began landing from the Sixth Fleet. And Britain put air units into Jordan. Unlike Suez, this intervention came at the request of the government and came promptly. But like Suez, it was harder to stop than to begin, more complex to withdraw than to mount. What ultimately made possible a graceful American withdrawal was a Lebanese compromise by which the commander of the Lebanese army, General Faud Shihab, agreed to become president of the country, and the incumbent agreed to step down.

In Iraq Abdul-Karim Qasim's new government, born of a violent coup and conceived in a social revolution, differed markedly from that of Nasser in Egypt. The king, the crown prince, and the prime minister were hunted down and shot, amidst scenes of great brutality and mob hysteria. The military forces which had seized power quickly split amongst themselves. The moderate, nationalist forces which had set the tone of the movement in the fall and early winter were replaced in 1959 by groups which moved more and more to the radical left. A countercoup was tried in the spring of 1959; when this failed, it was followed by a savage repression in Mosul and Kirkuk. The government became paralyzed, and the development program ground to a near standstill as the government failed to move on new contracts and defaulted on previous engagements.

The Kurdish followers of Mulla Mustafa Barzani rose against the Iraqi government in the late summer of 1961, rapidly seized the whole of the mountainous area of northeastern Iraq, Kurdistan, and prevented government forces from moving off the plains. In reply Qasim's government bombed Kurdish villages and issued an endless stream of communiqués announcing that the revolt had been completely crushed or soon would be or both. In August 1962, to show the world—and the Iraqi people—their power, the Kurds blew up the oil pipeline which connected Iraq to the Mediterranean. The inability of the Iraqi army to put down the revolt reflected both the lack of trust in the line officers on the part of Qasim, who insisted on controlling all operations, and the inability of his regime to act decisively. Finally, this issue, in conjunction with the other mistakes he had made, was to precipitate a coup which on February 8, 1963, resulted in the fall of Qasim's government and his own execution.

In Syria the United Arab Republic was not destined to last as it had originally been constituted. On September 28, 1961, a junta of army officers revolted, established a national government, and ordered all Egyptians to leave the country. On October 19 Syria was readmitted to the Arab League. On December 1 a general election was held, but on March 28, 1962, the new government was overthrown by a military coup.

Yemen, the most isolated and backward of the Arab countries, had experienced many coups and attempted coups in its bloody past. In 1948 the then ruler of the country, faced with rebellion, had called in the tribes of the north to sack the city of Sanaa. In March 1955 an attempted coup against the imam failed. Those involved in plots against the government were always few in number and were ruthlessly, often savagely, put down. Finally, on September 19, 1962, the old Imam Ahmad died of natural causes. His son, Crown Prince Badr, who was widely thought of as a comparatively liberal man and by some as a friend of President Nasser, became imam. Then on September 27 the chief of the army, Abdullah Sallal, a man of humble origins, led an attack on the palace, narrowly missed capturing the new imam, and proclaimed a republic. The imam himself fled from Sanaa to the tribal territory in the north from which he has organized and commanded a guerrilla army since that time. Meanwhile, Sallal, with few troops loyal to the government in comparison to the numerous and well-armed tribes, and with fewer other resources, appealed to President Nasser for help. Egyptian troops began pouring into the country to fight in the war against the supporters of the imam, and Egyptian technicians to help "bring Yemen into this century." No end to either effort seems in sight.

It can be said that the first decade of the "new era" of Arab freedom, neutrality, and assertiveness ended as it began, with the major questions of national life yet to be answered. In the interval, major changes had occurred in the society and the economy of the Arab world and to these we shall now turn.

PART FIVE THE MATRIX OF THE NEW ARAB

XIV. The Accelerating Social Revolution: The New Men

In the Arab World are many divisions. Traditionally, the bedouin have thought of mankind both in terms of kinship, with all mankind viewed in a pyramid of kindred from the family to the clan to the tribe to the races descending from the sons of Noah, and in terms of social economy with the bedouin sharply distinguished from the settled peoples. In the Koran men are divided religiously and by language. We in the West tend to think of divisions by income and class. But in analyzing the nature of the social revolution in the Arab countries, it is more useful to distinguish men of the traditional society from the "new men."

Both the new men and the traditional men can be seen in all social, religious, and economic groups and at all levels of society. The new men form a sort of "vertical" society, composed of all classes. They have an inner similarity and share certain values despite the obvious differences in economic, educational, and political attainments of their members.

The growth of this core within Middle Eastern society is one of the most significant changes in recent years. But viewed historically, what we observe today can be seen to be but a recent phase in a much older process.

The traditional society is not, of course, completely static. Contemporary hallmarks of conservatism in the traditional society were, in their way, often marks of social or aesthetic advance.

This is as true of social values as of such superficial signs of social usage as the wearing of a fez or tarbush. Regarded by recent reformers as the very symbol of reaction, the fez was a revolutionary innovation when introduced in the third decade of the nineteenth century to replace the more cumbersome and time-consuming turban. When the Lebanese Amir Bashir put aside his turban and effected the fez, he was symbolizing his entry into a new age; when the Egyptians later banned the fez they meant this as a symbolic step toward secular modernization. Likewise, on a more profound level, Islam was in its youth certainly revolutionary, with new ideas on the status of women, the brotherhood of believers, and the role of government. Yet modern Middle Eastern nationalists and modernizers have found in Islamic values a barrier to rapid modernization and have sought in secular nationalism a replacement for some aspects of Islam.

Like the tastes and the ideas, so the new men of each generation tend to fade, relatively speaking, into traditional society as they are overtaken and surpassed by a new generation. This is not, necessarily, to say that their role as modernizers has ended; some have come to be appreciated only long after their times. Moreover, some of the most significant innovations in the Middle East have been brought about by men who were, personally, deeply committed to the old order.

To gain some perspective on the current situation, let us briefly review the nature of earlier social change.

Writing in the first half of the nineteenth century, that remarkable observer and student of Egyptian life E. W. Lane echoed the thoughts of many previous writers when he pointed to lethargy as a hallmark of the people of the Nile. Since the then three or four million Egyptians could so easily support themselves on their fertile land, lacked a major inventive to devote themselves to industry, and found their simple and often crude products satisfactory, they could afford the luxury of backwardness. The picture painted by Lane and others is of a people whose lives were minutely regulated by established custom and whose appetites were as yet unwhetted for the new and the exotic produce of the Industrial Revolution, for the stimulating if disquieting ideas of the Renaissance, the Reformation, or the Enlightenment.

In the Syrian hinterland and the Iraqi basin, likewise, the people had accepted traditional approaches to life. Every man had his place in society. If that place were not entirely satisfying, it was God-ordained. To attempt to change it was unnatural. Indeed, even the word "change" (*ghaiyara*) carried the implication of "to corrupt" or "change for the worse." What was, was right, and the limits of acceptable human endeavor were narrow. As Professor Joseph Schacht in *The Arab Nation* has written: "One ancient Arab idea, arising from the very core of the mental endowment of the Arabs . . . became the central concept of Islamic religious law and theology . . . The Arabs were, and are, bound by tradition and precedent; they were, and are, dominated by the past . . . Whatever was customary, was right and proper; whatever their forefathers had done, deserved to be imitated."

The facts of life lent weight to this natural bent toward conservatism. The bedouin already had a highly sophisticated approach to a most difficult environment. To change his pattern of life, the bedouin would be required to change his environment. Only by nomadism can the extensive resources of the desert be utilized. Significantly, one of the Arabic words meaning "to settle" (*qantara*) also means "to possess a hundred-weight," for when a man becomes acquisitive, he must settle.

The villager, tilling a small plot of land, consuming most of what he produced, in need of only the most rudimentary weapons, tools, and consumables, and fearful of outside influences, was content within his small world. Much of his culture, the villager shared with the bedouin, but whereas the nomad ranged widely over vast, if not markedly different, expanses of the world's surface, the villager stuck close to a narrow, confining world. Surrounded by kinsmen with whom he shared his means of livelihood, the villager was intent on *protecting* his water rights, marketplaces, and common pasturage. Deeply wedded to his land, the villager married within his village and called it his "nation" (*watan*). Oppressed or ravaged from the one side by the rapacious nomad and from the other by the equally rapacious tax collector, the villager sought to retain and enjoy rather than to expand his means of livelihood. Seldom it was that he attempted to market his produce or to communicate with people outside of the small autarkic clusters of villages which were the limits of his world.

The city dweller, likewise, was enmeshed in a world of narrow scope, but known satisfactions. The mosque was his school, his club, and his parliament. In craft and religious guilds and brotherhoods, his relations with his fellows were drawn tightly together. His neighbors, like those of his village cousin, were often his kinsmen. They and he were segregated from other neighborhoods by walls and were ruled internally by men at least in part of their choosing. In the city as in the village or the tribe, man was never isolated but was able to find a stable, understood, and reasonably satisfying pattern of life.

The government was distant and its local agents were often foreigners, partaking of little of the local life and adding less to it. The government agent was himself a sort of nomad, camped in his headquarters, but little concerned with the life around him except in the collection of taxes.

More exposed, less secure, and less integrated were the minority groups. Some of these groups shared religions or languages with foreigners. Not the Muslim, therefore, but usually the members of the minorities were most open to change.

The British agent Dr. John Bowring, in his report on the "Commercial Statistics of Syria" in 1839, said that he found the Muslims to be the most backward as a group since they "accumulate little capital and fail to practice the arts progressively" whereas "most of the commercial establishments . . . (were) in the hands of the Christian or Jewish population." The merchant, he wrote, "is rarely an honored being—the power of the sword and the authority of the book—the warrior and the Ulema (religious leadership) are the two really distinguished races of society. All productive labour—all usefully employed capital is regarded as belonging to something mean and secondary."

The Christians, particularly of the Levant, had been in contact with European missionaries and many had studied European languages. The Jews were less aided by European powers or organizations but were freed from many of the inhibitions of Islamic politics and were somewhat affected by European contacts. Moreover, the Christians and Jews were able to enter into professions that the Muslims despised. In the Levant, for example, Jews and Christians were money lenders; the men who served as the equivalent of ministers of finance to the pashas of Saida were Jews and Christians, and the prevalence of such names as Katib, Haddad, Najjar (scribe, blacksmith, and carpenter) among the Christians testifies to their economic activity. The rulers of Egypt traditionally used the Copts as their tax collectors and as the cadres of their civil service. As late as 1910 almost half of the civil service of Egypt was drawn from the 15 percent Coptic minority.

Traditionally, in Islamic countries, education was not a function of the state but of the Islamic institution. In Egypt it was not until 1869 that the government tried even to inspect the schools, and only in 1925 did the state open half-day primary schools.

Egypt has been a pacesetter for the Arab countries in recent generations—even today half the literate Arabs are Egyptians —so it is instructive to observe trends there in some detail.

Between 1913 and 1945 school attendance in Egypt rose from 206,000 to 477,000 boys and 26,500 to 418,000 girls. In 1931 six public schools catered to 2500 secondary students of whom none were girls, whereas in 1945 fifty-three schools enrolled 33,000 boys and 3000 girls. During the same period the number of private schools increased from five to seventy-four. Higher schools increased their enrollment during that period from 1500 to 15,000. In 1952 only 45 percent of the children of proper ages attended schools, but following the 1952 revolution the figure rose to 65 percent and present plans call for facilities for all children by 1969. Total enrollment in 1950–51 was 1.5 million; by 1960–61 it had reached 3.1 million; it is expected by 1970 to reach 5.4 million. During that same period, university-level technical students almost tripled in number, and the secondary schools graduated more students yearly than the total enrollment in 1945–46.

In Iraq, one of the key factors when the British established their control in the last stages of World War I was the need to create a sufficiently large cadre of skilled men to administer the country and to work its industry. Particularly after the expensive revolt of 1920 had raised serious protests in London it was decided that economy must be the rule. Therefore, the British were anxious to pull out their relatively expensive foreign personnel as rapidly as possible. The Indian clerical help the British had imported during the war was, for political reasons, not regarded as a feasible alternative. However, India could be taken as a model for the small core of senior British officials who set policy for Iraq and supervised its execution by a local staff.

In Iraq as in India, the British faced what ultimately was an insolvable dilemma: they needed a skilled bureaucracy but deeply distrusted the urban literati who were its only native source. They felt that if this superficially Westernized group were allowed to gain control, it would corrupt the simple nobility of the "good Arabs," the bedouin, and would further impoverish the miserable peasantry. In any event, British interests would suffer. Therefore, a fine line had to be drawn between training for bureaucracy and education for government. The British therefore put major emphasis on primary schools. Their plan was to restrict secondary education to the "select few" needed by the administration.

In Kuwait, the coming of oil can be seen graphically in the rise of the education budget from $90,000 in 1942 to $33 million in 1960.

Other states are making major strides. Yet serious education problems remain. The population of the Arab states is still largely illiterate, and even that part of the population which is "educated" is still largely untrained in disciplines which are readily employable. But the efforts of the modernizers in Middle Eastern countries to educate the next generation for industrial and technical occupations are already showing results. Though statistics vary for the different countries, they all show the same emphasis on expansion of the technical qualifications of Arab society. In 1960–61 enrollment in preparatory and secondary vocational schools in four countries was as follows.

	Schools	Students
Egypt	181	114,693
Iraq	34	6,732
Jordan	14	1,281
Syria	32	6,830

And Saudi Arabia had 1081 abroad in schools. These figures do not include trainees in industry or apprentices, such as those in oil installations or other plants throughout the area. Occasionally, this kind of training has been on a massive scale. For example, the British forces in Egypt employed some 80,000 skilled or semi-skilled workers in World War II.

Today the emphasis placed on science and technology, in the schools and out, has greatly increased as several countries have set out to industrialize. It was estimated in 1961, by the Higher Council for the Sciences, that 38,000 Egyptians had graduated in the natural sciences and technology from Egyptian faculties. Of these 10,000 were engineers, 9700 agronomists, 9000 physicians, and 5000 scientists.

In addition to the more formal education in schools there was, of course, a major if less formal educational development in the increasing awareness of the outer world which was fostered by the presence in Iraq, Lebanon, Syria, Jordan, the Palestine mandate, and Egypt of large numbers of foreigners who brought with them distinctive habits. The goods and services which these foreigners imported, the administrative structures which they built, and the industry and commerce in which they engaged tended to impart education in the broader sense of the word to the native populations.

It is instructive to compare the former mandates and the colonial countries of the Middle East and other areas with those which have not had the disruption and benefits of foreign rule. A wound has been inflicted in the former colonial and mandate states' "national psyche." On the other hand, such countries as

Yemen, in which there has been no outside rule, have missed the beneficial aspects of foreign tutelage. Foreign powers did leave a sense of "structure" or organization and set styles for the new men who alone could run them.

In Iraq, there was an early recognition that the army was a school of nationalism. In its report to the League of Nations in 1926 the mandate government noted that "the army is proving a valuable means of fostering a true national spirit." Even the paramilitary groups, including the Boy Scouts, played an important part in the growth of national identity on the new model.

It was this same spirit which subsequently caused an Egyptian army officer, Sharaf ad-Din Zabalawi, to write in an article entitled "Military Education and Character Training": "Military life is the school of the people; it is an advanced school in public, social and national aspects of life, for the first lesson that a young soldier learns is self-denial and to exert all his efforts toward a noble cause. It is the repudiation of personal interests in favor of the public interest. The individual becomes a sound ideal citizen."*

It was logical that modernizers should assign this role to the army. We have seen that in the time of Mehmet Ali the army was in fact a vehicle as well as a reason for reform.

Today in many of the Middle Eastern countries the army is viewed as the guardian of national virtue, the sole force capable of and interested in pushing forward those reforms which alone will give dignity, strength, and justice. In part the army and modernization programs fulfill the role of creating the "image" which the military modernizers would like to project to the world —an industrialized, militarily powerful, state, respected in the world community.

Traditionally, of course, this was not the case. The military establishment, as we have seen, was restricted to a very narrow stratum of the society. In Egypt it was an alien force which did not even share the language or customs and certainly thought little of the well-being of the population. Egyptians only grad-

---

* Quoted in Morroe Berger, *Military Elite and Social Change* (Princeton, 1960).

ually won admission to its service and then, in the time of Mehmet Ali Pasha, usually as common soldiers. Indeed, it was not until 1936 that the Egyptian government opened the military academy to all social ranks. The nature of the change of the social composition of the army, as it grew larger and more "national," has been well expressed as one "from Praetorian Guard to Advance Guard." The armies, alone among the institutions of the societies, were organized along nationalist, modern, and secular lines without commitments to the past. The military alone has a defined code, a clear line of command, channels of communication, mobility, force, and, ultimately, will. The better an instrument of the state it became, the less committed it was to the state. As Professor Halpern in his *Politics of Social Change* has perceived: "The more the army was modernized, the more its composition, organization, spirit, capabilities, and purpose constituted a radical criticism of the existing political system . . . In civilian politics, corruption, nepotism, and bribery loomed much larger. Within the army, a sense of national mission transcending parochial, regional, or economic interests, or kinship ties, seemed to be much more clearly defined than anywhere else in society . . . As the army became modernized and professionalized, the traditionalist elements within the civilian sector found army service less to their taste."

Whereas in Western society the army has tended to be equated, at least in part, with the middle class, in the Middle East until recently this has not been the case. In the first place what we would call, on economic grounds, the middle class was often in large part composed of non-Muslims or even alien minority communities. This was particularly the case in Egypt where the Copts and large foreign communities of Greeks, Italians, and others predominated in the middle reaches of the economy and society. The Egyptian middle class in 1947 was estimated to comprise only about 6 percent of the population or half a million people. Of these about 51 percent were thought to be merchants, 26 percent clerks, 19 percent professionals, and only 4 percent businessmen. Very few were the new men who sought to remake the country.

In part, at least, the role taken upon itself by the Egyptian army has been the *creation* of a middle class. The middle class, composed of managers, administrators, teachers, engineers, journalists, scientists, lawyers, and army officers are, for the most part today, employees of the state. Where new state organs have been established, they are often staffed by men who were recently army officers. This is true of the Suez Canal Authority and the oil refinery and many of the nationalized business concerns.

The middle class in the modern Middle East is rather different in several ways from the Western middle classes we associate with the Industrial Revolution and democratic government. It is not distinguished by a dedication to private ownership, rights of self-expression, or a particular political credo. It uses and agrees to be used by the state for whose well-being it strives. And the new middle class is highly pragmatic in its approach—espousing "socialism" or whatever seems to offer solutions to baffling social problems. In these ways it differs significantly from the traditional sector which shares its "middleness" in economic terms, for example, the landlords and merchants.

Today the lack of a technical education effectively blocks the forward progress of men even within the middle class. Men who are well trained but trained in the traditional subjects do not have the assets to move upward socially and economically. Significantly, the acquisition of a foreign education, preferably at the source in a Western university, not a man's social rank or wealth, is the surest passport to advancement. This is the field of education in which one can note the most spectacular progress in the years since World War I in several Middle Eastern countries.

To take Iraq as an example, in 1921 nine Iraqis were sent abroad to acquire a Western education; by 1928 the number had risen to 93; by 1939 it had reached 238. By 1931 over 200 young men had spent periods of study abroad and had returned; by 1950 the number had reached almost 2000. In the one year of 1962 nearly 7000 were abroad at Western schools, colleges, and universities. As increased numbers were sent, and as governments committed higher proportions of money to education both on the lower and the higher levels, the young men and women were drawn from more humble social strata. Thus, in education as in the army, social class origins became less important. And, perhaps more significantly, whereas education *inside* an Arab country involved a limited exposure to the West in an Eastern context, the student on a mission abroad might spend upwards of eight years living in the West, acquiring new habits of life and far higher expectations; upon return, a sense of bitterness, extreme criticism, and frustration were common.

Curiously, this sort of contact with an alien society seems to have affected the humble more strongly than those at the top of the social ladder. Perhaps it was partly that the young man from a humble family could more fully commit himself to a new life and, because less bound, more readily accept its ways and values, and partly that upon his return from a relatively comfortable well-paid, and challenging experience, he viewed his own former position more bitterly, having less means of action and less protection—in family and money—from a harsh adjustment.

But those who went abroad and learned, at the prestigious source, a profession or new technical field were able to move ahead economically, politically, and socially more rapidly than those who stayed behind. Thus, even men of wealth and family who stayed behind gradually became socially inferior to those of more humble origin who went abroad and returned with a marketable skill. The graduate of a Baghdad college was destined for inferior jobs, perhaps as a primary or secondary schoolteacher, whereas the graduate from Oxford or Harvard could teach in the colleges, practice his profession, or take a responsible government position. Here it is possible to see the very sharp differentiation between the new men and the more traditional.

Likewise, one can observe this differentiation among the groups which we would categorize as lower class. In their study *Human Resources for Development in Egypt*, Harbison and Ibrahim distinguished several groups of workers. The largest is unskilled, landless, and without capital. The second, much smaller, consists of skilled or semiskilled traditional artisans who are technologically increasingly unemployed. The third group, perhaps now less than 10 percent, is made up of men with some degree of modern skills. Although all would be lower class because of the sharp contrast they present to men of the rest of the social order, they are clearly distinguished from one another by salary, regularity of employment, and morale. In Egypt, where, as in most countries of the underdeveloped world, unemployment and underemployment are common, a mechanic, for example, earns three times as much per diem as a day laborer and is assured of continual employment—so his real wages may be many times that of the day laborer. Everywhere the differential has been very high, and apparently the aim of a number of the Arab governments is to increase it.

Aware that a technologically backward and poor population is unable to form a solid base for the growth of national dignity and power, the two cherished goals of the modernizers of the Middle East, both the Iraqi and the Egyptian governments in the 1950's embarked upon programs to create new men not only in the cities but also in the countryside. This was the essence of the "Liberation Province" scheme in Egypt and the resettlement and housing experiments in Iraq.

Roundly, and perhaps rightly, criticized as an economic fiasco or as an example of ambitious political planning without the requisite technological and economic foundation, Liberation Province does give a clue to how the government felt about the need to build a new Egyptian. In the words of the director of the Social Affairs Department, M. Gamal Zaki: "Settlers are selected scientifically on social, medical, psychological tests. As social qualifications, applicants must possess one wife, no dependents except children, and no property; they must have been married only once, and must have finished their military service. Of 1,100 applicants so far, all have the right social qualifications, but only 382 families were accepted medically, because while most of the men were healthy enough, the women and children fell far short of the standard. Only 180 families survived the psychological test . . . of these 132 are now undergoing a six-month training, which included a three-month probation period. We must consider both people and land to be under reclamation."*

* Quoted in Doreen Warriner, *Land Reform and Development in the Middle East* (London, 1957), pp. 50–51.

The new man of Liberation Province was marked off from the traditional Egyptian peasant by a new standardized uniform in place of the traditional gown—the new version of the fez for the turban or the cap for the fez—by a much higher caloric intake of food, and by a salary four times the average rate in Upper Egypt. In addition, the workers were to put their children into a boarding school, as in the Israeli kibbutzim, which presumably would enable teachers to ensure a better and modern upbringing for the children. Moreover, like the rest of Egypt, Liberation Province was to become a mixed rural and industrial economy with factories interspersed throughout the agricultural area.

Liberation Province has had a stormy career and has certainly fallen short of goals intended for it, but the purpose was clear, and one may see this purpose, if less clearly specified, perhaps much more uniformly carried out, in certain other ways. For example, as mentioned above, the army has long been regarded as a school in civic virtues. In addition, today the army has also become a school to impart modern skills, a hospital to cure the ills of society and turn out healthier men, and a source of discipline. Each year approximately 20,000 Egyptians are inducted into the army for three-year enlistments; in Syria about the same are called up for two years. From 1957 to 1963 perhaps as many as 130,000 Egyptians have passed out of the armed forces into civilian life. When one considers that larger-scale, modern Egyptian industry in 1961 employed roughly 250,000 workers, the impact of this group of ex-soldiers can be appreciated.

Not very much is known about these new men when they return to civilian life. It is clear, however, that they are possessed of a rudimentary technical training, a sense of discipline, an indoctrination in nationalism, and certainly a far higher standard of health than are those who have not had army experience. All of these things are rare and prized possessions in a rapidly evolving and industrializing society.

At the upper echelons, the former army officer is the "doer" of the new order. He may aspire to cabinet rank, or take a key managerial job in the apparatus of government-run industry or commerce. As a factory manager or a senior bureaucrat he will play a dominant role in modernizing the country. In the middle levels, it is probable that the former noncommissioned army officers and junior officers take on lower-level administrative and industrial functions and former private soldiers are probably readily absorbed into industry. It is doubtful that many return to village communities where their skills are not in demand and where the life they have learned to lead, or at least aspire to, is impossible. As yet little is known in specific terms, but, in the round, it is possible to see that in the making is a multiclass, nontraditionalist, as yet politically or philosophically uncommitted, pragmatic, disciplined, privileged core of new men.

XV. The Economy of the Arab World

The economy of the Arab World is profoundly affected by international politics and can only be understood in this perspective. To illustrate this point, it may be useful to think in terms of a piece of real estate. To a homeowner the value of property depends largely upon the comfort, income, or other satisfactions it gives, but for outsiders the value may be largely a matter of location and the virtues of the building may count for little or nothing.

Historically, the "real estate" of the Arabs has presented them with an irony. In it, they have found little of the ease of life to be gained from ample water, a moderate climate, or a balanced endowment of minerals. However, the Middle East, athwart the trade and communications routes joining Europe, Asia, and Africa, with important religious and cultural influence in Africa and Asia, with an agricultural season different from Europe's, and, in this century, with the discovery of vast deposits of oil, has been of great strategic value to others.

Until recently the contrast of inner poverty with strategic value worked to the disadvantage of the Arabs. Now, it has become a major asset if not the major hope for the Arab's future. The contrast of the present with the past is evident in commercial relations. One side of the coin is the Suez Canal, which was dug by Egyptian labor, is located on Egyptian territory, and was largely paid for by Egyptian capital, yet from which Egypt received almost no return for this first sixty years of its operations.

The other, bright, new side of the coin is oil. Foreign companies have paid vast treasures simply for the privilege of being allowed to explore some of the most inhospitable and barren land on this planet. When petroleum was found, as it usually has been in vast quantities, they have paid enormous and increasing revenues to the lucky government, providing fringe benefits in public services and employing local citizens in the facilities which inevitably grow around oil fields.

The really striking change, however, is in the actions of the outside powers. That great figure of nineteenth century Egypt Mehmet Ali Pasha opposed the digging of a canal at Suez because he rightly perceived that it would make foreign domination of Egypt inevitable. Mehmet Ali's attempt to industrialize Egypt was opposed by a Europe which sought markets for its own produce. And the European powers threw the full weight of their power behind their bankers and merchants even when they were committing what amounted to grand larceny. Today, not only the United States and the Soviet Union but also Britain, France, Germany, and Japan are willing to assist the Arab countries with grants, loans, special trade arrangements and technical assistance on an unprecedented scale to develop local industry and agriculture. They also give or sell great quantities of military equipment to enable the Arabs to protect what they have. The fact is simply that the strategic value of the Middle East has now become a major natural resource.

In the years since 1945 the United States has granted $795 million, lent $583 million, and given military equipment worth $88 million to the Arab states. During this period the Soviet Union has given or lent about $1.2 billion in economic aid and in excess of $1 billion worth of military equipment. Other Western states have lent or given the Arab states about $700 million worth of aid.

The domestic resources of the Arab World, as we have seen, are extremely meager. Only in a few places—mainly in the north of Syria and Iraq—does sufficient rain fall to sustain agriculture. In the Arabian Peninsula, an area a fifth as large as the United States, only one tenth of one percent—an area about twice the size of Long Island—is arable. Egypt, as Herodotus said, is the "gift of the Nile"; without the Nile the 3 percent which is now arable would be as barren as the 97 percent which is now desert. Iraq owes most of its agriculture to the Tigris and Euphrates rivers which rise in the Turkish and Kurdish highlands where more than eight inches of rain falls. Elsewhere, agriculture areas are islands in a vast, waterless sandy "sea."

The economy of the Arab countries of the Middle East has gone through three discernible stages and is now in the early stages of a fourth, characterized by major efforts at development. In the first, which lasted until the 1820's in Egypt, the 1830's in Syria, and perhaps the 1860's in Iraq and the 1930's in Arabia, the economy was largely fragmented into clusters of villages and tribal groups which, in the main, were self-sufficient and in which a balance existed between nomadism, agricultural life, and small-scale urban industry. This first phase was followed by a second characterized by the rapid introduction of cheaper Western goods and more attractive Western styles as a result of the European industrial revolution, of the development of public security, and of the weakness of the Ottoman sultans who, in the commercial code of 1838, virtually turned over to Europeans the commerce of the empire.

In the third phase, which began in Egypt at the end of the First World War and later in Iraq, Syria, and Lebanon, and is just starting in Arabia, the Arabs set about creating an industrial base. As described above, a false start was made in this direction in the 1820's and 1830's in Egypt, when Mehmet Ali tried to create an industry, but Egypt lacked both the skilled manpower and the resources to sustain the development. It is possible that this attempt set Egypt back by shutting out private initiative. It did definitely channel all efforts into monopolies which were politically unworkable. A somewhat different attempt was made later in the century, under Ismail Pasha, to create the "social overhead" or infrastructure of development. This was successful, but the results were long delayed and too costly.

The feeling has never died that until the Middle East has its own industrial base, it will be nothing more than a "country cousin" of Europe. Moreover, it was clearly not acceptable in terms of national self-respect merely to have industry *in* the Middle East. The British and French had filatures in Lebanon and small-scale factories in Egypt before World War I, but leading Arabs felt strongly that the institutions of modern capitalism must be in part native. So strong was this feeling that an Egyptian trade and industry commission secured major government support in 1920 to found the first Egyptian-owned and Egyptian-directed financial and industrial promoter, the Misr Bank.

Egyptian industry never was able to match Egyptian agriculture in competition for private capital, however. Cotton was king. Any Egyptian with money put it into land. Egyptian industry was new and untried, and with international commitments preventing the government from creating tariff barriers, infant industry was not an attractive investment. By 1927 only about 5 percent of Egyptian gross national product came from industry and mining. In the 1930's, however, the collapse of cotton prices and the continued rise in Egyptian population without compensatory rises in agricultural area or production led to a renewed interest in industrialization.

Textiles were the front runner in Egyptian industrial growth. Production increased from 9 million square yards at the end of World War I to 20 million in 1931 and 159 million in 1939.

But it was not really until the Axis blockade during World War II and the presence of a huge Allied army—whose expenditures totaled 25 percent of Egyptian National income—that the major stimulus to local production was felt. In Egypt 80,000 skilled and semiskilled workers were employed to supply the British Eighth Army.

A major part of the activity of Egyptian industry was stimulated by the Misr Bank, which participated in the founding of some twenty-seven companies. But the bank was always short of capital, even though used by the government to pump loans into industry, so in 1949 the government founded an Industrial Bank in which it owned 51 percent of the stock. Even though somewhat freer in the lending of capital, this institution fell short of the needs of the economy and tended to accentuate the growth of larger-scale industry to the detriment of medium- and smaller-scale companies.

The Iraq government began in 1927 to allow the import of industrial equipment without duty and in 1929 passed a law to encourage industry by granting some tax exemptions if the industry to be started were above a certain size and used power-driven rather than hand-powered equipment. In 1933 Iraq imposed high tariffs on those industrial goods which could be supplied locally. And in 1936 an Agricultural and Industrial Bank was formed to initiate industrial schemes.

The war made a major impact in Iraq as elsewhere. The military expenditures of the Allied forces there in 1943 were about three times the size of the government budget for that year. The existence of ready cash and the lack of imported goods caused a wartime spurt of industrial activity.

Not only was the war a short-term stimulus to industrial activity in the Arab countries; even more significant was the long-term impact it left as a school in fiscal and commercial control. This "school" was the Middle East Supply Centre. The Supply Centre was established by the British government in 1941 (and made a joint Anglo-American project in 1942) to ensure that the population of the Middle Eastern countries would continue to get essential supplies despite the wartime shortages of goods and shipping space. Essentially, the Allies sought to cut imports and particularly those whose bulk or shortage was a critical factor. The key measure of success in Allied strategic terms was the reduction of imports from about 6 million tons in 1939 to 1½ million in 1944.

The principal means of accomplishing this reduction were two. In the first place the advice of experts was sought on means to expand local production. Since the major bulk imports were agricultural and the primary danger was famine, a premium was put on agricultural development. Investments were made in studies, farm extension programs, and means to control the distribution of fertilizer, resulting in considerable short-term increases. The most lasting results, however, lay in the second major means available to the wartime military authority: government regulation of industry, commerce, and agriculture. As elsewhere, so in the Middle East, the war provided a justification and a need for forms of government activity which were continued long after the war ended. All import goods had to be licensed, currencies were controlled, and elaborate plans and machinery were established to allocate goods and services. Even for those who assumed that the purpose of the Middle East Supply Centre was to exercise foreign control over the area's economies and that its heavy emphasis on agriculture was motivated by a desire to keep the Middle East backward, the principle of central control was not abhorrent. At least in part the Middle East Supply Centre was a school in the fundamentals of state economic control.

In Iraq, Syria, and Lebanon, meanwhile, little industry had been started until the end of World War II. Characteristically, textiles led the way. In Iraq the oldest plants processed cotton and wool which were sold in large part to the government for army use. What little industry there was in Syria before World War II was primarily handicraft, but the shortages and high prices of the war and immediate postwar years served as a stimulus to the development of native industry. This, in turn, was encouraged by the newly independent government as a means of achieving economic independence to match political independence. Protective tariffs were introduced in 1949 alongside low-interest, state-guaranteed loans for industry. In 1952 the importation of a number of articles that could be manufactured in Syria was prohibited and import quotas imposed on others.

The problem faced immediately in Syria and Iraq was the creation of industry in the general absence of capital or skills in the population. Whereas in Egypt both had evolved over a number of decades, Syria and Iraq wanted to find short cuts to catch up with the West. In Syria the government was further hampered by the fact that the little capital it had was channeled through the Banque de Syrie et du Liban, then controlled by France.

But everywhere in the Arab countries, industry was a small part of the economy. Just what it amounted to in terms of gross national product of the several countries is at best a guess before recent years. In fact, relatively little was known of the economy of the Middle East as a whole, despite the efforts of the Middle East Supply Centre, until the Palestine War posed, in the displacement of nearly a million Arab refugees, economic problems of such magnitude and immediacy that a special United Nations Economic Survey Mission, the Clapp Commission, was created to study the problem.

The report of the commission, published in December 1949, pointed out that "the solution of the problem of the poverty and unemployment of the refugees is . . . inseparable from a solution of the problem of poverty and hunger as that already affects a large section of the population of the Middle East." Apparently affected by the talks with the new nationalist officials they met on their travels, the members of the commission felt called upon to say in their introduction that a "higher living standard cannot be bestowed by one upon another like a gift. An improved economy does not come in a neat package to be sold or given away in the market place . . . The highly developed nations of the world did not make their way by wishing. By work and risk they forced the earth, the soil, the forest and the rivers to yield them riches. They pooled their energy and resources by taxation and mutual enterprise . . . There is no substitute for the application of work and local enterprise to each country's own resources. Help to those who have the will to help themselves should be the primary policy guiding and restraining the desire of the more developed areas of the world to help the less developed lands."

The report pointed out that the area is "and for a long time to come will remain, agricultural." The first requirement was said to be the need to develop its potential to feed its people and increase export crops. Only limited industry was seen to be immediately required. Needs apart, besetting any large-scale projects were many obstacles. "The region is not ready, the projects are not ready, the people and Governments are not ready, for large-scale development." The conclusion was that pilot projects should be begun, with international assistance, while governments of the area organized themselves to mobilize their resources and focus their talents on national development plans and agencies.

The advice given to the Arab governments had two immediate effects, one good and one not. On the one hand the report pointed out the potentials of the area and indicated a road toward their realization; it encouraged local enterprise and promised external help; and, while eschewing unrealism, it underlined projects that could be undertaken immediately in the interval before larger developments could be launched. This was a valuable endowment. On the other hand, the mission was viewed with a jaundiced eye by the critical and suspicious Arab, suffering from the humiliation of the Palestine War. He saw external assistance as a means to salve the conscience of the West for the fate of the Arab refugees while emphasizing agricultural development to keep the Middle East merely the "farm" for Europe.

The first country to profit from the advice offered by the Clapp Mission was Iraq, which in 1950 created a Development Board charged with the planning and execution of schemes to develop the country. To carry out its projects, the board was to receive 70 percent of the government's revenue from oil. At that time this sum was about $12 million; it rose rapidly over the next few years to nearly $180 million yearly. Recognizing its need for large-scale technical assistance, the government of Iraq began to recruit foreign experts and asked the International Bank to send a team to study the economy. Upon the report of this group, the first development plan for the period 1951–56 was based.

At the time, also, Iraq entered into an agreement with the United States government under which the United States gave Iraq technical advice on the development of its resources. A part of this project led to a further broad study by a technical consulting firm on industrial development and to a myriad of project plans by other consultants. Indeed, while much useful work was done in the many studies and plans, planning became virtually an end in itself as the headquarters of the Development Board commissioned whole teams of contractors to design facilities which required or catered to talents and personnel not then available in Iraq.

But Iraq was fortunately situated between the two extremes of the Arab countries, those with dense population and shortage of capital, led by Egypt, and those with proportionally vast capital resources but little into which to invest it locally, typified by Kuwait.

Among the many problems associated with development is the acquisition of sufficient foreign exchange to hire or buy the equipment and skills needed to build the physical plant and train the personnel for modern economic activity. In the Middle East, during the past three decades, oil has been the magic source of this foreign exchange.

Used on a small scale for thousands of years where it bubbled to the surface, as at Nebuchadnezzar's "fiery furnace" near Kirkuk, oil was first discovered in commercial quantities in Iran in 1908. Since at that time the Royal Navy was changing from coal- to oil-burning ships, the British government, at the insistence of Winston Churchill, on the eve of the First World War acquired 51 percent of the stock of the corporation set up to exploit Persian oil production. In large part it was the existence of the Iranian oil fields and the need to protect them from the Turks that led to the Anglo-Indian invasion of Iraq in November 1914. While American and other companies acquired leases in the Ottoman Empire, the government of India arranged with the Arabian shaikhdoms under its protection to withhold concession rights from any but British nationals. An Anglo-German enterprise, the Turkish Petroleum Company, acquired a concession in Iraq on June 28, 1914.

After the war it was in part the desire of the Turkish Petroleum Company to control the areas around Mosul that led the British government to get French agreement to a revision of the Sykes-Picot Agreement which had awarded Mosul to French-controlled Syria. In return for the inclusion of Mosul in Iraq and transit rights across Syria for oil, the British agreed in the San Remo Conference to let French interests take up a part, later reduced to roughly a quarter, of the combine which later became the Iraq Petroleum Company. Turkish acquiescence to the inclusion of Mosul in Iraq was purchased for a consideration of 10 percent of Iraq's oil revenue for a 25-year period.

In America, at this time, there was a panic over oil, with talk of American reserves being depleted in four to six years; the government was, in fact, so alarmed that it considered entering the oil business itself as the British government had done. But American companies, some of which had concessions from the now defunct Ottoman regime, were excluded from areas of British and French influence. After long and somewhat acrimonious diplomatic negotiations, the British agreed to let American companies operate in the Middle East, and in 1925 American companies took roughly a quarter of the stock of the Iraq Petroleum Company. With the major oil interests included, in 1928 a monopoly area of the Middle East was created for the Iraq Petroleum Company alone.

Meanwhile, American companies not a part of the 1928 agreement tried to get concessions in the Arab areas. In 1932 the Standard Oil Company of California, having found a loophole in British restriction on foreign enterprise in the Persian Gulf by establishing a Canadian company, struck oil on Bahrein Island. Stirred by this enterprise, it acquired a concession in Saudi Arabia in 1933. Joined by the Texas Company, which had a stronger market for oil, it struck oil in Saudi Arabia, near Dhahran, in 1938. Meanwhile, in 1933, the Gulf Oil Company in partnership with the Anglo-Iranian Oil Company, which held the concession in Iran, acquired a concession in Kuwait and struck what eventually became recognized as the world's richest oil field, the Burgan Sands, an area of thirty square miles, fourteen miles from the coast, and only 3400 feet deep in 1938.

World War II interrupted the development of Kuwait's oil before it had achieved commercial production. The real stimulus came in 1951 when Anglo-Iranian Oil lost its concession in Iran and turned to Kuwait in search of another source of supply. From 1950 to 1954 Kuwait production tripled and additional oil was discovered. Today it is estimated that Kuwait has proved reserves in excess of 62 billion barrels or 25 percent of the world's total. Near the surface, adjacent to the sea, and of extremely high quality, this oil has made Kuwait a golden land. At the present time oil revenues are approximately $500 million yearly in a country whose population totals only 340,000. In past times Kuwait had small trading and pearl-fishing industries, which in 1938–39 earned the government about $290,000, but these were literally forgotten in the incredible deluge of prosperity. From a prewar gross national product per capita of about $40, the current rate has risen to $3360. Kuwaitis rapidly became the landlords of Cairo, Beirut, and Lausanne apartment houses, and Kuwaiti deposits in London became an important factor in the stability of the pound. Yet the country was so poor in resources as to have to import not only all its drinking water but even the labor to work the oil facilities and build the labyrinth of Western-style suburbs which grew up around old Kuwait Town.

Kuwait quickly came under heavy criticism among the Arabs for its inability to spend its vast riches to their satisfaction. Iraq, in serious financial trouble, in 1958 resurrected the claims made repeatedly by successive Iraqi governments that Kuwait was a part of Iraq. In the face of a threat to invade the country, Britain rushed in troops and equipment in 1961 until the Arab League took action to replace them with a mixed Arab force. For the Kuwait government the lesson was clear that it must give other Arabs collectively a stake in its security. Thus, Kuwait created in 1962 an Arab Development Fund, with assets now totaling nearly $1 billion, to lend to other Arab states.

The Iraq Petroleum Company is one of the world's great cartels. Among its owners are Royal Dutch Shell, British Petroleum (which is 56 percent owned by the British government), Cie. Française des Pétroles (35 percent owned by the French government), and a consortium of American petroleum "giants." The Arabian American Oil Company is jointly owned by California Standard, the Texas Company, Standard Oil of New Jersey, and Socony; the Kuwait Oil Company is jointly owned by Gulf and British Petroleum. The maze of interlocking and separate research, refining, marketing, shipping, production, and exploration companies controlled by these groups and their vast assets and armies of employees make them literally empires within the petty states of the Middle East and silhouette them bleakly against the simple economic horizons of the countries in which they operate. Irrespective of the enormous contributions to Middle Eastern development and the usually enlightened public relations policies of the companies, this fact has created a highly charged political atmosphere both for the governments and the companies.

As the governments have begun to develop cadres of men with some knowledge of the petroleum industry, they have naturally aspired to control and exploit this single national resource of worldwide importance. They have found that the companies usually can afford to pay almost any demand, after a decent period of bargaining, because the stakes are so enormous: the goose has been hard to kill and the golden eggs seemingly unlimited. Oil royalties have gone up from token payments in the 1930's to a flexible definition of a 50-50 split today with higher charges in special circumstances. The Arabs have concerted with the other members of the Organization of Petroleum Exporting Countries (OPEC) to find ways further to increase their income from petroleum. A favorite idea of some Arabs is that fully integrated companies—"from the well head to the gas station pump" —should exist to give the Arabs a share of profits at each stage of the operation. However, discovery of oil in North Africa and increasing Soviet exports of oil have tended, to a degree, to inject into company-country discussions a note of caution on the health of the goose. It is clear that the relations between companies and countries today are far more healthy, in inverse proportion to that of the industry, than some years ago. Nevertheless, so long as the oil industry is *the* Middle Eastern industry, its political position is exposed and dangerous.

Leaving aside the oil boom, the basic economy of the Middle East is still agricultural. In most of the Arab countries roughly two out of every three people are directly dependent upon agriculture for their livings. Moreover, most of the foreign currency earned by the nonoil countries is from agricultural production. Yet agriculture accounts for one quarter to one third of the gross national product of Iraq, Syria, Jordan, and Egypt.

Agriculture is lacking in both social and political prestige. The nationalists of the Middle East do not propose to be Europe's farm, and the Arabs traditionally have despised the menial lot of the peasant. However, since the major foreign exchange earner apart from oil and strategic location (which earns revenues in aid and in rental of the Suez Canal, transit facilities for oil, and so forth) is agricultural produce, economic development is largely dependent upon its sale on the world markets. The infant industries of the area simply cannot yet compete on the world markets whereas cotton, dates, and other commodities can.

Ironically, one must conclude, the more successful the Arabs are in their industrial projects, up to the time they became capable of competing on the world market, the more they will depend upon agriculture, since more raw materials, more components, and more machines will have to be imported at greater and greater cost in foreign exchange. This means more strains on the agricultural base which furnishes the bulk of the foreign exchange.

Further, the economic and political situation is dynamic: yesterday's dream is today's norm and tomorrow's failure. The "revolution of expectations" is continuing and accelerating. The "new man" in part brings about and in part is a result of the growth of industry.

Improvement in agricultural output and marketing, therefore, is vital to the success of the development effort. How possible is it? The answer cannot be given in purely economic terms.

For many centuries the *fellah* or peasant had been treated as a domestic animal, a part of the sultan's flock, to be shorn of his yearly produce by tax collectors, usurers, and casual robbers under various titles. His attitude toward government was one of sullen hatred, fear, and—when one of his many ruses succeeded—contempt. For him, as for the very rich, the best government was the least government. In no way did the government benefit him. Regulation of his personal affairs, guidance in matters of law, and what little succor or education he received came from the religious establishment, from the village custom and its council of elders, or from his own numerous kindred.

The villager and many of his city cousins lived apart from government and according to rules different from its formal laws. In the eyes of the government the village lands belonged to the state and the villager enjoyed an insecure tenure upon payment of various sorts of taxes and fees to someone rich or powerful enough to contract with the government for the right of a tax farm (*iltizam*). The tax farmer obligated himself to pay a fixed fee or render military service to the government in return for the right to extract anything he could from the peasants.

Let us take Egypt as the example as the history there is the most precise. When Mehmet Ali became pasha of Egypt in 1805, he was in conflict with the previous ruling group, the Mamluks, and undertook to undercut their authority in various ways. One way was in the abolition of the *iltizam* titles. As in his military reforms, he had to move somewhat slowly and it was not until after his massacre of the Mamluks in 1811–12 that he was able to destroy the system.

In 1812 the *waqf* lands—lands devoted to a foundation though the former owners continued to enjoy the produce—in upper Egypt (and shortly thereafter in all Egypt) were confiscated and their former beneficiaries given compensation. Lands were then turned over to village communities, in accord with the customary, as distinct from formal, law in many parts of the empire; the villages became responsible for the payment of taxes to the state. What the individual "owned" was the right to cultivate certain plots of land, and this right was passed from father to son.

Having destroyed the "feudal" class and established a direct relationship between the state and the land, Mehmet Ali began in 1829 to encourage the development of uncultivated lands by granting tenure to army officers, merchants, and others willing to invest in them. Apparently, he also sought in this way to create a new landed aristocracy. Gradually, over the years, as the role of the state in the economy declined, laws and degrees converted tenure rights into something approximating full ownership. Then as crops for export, notably cotton, became more common in Egypt, title to the land became more firm.

Meanwhile, great improvements in land productivity were made. After the introduction of cotton in 1821 the rich lands of Egypt became golden. The American Civil War, which took American cotton off the world market and produced a financial panic in industrial England, made Egypt prosperous and lured to the land large amounts of capital. Finally, even a peasant could own and sell or mortgage his lands.

What this did to the peasant is clear: he achieved more mobility, but his ties to the land were weakened so that in bad years he risked losing both his new title and his age-old usufruct. In the slump following the end of the American Civil War the smaller operators in Egypt went heavily into debt or lost their lands to larger companies. As the government became desperate for revenue, particularly in the days of Ismail Pasha, it was willing to play fast and loose with law and tenure, so that the wealthy were able to buy titles to land, and rights over the peasants on them, by the payment of back taxes.

Foreigners were encouraged even in the time of Mehmet Ali to invest in the land of Egypt, and by 1901 they individually and through land companies had acquired about 11 percent of the agricultural land of the country.

As dams and canals were built by the state, marginal lands came into production and passed into the hands of larger capitalists and land companies.

The amount of land devoted to agriculture increased from 4.8 million acres in 1893 to 5.4 million in 1906. It has undergone little lateral expansion since, although more control over flooding and irrigation has resulted in double cropping (vertical expansion) and thus more real agricultural area.

Perennial irrigation, however, decreased productivity since it halted the infusion of large amounts of silt which had yearly renewed the fertility of the lands and required heavy use of fertilizers which the peasants could not always afford, often did not know how to use, and periodically, as in World War II, could not obtain. Moreover, the steady waterlogging of the delta has presented major problems of salting and so required expensive canals. And the constant availability of water has promoted the spread of the debilitating disease of bilharziasis and various sicknesses spread by flies and mosquitoes.

The lot of the peasants was always difficult at best. If the year was bad—in Egypt the key factor was the size of the Nile flood

—the peasant had little to eat, and as the crop became specialized, usually in cotton, he could not even eat his produce. (For this reason peasants bitterly opposed extension of cotton plantations.) If the year was good the unit price for his goods fell and the state demanded higher taxes from him.

In Egypt as in Syria and Iraq men fled from the land when the government or the landlords pressed too hard. Conscription or forced labor (*corvée*) were added incentives for men to quit the land or to migrate to protected lands or to the lands of those who could protect them from what amounted to kidnapping for army service or labor gangs. Moreover, due to the Islamic laws of inheritance, there was a steady tendency to subdivide lands, resulting in plots too small to support a farming family. In Egypt in 1910 6.7 percent of the agricultural land was in units of one acre and 18.3 percent in one- to five-acre plots; by 1950 13.1 percent was in units of one acre and 22.2 percent units of one to five acres.

The policy of the government, in Egypt as in Syria, was to force bedouin tribes to settle on the land. To lure the tribes, tax exemption and land ownership was offered. In Egypt as later in Iraq the bedouin shaikh normally became in law and gradually in custom the landlord while his formerly equal tribesmen became his peasants.

By the end of World War II conditions in rural Egypt had become unbelievably bad. At the end of a careful survey in 1946–47 the English economist Doreen Warriner wrote, in *Land and Poverty in the Middle East*, "Near starvation, pestilence, high death rates, soil erosion, economic exploitation—this is the pattern of life for the mass of the rural population in the Middle East. It is a poverty which has no parallel in Europe, since even clean water is a luxury. Money incomes are low—£5 to £7 per head per year—but money comparisons alone do not convey the filth and disease, the mud huts shared with animals, the dried dung fuel. There is no standard of living in the European sense —mere existence is accepted as the standard."

The man-land ratio declined drastically, as population rose from 6.8 million people on 4.7 million real acres or 6.2 million crop acres (since some land produced two crops) in 1881 to 12 million people on 9.7 million crop acres in 1914 to 16 million people on 8.4 million crop acres in 1937 and 19 million people on 9.1 million crop acres in 1948. Today the population is about 28 million and the agricultural area has increased only slightly to 10.3 million crop acres. Little further increase is possible from the Nile waters, yet the population is doubling each 25 years. This has resulted both in a massive migration to the cities, whose populations are rising at a rate beyond that of the country as a whole, and the conversion of the Egyptian countryside into a quasi-urban area with population densities of approximately 2000 per square mile.

Miss Warriner went on to say that while "it is fashionable to praise the Egyptian fellah for his industry and frugality, in fact the conditions of his life are of unrelieved horror. The fellaheen are physically wretched . . . they are an almost slave population." It was partly to alleviate the horror of rural wretchedness and partly to break the power of the landlord class (as in 1812) that reforms, including the change of titles to the land, were undertaken in 1952 by Nasser's new regime. To the surprise of the government it was quickly discovered that only about 8 percent of the land was held in blocks of over 200 acres and that a real increase in the standard of living of the people could not be achieved simply by cutting out the big rich. Redistribution was undertaken, however, and by 1962 nearly one sixth of the agricultural land of Egypt was made subject to the program and nearly 240,000 farmers had received land. Since an acre of delta land yields about $150 net profit yearly, this injected into the agricultural sector of the population a considerable potential for new income.

In the interval, there has been a major increase in the well-being of the people in large sections of the Arab countries. Disease has fallen and public health facilities—rudimentary by Western standards yet revolutionary in local terms—have been exported from the cities to the rural areas.

The problem posed by the social history of the rural Arab, however, may require solutions which are unconventional by

Western standards. It is true that acre for acre, American methods of cultivation produce more than do those of the Arab peasant, but the American methods depend on a level of technology that is not matched in the Middle East. Thus while in American terms "vertical expansion" and the use of better seeds, fertilizers, and methods are more economic, these may not produce the same results in the Arab countries. Not only is the peasant poor and uneducated but he is suspicious of government, unwilling—perhaps sensibly so—to experiment with methods he does not know and cannot understand, and prizes above all else the acquisition of additional land. "Horizontal" expansion of agriculture, even when this involves heavy investment in dams, irrigation and drainage canals, and eventually desalination facilities, may therefore offer the best hope for a higher agricultural output in the near future.

Meanwhile, every Arab government is planning its future. And in every plan the emphasis on expansion of industry is paramount. Industry is a thing of the modern world; to be modern, it is thought, one must industrialize. The index of success, therefore, is the speed with which each state can acquire an industrial plant. In Egypt, for example, between 1939 and 1947 the value of industrial production rose 50 percent, from 1947 to 1954, 40 percent, and from 1954 to 1960, a further 50 percent. Yet this was mainly a result of increased capital investment per worker. Industry has, as yet, proved unable to absorb the large numbers of unemployed and underemployed people for whom there is insufficient land. A serious political problem is thus to find a means of increasing the number of jobs created by industry. Shorter hours and emphasis on industry requiring a higher input of labor is a partial answer. But often the pressures behind the urge to industrialize work in the opposite direction: it is the huge steel factory, which requires a high capital input and little labor, rather than the consumers' goods factory, requiring little capital and much labor, that gives prestige.

Lastly, it must be said that the building of an industrial plant and the infrastructure of the modern state will not sustain a developmental revolution: none of the Arab states has found ways to create markets—which alone will make possible a sufficiently large-scale production to encourage their infant industry. The great economic problem of the Arab countries is not how to build factories and get men to run them, or "build better mousetraps," but how to get people buying the goods of their industry, so that the economy, in Walt W. Rostow's famous phrase, can "take off."

XVI. The Arabs and the World: A Quest for Identity and Dignity

Arab politicians and thinkers have set out to answer two basic questions: "who are we?" and "how can we get the world to respect us?" These have been implicit in most of the speeches, books, and actions of the Arab leaders since the end of World War I, and are still burning issues today. It was not very long ago that they were explicitly stated in all significant Arabic-language books. Most began with an attempt to define who the Arabs are: Are Egyptians to be considered Arabs? If so, to the same degree as men of Arabia? Are Christians *really* Arab or must an Arab be a Muslim? Is a man of Damascus more an Arab or more a Syrian? How does the Westernized Lebanese compare in "Arabness" to the isolated Yemeni? Is there *one* Arab nation despite the obvious diversity and conflict of the several Arab states? And, if so, how can the Arabs so express this nation in political, economic, and social terms to give it reality?

The political experience of the several Arab countries, as we have seen, has been remarkably different. This fact has profoundly colored both Arab reactions to the situations in which they found themselves and their intellectual formulations of their goals. The surer road to understanding starts from a description of the Arab situation than from an analysis of the ideas. Many of the ideas were borrowed from Europe and are, in reality, more in the nature of flags of convenience than precise ideological formulations.

Egypt was geographically and culturally the most coherent of the Arab states. Compressed into the Nile Valley, cut off from the other Arabs by great distance, and after 1805 ruled by a strong national, if not Arab, government and after 1882 by a British government, Egypt was subjected to intense, beneficial but intellectually disquieting Western influence. Thus it was to achieve, more surely and easily than the other Arab states, an awareness of itself as a separate entity. Not only were other Arabs far away and living at least economically very differently from the Nile dwellers but the Egyptians, living in the shadow of monuments of their ancient grandeur, developed a sort of Aïda complex. Egypt as Egypt, rather than as an Arab country, had a continuous and recorded history for 4000 years, and whatever changes the successive invaders had made, each layer of foreign influence was built on the same Nilotic core. In contemporary squalor and weakness before foreigners, Egyptians were awed by the majesty of the past, their past, a non-Arab past. These feelings were accentuated by the exciting archaeological discoveries of the late eighteenth and the nineteenth centuries, particularly when the decipherment of hieroglyphics suddenly opened a wide window on the ancient civilization.

Nevertheless Mehmet Ali's attempt to create an Egyptian power failed in 1841 when the European powers forced Egypt to give up its military machine and the economic organization which had sustained it. Thereafter, Egypt "slowly went to sleep again" as Europeans took over more and more aspects of the national economic and cultural life and the more energetic and better educated Egyptians competed in becoming European.

By the 1870's Egypt had no real "line of defense" against the West in political, economic, or even cultural affairs. It was at that time that Jamal ad-Din al-Afghani came to Egypt, inspiring all he met with the notion that Islam could offer a coherent and powerful identification and means of defense. As a result of his influence and that of his disciple Muhammad Abdu, the hope of a revival of Islam and the identification of Egypt as a part of the enduring Islamic civilization became cardinal elements in successive Egyptian efforts to achieve a sense of identification and dignity.

A contrary force was evident, however, in the extensive Westernization of urban Egypt. This was evident in the political movements before World War I and was codified, in the 1930's, by the Egyptian scholar, novelist, and statesman Taha Husain, who stressed the Mediterranean base of Egyptian civilization and urged Egyptians to think of themselves as having a culture in common with Europe rather than with Africa or Asia. Even on the eve of the foundation of the Arab League, Egyptian statesmen echoed this sentiment and described the role of Egypt as a bridge between East and West. But the East was not exclusively the Arab East. If East and West could not meet in Kipling's Suez, they might in Taha Husain's Cairo, which was, in fact, a remarkably cosmopolitan city in a remarkably discrete land. This tendency in modern thought was in the main stream of the urban, polyglot, tolerant, cosmopolitan tradition of the golden age of Islam.

In Syria the environment was quite different. In the first place, before World War I the government was the Ottoman Empire, an Islamic state, so that Islam offered no means of achieving a separate identity. Moreover, a number of the pioneers of nationalism were Christians. Obviously, the Christian minorities could not hope, except to a limited extent in Lebanon, to achieve power or even security as Christians. The only things which they shared with their Muslim neighbors were the Arabic heritage and Syrian residence. In historical memory the shared residence achieved major importance only as the seat of the Umayyad Arab kingdom. That kingdom was not only little associated with Islam but was viewed by many Muslims almost as a secular, indeed as a pre-Islamic, pagan Arab state. The post-Umayyad Arab heritage had, of course, become intertwined with Islam. Thus to avoid the divisive religious issue and to capitalize on such elements of Syrian "nationalism" as existed in the Arabic heritage, modern Syrians had to go back to pre-Islamic Arabism to find a common base. That base could only be the notion of folk nationalism (*qawmiyah*) with a glorification of Arabism (*Arabiyah*).

In Iraq, for reasons quite different from those in Syria, the emphasis was also placed on Arabism. Like Egypt, Iraq had a rich and long past; unlike the Egyptians, however, the Iraqis were not so conscious of their pre-Islamic, pre-Arab past as to find in it the basis of a separatist nationalism. Like the Syrians, the Iraqis could not oppose the government, the Ottoman Empire, in the name of Islam since the Ottoman sultan was also the Muslim caliph. Unlike the Syrians and the Egyptians, however, the Iraqis had not one but two Islams: whereas the Syrians and Egyptians were almost exclusively Sunni or Orthodox Muslims, the Iraqis were divided between the Sunnis and the Shiis. Many of the Shiis were Persian or culturally oriented toward Iran and differed profoundly from the Sunni Arabs, who, in turn, differed significantly from the Sunni Kurds. Iraq also had a sizable Jewish population, some of whose leaders were active in the process of building the state—a good deal of the prosperity of the Iraqi state was due to the wisdom of a Jewish minister of finance—before the violent clash between the Arabs and Zionists after World War II. All of these factors tended, as in Syria and Lebanon, to de-emphasize religion as a basis of national identity. Consequently, as in Syria, nationalism came to have an ethnic and cultural coloration.

Arab nationalism received its first major challenge in the Middle East in Palestine; there a competing ethnic nationalism, Zionism, was the challenger. Impressed as they were by the vigor of this challenger, Arab writers, particularly of the 1930's, sought to meet the strengths of Zionism point by point in a revival of Arabism. And it was just at this time that the spread of public education, made possible in large part by the mandate system, required authentic Arabic cultural materials to form a humanities program for the increasing numbers of students. What could this program be? It could not, with Western notions of the separation of Church and State and with serious religious cleavage within the Arabic-speaking population, be Islamic. Whereas Islamic schools had taught pupils to read by reciting the Koran, public schools could not. There was no modern literature. The only acceptable answer was, therefore, pre-Islamic. This was the classical basis of the culture of all Arabic-speaking peoples of whatever religion or whatever region. Thus it was, with little thought of the political consequences, that the public school system injected into the population on a mass basis the elements of pre-Islamic, pan-Arab values as embodied in classical Arabic literature.

Meanwhile, inhabitants of the Arabian Peninsula, cut off from the disturbing intrusions of foreign thought, relatively secure from the tyranny of the Ottoman Empire and the imperialism of the European powers, and almost completely Sunni Muslim, were little concerned with what the outside world thought of this culture. They knew themselves to be tribal, Muslim Arabs and, like members of a small club, never were concerned with identifying badges.

The mandate system posed new barriers between the separate units of the Arab World. The young man of Iraq acquired English as a second language and was influenced by European formulations of ideas and information as these were filtered through English thought and institutions. The Syrian, to the contrary, viewed the world through a French window. The Egyptian either attended one of his own national universities, the first founded in the Arabic-speaking areas, or picked freely from Italian, French, English, German, or American institutions. Culturally he was apt to be influenced by France, but politically he dealt with the English. The Saudi Arabian usually went to an American school, often under the sponsorship of an American oil company, but was less motivated to learn foreign ways than his Iraqi, Syrian, or Egyptian cousin since, he discovered, his oil made foreigners willing to learn his own difficult language and to respect his customs.

Ironically, in this diversity was a force for unity. Arab students meeting in London or Paris were impressed by their foreignness from the English and the French and with their common identity as Arabs. Measured by their cultural distance from the Europeans, their differences from one another as Syrians, Iraqis, Saudis, or Egyptians paled into relative insignificance.

Meeting in Brussels in December 1938, a group of Arab students tried to reach an agreed definition of "Arab" and "Arab Homeland." The very cumbersomeness of their definition provides an index to the seriousness of their problem. An Arab, they decided, is anyone "who is Arab in language, culture and *wilā'*," the last term being defined in a footnote as one who has "nationalist sentiments" (*ash-shu'ūr al-Qawmi*) while nationalism (*qaw miyah*) is defined as "sensitivity to the existing necessity of liberating and unifying the inhabitants of the Arab lands in view of the unity of the homeland and language and culture and history." Interestingly, a decade later the Syrian Baath party, in many ways the most ideological of the Arab political movements, had not got much further with an attempt at definition. It regarded as Arab one who lives in an Arab country, speaks Arabic, and believes in his connection with the Arab nation.

The desire on the part of the several Arab governments to cater to the popular sentiment for some degree of Arab unification, added to their determination to improve their own bargaining position, impelled the Arabs to organize the Arab League during the later phases of World War II. The principal test of that organization came in the Palestine conflict, and that test, as we have seen, was a trauma for the whole Arab body politic. The Palestine War severely challenged the previously acceptable concept of separate states in a loose confederation; consequently, great stress came to be placed upon the unity of the Arabs. Disunity was branded as a holdover from the bad old days of Western colonialism.

Yet long after the departure from the Middle East of instruments of Western influence and power and even after the overthrow of the government of Nuri Said in Iraq and the withdrawal of Iraq from the Baghdad Pact, unity was still unattained. The union of Egypt and Syria was short-lived, and its disintegration clearly had nothing to do with Western policy or pressures.

The fact is that the "artificial" states into which the Arabs have been divided have their separate existence enshrined in the whole complexity of Middle Eastern life. Consequently, however profoundly united the Arabs may feel themselves to be culturally, they have not been able to formulate even intellectually an acceptable basis of political or administrative unity.

There can be no simple answer to the question "what is an Arab?" or, as phrased in the beginning of this chapter, "is a man of Damascus more an Arab or more a Syrian?" In his political acts he shows himself to be both—and many other things, which impinge upon the precise frontiers he would put around *his* Arabness.

In this book on the Egyptian coup of 1952, *Egypt's Destiny*, Muhammad Nagib, the first president of Egypt, said, "We seized power because we could no longer endure the humiliation to which we, along with the rest of the Egyptian people, were being subjected." Another figure of the revoluion, Anwar Sadat wrote, similarly, in his *Revolt on the Nile* that "the humiliation, frustration and anger aroused by the incompetence of the men who had led Egypt to defeat instead of victory, provoked a passionate desire to overthrow a régime which had once again demonstrated its complete impotence."

Remarks of this sort filled the press in the Arab states in the aftermath of the Palestine War. It had been clear to some intellectuals since World War I that the West had not taken the Arabs seriously. Periodically—as in Egypt following the murder of Sir Lee Stack in 1923, or in Iraq in putting down an anti-British government in 1941, or in Syria in bombarding the capital city in 1925 and 1945—the new national pride of the Arabs was wounded. But it was in countless smaller ways that Westerners hurt the Arab pride the most. The facts that Egyptians were not allowed in the British sporting club in Cairo and were subjected to continuous and biting satire in cartoons, songs, and books were particularly galling.

The "quest for dignity" has, therefore, been at the heart of virtually every political movement in the area. But what gives dignity to a people? Obviously, there are many answers. No one answer is acceptable to all Arabs. But, there are three points on which there is a striking degree of agreement. One is negative and the others positive.

First, none of the modernizers of the Arab lands is prepared to accept the coherence of traditional society as the source of dignity. The "dignity" of a village elder or a Muslim shaikh or the haughty pride of a bedouin, so often admired by Western visitors, seems to the modernizer a consequence of ignorance. The attitude of the Westerner toward these people, moreover, seems to the modernizer to be compounded more of condescension than admiration. In short, the modernizers regard the "colorful bedouin" or the "quaint villager" in the same light as American Negroes regard "Uncle Toms."

Second, the Arabs must be united in order to achieve the strength and coherence which causes others to respect them. This was the lesson of the Palestine conflict. Unity is a complex quality, however obvious may be the manifestations of disunity. The failure of the union of Egypt and Syria showed just how fragile the elements of unity were. Clearly, the lack of unity was not simply a factor of foreign opposition or the lack of agreement between Arab rulers—although both are believed by Arabs to be significant—but depended in part on many other factors: economic organization, political orientation, trade, military doctrine, relations with outside powers, and so forth. It seemed manifest, after the breakup of the union of Egypt and Syria, that only when the Arabs became united in a myriad of cultural, economic, social, political, and military ways could this unity be expressed in a governmental form, and that the expression of the form would not necessarily give reality to unity. Thus, while all Arabs remain vocally committed to union, they differ on questions of the terms, the leadership, and the speed and the profundity of the measures.

Third, most if not all of the modernizers are willing to use the full apparatus of the state to carry their reforms into effect. This does not, in the Middle Eastern context, imply the same sort of ideological commitment as it would in Western Europe. It is not, as some observers aver, pragmatism—a willingness to experiment with various answers to problems—but is a commitment to use all available power. It is this which links Mehmet Ali Pasha to Gamal Abdul Nasser. On this basic point there is no significant ideological disagreement.

Why should this be so?

We in the West are so conscious of our own norms as often to seek to use these too precisely as measures for the actions of others in different cultural patterns. The split we find to be normal between Church and State, for example, we do not find in quite the same form in Arab society. Nor has there been in the political and economic spheres of life in Arab society the sharp distinction between the state and individual endeavor. It is important to be clear about this.

In the great river basin economies of the Near East, the role of the state in economic life was not only predominant but both minute and active. The state controlled water, the state set the standard in taxation and rent of land, the state decided what should be planted and when; in industry, the state owned the factories, bought the raw materials, employed the workers, set output quotas, and collected and distributed the production; in commerce, the state was often the sole merchant, monopolizing virtually all distribution of imports and exports. This was a pattern common to the ancient pharaohs, the Mamluks, and Mehmet Ali and is today the pattern adopted by "Arab socialism."

In this pattern there is no major role for the initiative of the individual, except as he operates within the state machinery, and no respect for or toleration of separate bases of power. Private property is not deeply rooted in either the Islamic or the Middle Eastern past: men have traditionally had usufruct of income producers but the state retained ownership. Land, for example, was the possession (*mulk*) of the state even though individuals either as favorites, payers of taxes, or holders of office, ex officio, had rights to some of the revenue of the land.

Property, per se, was regarded as exploitive rather than creative. It was what God did, through rain and sun, that made land yield under the hand of the peasant, himself virtually a "natural resource," rather than what a manager or investor did that gave value.

In nomadic society the land was the gift of the superhuman forces which control the fall of rain and the changes of the seasons. Herds of animals depended upon teams of men, the clans, for their guidance and protection. No man could accumulate very much because he could neither protect nor use more than a certain amount. For the individual real wealth and power came from membership in a rich and powerful "nation-state," his clan. The peasant often had an understanding with his fellows on allocation of resources for he, like the nomad, could not exploit or profit from more than a certain amount of land and water. Even less than the nomad could he protect wealth. Consequently, in many parts of the Arab World, as in the Russian village commune, the *mir*, land was periodically reallocated. It was less in a particular plot of land than in a village community that the farmer had a share. He had, of course, no major incentive to invest in the particular plot that was his this year and might be someone else's next. When he had to invest, as on the mountain sides of Lebanon where terrace walls had to be built and maintained, property tended not to be reallocated and tenure to be clearly defined.

The landlord, similarly, could not count on possession of land for long periods. The estate which he "owned" came to him primarily in his capacity as tax collector for the government or to give him an income while he exercised an office or supplied soldiers. His relationship to the land was thus that of an exploiter rather than an investor or entrepreneur.

Finally, the merchant and manufacturer lived on the bounty and at the whim of the governor. It was essentially the control of competition, through the customs and marketing outlets, that decided success or failure of a venture. The business man, therefore, became a sort of agent of the ruler rather than an independent contributor to public prosperity.

Thus, as tolerant as Islam and pre-Islamic society have been of religious or kindred diversity, they never found congenial the notion that ownership of property or creation of wealth alone entitled men to any special toleration. Nor did they understand or condone the division between the individual and society or the individual and the state in ways familiar to us. These are factors of major importance in understanding the Arab Middle East of today.

Two other factors contribute to the emphasis on the role of the state in economic affairs. On the one hand, the modernizers in Egypt, Syria, and Iraq, particularly, came to power to speed up the modernization process. Their competitors for power were the men of the existing regimes, and these men, under the liberalizing influences of European mandate or guidance, had tried to diminish the role of the state and to foster the rise of private business initiative. Ownership of property had not yet created a vigorous, reforming "middle class," but had been adopted as a protection of privilege by the old power elite. The landlords of Iraq and Egypt and Syria had seized control of parliaments and had used their power to evade taxation and to tighten their control on the rural areas; to break their power the revolutionary regimes logically as well as sentimentally turned to programs of land distribution and sequestration of property.

Secondly, the "new men" wanted to move quickly and dramatically to catch up with the industrialized West and to solve problems of unemployment. They needed investment of a sort that private capitalists were unwilling to make. What the nation needed, in the eyes of the new men, was not necessarily, or even probably, going to have a good investment-profit ratio. What Egyptian capitalist could be Egypt's Carnegie to build the Helwan steel mill? With Iraq's oil fields already farmed out to the international consortium, the Iraq Petroleum Company, Iraq had no scope for a Rockefeller.

Moreover, if the Arabs are to catch up with the industrial areas of the world, they are going to have to make massive investments quickly in "social overhead" facilities which are traditionally, even in Western society, the domain of the state. Schools, hospitals, dams, and bridges are a felt need for the present, and in most of the Arab countries these have virtually been begun from the start in the last generation. Not only was the state, therefore, the organizer and motive force but it had to operate on a scale and in a period of time which made it preponderant: the Arab World has not had time for an Oxford, much less a Harvard or even such a new university as a Stanford, to evolve; what it needed, it needed quickly and on a huge scale.

Over the course of sixty years, for example, the Egyptian educational system has moved from no government schools to a
system which, by 1970, will enroll five million students, from the
first grade to postdoctoral work in nuclear energy. Only the state
could make such progress; in this, men as different from one
another as Lord Cromer and President Nasser have agreed.

Contributing to this emphasis on the role of the state, also,
was the other major impulse of the modern Arab scene, the need
to acquire military power. Clearly, this was a proper role for the
state. Private armies did exist in Egypt until about 1805, and, in a
sense, still today exist in Saudi Arabia, but these guards units and
"White armies" do not and cannot command the plethora of
expensive and complex equipment which distinguish modern
armies. Only a state can afford to buy and maintain a Mig-21 or a
T-54 tank. But, as Mehmet Ali realized long ago to own the
machine is very different from having power. Power comes from
control over production of the machines, the generation of economic capability to sustain them, and the training of men to use
them. Thus, the growth of military establishments has led most
of the Arab states into the myriad of associated problems of
logistics, creation of maintenance facilities, and, ultimately, the
development of factories to make all the tools of modern armies
and air forces. In Egypt this has now reached the point of developing and building rockets and jet fighter planes. These efforts
have led the state into many activities which in earlier, less complex times in the West contributed to the establishment of a
sphere of economic activity in which the state played a lesser,
more detached role. There is, therefore, no place for a Du Pont,
a Krupp, or a Nobel in the Arab World today.

On this basic point of the role of the state there is today very
little difference between any of the Arab governments, whether
monarchies or revolutionary "new men." What then are the principal points of difference?

The major differences are in the tactics to be adopted to
achieve agreed aims: the speed and control of the modernization
process and the political involvement of the individual in the
state. On these points there are profound differences of emphasis

and direction particularly between the "postrevolutionary" or "intrarevolutionary" states of Iraq, Syria, and Egypt (and Algeria in North Africa) on the one hand and on the other the more conservative, nonrevolutionary states of Lebanon, Jordan, Kuwait, and Saudi Arabia (joined by Libya, Tunisia, and Morocco in North Africa). Neither group feels safe as long as the other continues its programs and both have made strenuous efforts to persuade or force the other to adopt its model.

Involvement with outside powers likewise distinguishes the Arab states. From membership in the Baghdad Pact in the spring of 1958 Iraq swung very close to the Soviet Bloc in the spring of 1959; Saudi Arabia and Jordan depend heavily upon the West; Lebanon and Kuwait are usually able to call their own terms but each has ultimately shown to all that its security rested upon Western protectiveness. Egypt and post-Qasim Iraq have charted a more or less middle course which has been termed, by President Nasser, "positive neutralism." Essentially, this involves two elements: maintenance of political independence and extraction of all possible aid and assistance from both sides in the Cold War. Egypt, to date, has managed to get nearly $1 billion worth of arms and $1 billion worth of economic assistance from the USSR while banning the Communist party in Egypt, and while nationalizing foreign and domestically owned industry convinced the United States that it was to the American national interest to assist with a large aid program. The reasons for this willingness of outside powers to help Egypt, despite the unwillingness of the Egyptians to cater to foreign desires, are clearly not transferable to other areas and other peoples. Nevertheless the Egyptian program of neutralism has exercised a strong attraction not only in the Arab World but all over the Tropical belt of modernizing nations.

These are, obviously, tremendous areas for disagreement. They are the elements of Arab politics and interstate relations today, but as important as they are they come after a basic agreement that *the* objective is the achievement of a place of dignity for the Arabs in the world.

PART SIX THE UNITED STATES AND THE ARAB WORLD

XVII. A Decade of Discovery

Two aspects of United States relations with the Arab World call for our attention. Essentially these are merely different ways of approaching the same subject. The first is the history of the relationship and the second is a catalogue of what the United States seeks.

Unlike Latin America, Europe, and the Far East, the Middle East held little commercial or political interest for Americans in the nineteenth and early twentieth centuries. It was the missionary, for whom the Middle East was the Land of the Bible, who set the style of American involvement there. But the early missionary found its people so ignorant of their heritage and so borne down by the ills of this world as to be unwilling and unable to aspire to a higher calling. Consequently, starting in 1823, small bands of American missionaries began laying the foundations of what by the end of the century grew into a network of schools, colleges, and hospitals in Syria, Anatolia, and Egypt. In times of crisis, the Americans were sustained by British consuls. Rarely was much notice taken of them by the United States government except that it occasionally augmented its own small diplomatic corps by appointing missionaries as part-time consuls.

The United States did not declare war on the Ottoman Empire in World War I. But during the war President Wilson's declarations on self-determination led to a belief on the part of others that the United States would accept a large measure of responsibility for the achievement of a just and enduring peace in the Middle East, based upon the applications of its own domestic political ideals. There was a period in which the United States seemed to be moving in this direction. At one time she was deeply involved in the Armenian question. Suspicion of the intentions of Britain and France caused the United States government to send to the Middle East the King-Crane Commission to ascertain the desires of the native populations. At the Peace Conference an American Zionist delegation persuaded President Wilson to urge the application of the Balfour Declaration. But with the American return to isolationism, these efforts amounted to little. A bill urging an American protectorate for Armenia was killed in Congress; the report of the King-Crane Commission was probably never seen by Wilson, was not published in the United States until the end of 1922, and had no perceptible effect in the Middle East; and though the American Congress passed the first of several resolutions approving the Balfour Declaration, it was unprepared to commit the power of the United States to realize its terms.

The return to isolationalism was not, however, complete. Oil interests, already grown strong within America, were pressing for free entry into the new and promising field of the Middle East while their British, Dutch, and French competitors were anxious to keep these areas to themselves. In this case, for the first time, the American State Department took an active part in securing American access to the area. But the chief motivation behind the United States action, fear that American reserves were near exhaustion, was weakened by successive petroleum discoveries on the North American continent. Consequently, the United States government took little further part in Middle Eastern affairs until the coming of World War II.

During World War II, with the notable exceptions of stimulating Saudi Arabian oil production and establishing the Persian Gulf–Iran route to Russia, America took a decidedly secondary role in Middle Eastern activities; the area was British, and the United States was otherwise occupied. Where useful, the United

States would associate itself with Great Britain, as in the Middle East Supply Centre or in the moves to evict France from Lebanon and Syria, but the United States was, as it traditionally had been, far more concerned with other areas.

At the end of the war the United States government resisted British attempts to draw it into a responsible position in Middle Eastern politics. With its own overseas might being severely contracted, its deep sense of involvement in the Far East and Europe, and its people's desire to return to their homes to enjoy the fruits of wartime prosperity, was joined the conviction that Great Britain had both the power and the experience to handle the problems of the Middle East. Few Americans in 1945 thought otherwise. Thus, though President Truman on April 6, 1946, warned of the area's weakness and instability and its importance to the West, he was willing to work only through the United Nations, as in the Iranian dispute, or to offer mediation, as through the Anglo-American Committee of Inquiry in Palestine. He was not willing to accept direct responsibility.

A situation was being created, however, which impelled America to intervene. The Soviet Union refused to participate in the supervision of elections in war-ravaged Greece in 1946 while the Greek Communist party led the rebels in civil war. Soviet territorial demands upon Turkey in 1945 and the prolonged stay of Russian troops in Iran into 1946, emphasized as these were by events in the Balkans, convinced the American government that America must—as Britain announced in February 1947 that it could not—counter Soviet pressure. As the President said: "If Greece should fall under the control of an armed minority, the effect upon its neighbor, Turkey, would be immediate and serious. Confusion and disorder might well spread throughout the entire Middle East."

It was because of the Soviet Union, then, that America first undertook direct and large-scale responsibility for events in the eastern Mediterranean. It did so in default of Great Britain, to whom it had preferred to leave responsibility for the area. And through its European commitments in Greece, America was drawn into an involvement in the Arab World.

Despite the intensity of interest which it had evoked, the Palestine problem was long in calling forth a clear expression of official American policy. The reasons are basically three. In the first place, the Palestine problem has involved, more than any other of the overseas endeavors of the United States, an extension of domestic American politics. Both American Zionists, with well-directed, large-scale campaigns to influence the public, and American liberals, shocked and outraged by the brutality of the Nazis and fearful of future anti-Semitism in Europe and America, have taken to heart the issue of the settlement of Jews in Israel. This interest clashed with that of other groups, particularly those with ties to the Arab World. In the second place, in relation to the growing American concern with the Soviet Union, the problem of Palestine seemed to challenge no basic and vital American interest; whereas the United States government was not prepared to allow Greece or Turkey to slip into the Soviet orbit, it was prepared, within limits, to tolerate hostilities in Palestine. In the third place, the Palestine issue, as it still faces the world, may be said to have been molded at a time when the United States was not responsibly engaged in the Middle East.

When Great Britain indicated that it was unable to resolve the Palestine conflict and intended to turn it over to the United Nations, the United States played a major role in pushing through the General Assembly, in November 1947, a modification of the latest partition plan. However, the United States government was unable to lend the United Nations the force which *might* have made partition possible without war. Its military establishment was depleted and those planning American policy believed that they could not count on congressional or party support for an active policy.

Unable to move forward with any confidence, the government on March 19, 1948, suggested at the UN that action on partition be suspended and that a trusteeship be established over all Palestine to delay final settlement. When this was refused, both by the Soviet Union and by Great Britain, the United States again strongly advocated partition and recognized the State of Israel within minutes after it was proclaimed. Meanwhile, the United

States urged the creation of the UN Palestine Conciliation Commission. When the Commission was established in December 1948, the United States, in its first direct acceptance of responsibility in Palestine, agreed to serve as a member (along with France and Turkey). To support and to resettle the Arab refugees, the United States cooperated in the formation of the UN Relief for Palestine Refugees.

Outside of the United Nations, the United States joined Britain and France in issuing the May 25, 1950, Tripartite Declaration on the security of Middle Eastern frontiers, out of "the desire to promote the establishment and maintenance of peace and stability in the area and . . . unalterable opposition to the use of force or threat of force between any of the states in that area." This undertaking has remained a part of American policy for fifteen years.

Returning from the Middle East in May 1953 Secretary Dulles said he had ascertained that the Arabs were "more fearful of Zionism than of the Communists" because they thought that "the United States will back the new State of Israel in aggressive expansion." The new administration clearly perceived that this fear, and the suspicion it promoted of pro-Israeli policies, inhibited American action in the Middle East.

Israel at this point of her statehood was dependent upon American governmental and private aid. Private aid was pouring into Israel in loans and U.S. income tax–deductible gifts. In the fiscal year 1953 American aid still accounted for an estimated 35 percent of all imports into Israel. The new administration saw this factor as one of considerable leverage in influencing Israeli policy and used it.

When, in the early summer of 1953, the Israeli government began to move its offices to Jerusalem from Tel Aviv the United States government protested that this violated the 1947 UN partition resolution which, inter alia, recognized Jerusalem as an international city. Shortly thereafter, the UN Truce Supervision Organization, acting on a Syrian protest, requested that Israel not undertake a hydroelectric project on the Jordan River at Banat Yaqub, but Israel in September refused to halt work. On October

14–15 the Israeli army raided the village of Qibiya and killed fifty-three Arabs. Joined by France and Great Britain, the United States brought this issue to the Security Council, and Secretary Dulles, noting that the United States had "played an essential part in creating the State of Israel," admonished Israel that "this was clearly an occasion to invoke the concept of decent respect for the opinion of mankind as represented by the United Nations." At the same time it was announced that since September 25 the United States had been withholding an aid allocation because Israel was acting in defiance of the UN. On October 27 Israel suspended work in the demilitarized zone, and the next day Secretary Dulles recommended a grant of $26,250,000 in economic aid for that fiscal year.

Plain speaking on the Palestine issue drew hostile comments from both Israel and the Arab states. Assistant Secretary Byroade in particular was criticized for setting out American policy in 1954 in the following terms:

To the Israelis, I say that you should come to truly look upon yourselves as a Middle Eastern state and see your own future in that context rather than as a headquarters, or nucleus so to speak, or world-wide groupings of peoples or a particular religious faith who must have special rights within and obligations to the Israeli state. You should drop the attitude of a conqueror and the conviction that force and a policy of retaliatory killings is the only policy that your neighbors will understand. You should make your deeds correspond to your frequent utterances of the desire for peace.

To the Arabs I say you should accept this state of Israel as an accomplished fact. I say further that you are deliberately attempting to maintain a state of affairs delicately suspended between peace and war, while at present desiring neither. This is a most dangerous policy and one which world opinion will increasingly condemn if you continue to resist any move to obtain at least a less dangerous *modus vivendi* with your neighbor.

Border tension continued to increase with clandestine raids on the one side and on the other the announcement and fulfillment of Israel's policy of retaliation. The February 28, 1955, attack on Gaza was the high point of these clashes; for it, the Security Council censured Israel on March 29. Since the Gaza raid may be taken as the key event in the build-up to the Czech arms deal, it will be useful at this point to leave the Palestine problem to turn to a second sequence of moves, the attempt by the United States government to improve the economies of the Middle Eastern states.

The experiment with "pump priming" under the New Deal was perhaps the most extensive government economic endeavor in American experience. Moreover, wartime spending accustomed the public to large outlays by the government of funds and the use of these funds for the creation of new industries. The first major application to foreign affairs of government economic initiative was in the 1947 Marshall Plan for European Recovery. The basic ideas there were elaborated and carried a logical step forward in the famous Fourth Point of President Truman's inaugural address in 1949: "We must embark on a bold new program for making the benefits of our scientific advances and industrial progress available for the improvement and growth of underdeveloped areas . . . Our aim should be to help the free peoples of the world, through their own efforts, to produce more food, more clothing, more materials for housing, and more mechanical power to lighten their burdens."

Already, in fact, between 1945 and 1950 Export-Import Bank loans to Middle Eastern and Asian states had totaled $266,110,000. Also the United States had already undertaken a share in the responsibility for the Palestine refugees' economic future.

The American government realized, of course, that the Arab refugees could not be permanently supported on an international dole and that a capital investment would be required if they were to be reintegrated into the economy of the Middle East. To this end, the State Department urged the UN Conciliation Commission for Palestine to send to the Middle East an economic survey mission under the leadership of Gordon R. Clapp, the chairman of the Tennessee Valley Authority. Out of the Clapp Commission report came the establishment of the UN Relief and Works Agency and, not less important, a broad scheme for the economic development of the whole area due to the recognition that "solution of the problem of poverty and unemployment of the refugees is . . . inseparable from a solution of the problem of poverty and hunger as that already affects a large section of the population of the Middle East."

The United States government undertook to assist in both programs. It contributed $45 million to the initial UN Relief and Works Agency and yearly since has met over one half of the agency's budget. The 1950 Act for International Development set aside $34.5 million for technical assistance, and the 1951 Mutual Security Appropriation Act set up a $160 million fund for technical and economic assistance and allocated $21.5 million for general Point IV aid. In addition the United States contributed $12 million to the UN technical assistance program for the eighteen months from July 1, 1950. In the following years these amounts have been generally increased so that by the end of the fiscal year 1963 the United States had advanced some $795 million in grants and $584 million in loans for economic and technical assistance to the Arab countries of the Middle East.

In presenting the argument for the Mutual Security Program for the fiscal year beginning July 1, 1952, the government stated that "Political unrest and intense nationalism characterize many of the countries in this area, and in part reflect deep-rooted social and economic ills . . . The poverty resulting from these factors together with a disease and illiteracy contributing to them, form a vicious circle which we can help to break by the application of technical skills." Given this analysis, the policy of the United States was to "assist the people and governments of the area to achieve not only greater military security, through the Middle East Command and limited military assistance, but also to assist responsible leaders in getting under way orderly reform and development, in which the energies of the people can find constructive expansion. Our purpose is to demonstrate to these countries, by concrete cooperative effort, that they themselves can achieve their desires for economic and social progress as a part of the free world. People who have evidence of this will not turn in desperation to Communism."

Initial reception in the area was good: Israel, Libya, Egypt, Saudi Arabia, Lebanon, Jordan, and eventually Iraq entered into Point IV or subsequent aid agreements.

The change of administration brought no drastic changes in American policy; the Middle East was not mentioned in President Eisenhower's Inaugural Address in January 1953. The tide of United States involvement ebbed in the Middle East but flowed in the Far East. Under the impact of the Korean War American thinking increasingly followed military paths in its quest for security, and American funds were forthcoming mainly for military projects.

From the period following the Palestine War American aid has been used to damp down intra-area hostility and to build economies strong and progressive enough to resist the lure of Communism. American policy planners never changed in their close attention to what they regarded as the overriding goal, to counter or contain the Soviet Union. The policy of containment had been closely linked with economic aid. In the Mutual Security Program recommended to Congress by President Truman on May 24, 1951, the union of these concepts was clearly spelled out. Aid to the Middle East was necessary, said the President, because the Soviet Union was applying to the area "steady and relentless pressure" which the area was unable, alone, to withstand. "Endangered by political and economic instability, the security objective in the area must be to create stability by laying solid foundations, now, of economic progress and by establishing, now, confidence that further advances can be made." But, increasingly, after 1952 money was to be put directly into the creation of military strength rather than into programs to build economic strength. Of the $540 million proposed for 1953 for the Middle East, exclusive of economic assistance given to Greece and Turkey, $415 million was to be spent on military aid, mainly for Greece, Turkey, and Iran. Even at this date the government was clearly most concerned with the military aspects of what Secretary Dulles was later to call the "northern tier of nations," and in September and October invited Turkey and Greece to make arrangements to join in the military planning work of NATO. Both accepted and in the following September were invited to join as full members.

The rest of the Middle East presented a pact-maker's nightmare. Iran, already in serious financial troubles, was involved in the dispute which ended in the nationalization of the oil company and so in conflict with the British government. It was, therefore, a most unlikely partner in a British-led pact. Israel was an unlikely choice since its participation would automatically exclude the Arab states. The center of military strength at that time was at Suez, and in British thinking Egypt was the pivot of Middle Eastern power. Therefore, Egypt seemed to be the logical place to start. Consequently, on October 13, 1951, Great Britain, France, Turkey, and the United States invited Egypt to help found the Allied Middle East Command. If Egypt were prepared to join and to permit the use of her facilities, including the Suez base, Great Britain would agree to suppress the Anglo-Egyptian treaty of 1936 and would withdraw all British forces not assigned to the Allied Command. Britain made clear, however, that Egypt's demands on the Sudan would not be met.

Given the political climate in Egypt, neither the formula nor the time was propitious. Prime Minister Nahhas' weak government, under attack for domestic corruption, sought to protect itself with safe patriotism. It was publicly committed to the "unity of the Nile Valley" and could hardly give its domestic enemies the weapon they could have fashioned from a Wafd deal with the British. Nahhas immediately rejected the proposal and then pressed a counterattack by abrogating, unilaterally, the 1936 treaty under which British troops were in Suez. Thus, not only did the West not get a better coordinated defense arrangement, but it seriously weakened, at least de jure, its existing position.

The United States government was not prepared to give up. Despite the Egyptian rejection and Soviet protests that the United States was trying to draw the Middle East into the "aggressive Atlantic bloc," the government tried to keep the project alive until the May 1953 visit of Secretary Dulles to the Middle East.

Returning from that trip, Mr. Dulles indicated that he had come to the conclusion that it was not then feasible to attempt to create a Middle East parallel to NATO. There was, he found, "a vague desire to have a collective security system, but no such system can be imposed from without. It should be designed and grow from within out of a sense of common destiny and common danger." No two senses could be further from the thoughts—and nerves—of the Arab states. Mr. Dulles found that American fear of Communism was paralleled by Arab fear of Israel. But in Greece, Turkey, and Iran, he took hope. The implications of this finding represented less of a new departure in American policy, which had throughout the period included heavy contributions to Greece, Turkey, and Iran, than a departure from the ideal strategic model of the British, based upon Suez, a concept, incidentally, upon which the Arab League Collective Security Pact has been partly based.

Extension of the "northern tier" concept into the Baghdad Pact was a development in which the United States government took the keenest interest without playing an overt part. It was thought in Washington that however much use of the carrot and the stick were required, the states involved must pull or at least seem to pull their own loads. By late 1953 the United States had begun to plan a military assistance agreement with Pakistan which materialized in May 1954; on April 2, 1954, Turkey and Pakistan signed a military pact. When Pakistan joined the Southeast Asia Collective Defense Treaty in September, it became obvious that in the making was a belt of defense treaties from Europe to the Far East. The United States extended military assistance to Iraq in April 1954. In February 1955 Turkey and Iraq signed the Mutual Cooperation Pact which was opened to all members of the Arab League and other states concerned with peace and security in the Middle East. The United Kingdom adhered to this agreement on April 4 and terminated the Anglo-Iraqi treaty of 1930; Pakistan joined on September 23 and Iran on October 11.

Since the new pact bypassed the Arab League and was based in Baghdad whose government was hostile to President Nasser, it brought about an immediate deterioration of American relations with those Arab states in which President Nasser had strong influence, first Syria, then Saudi Arabia, and for a time Jordan. This development, coupled with the growing tensions along the Arab-Israeli frontier, with the United States' unwillingness to supply arms on terms acceptable to Egypt, and possibly with internal pressures in the Egyptian army, caused Nasser to conclude the arms purchase agreement with Czechoslovakia. President Nasser announced the arrangement on September 27, and on September 28 an American emissary was sent to Cairo to reactivate and make more acceptable the earlier American arms offer. The Egyptians were not swayed, but the American response to the Russian move set what President Nasser was to regard as a precedent—the key to American motivations—when he came to negotiate aid for the Aswan High Dam.

As the United States government saw the Czech arms deal, it was sure to touch off an uncontrolled arms race; American arms, it was thought, would not, even if they were given to Egypt, since they were legally tied to specific uses. Furthermore, the United States pointed out, it estimated that the likely terms upon which the arms were acquired would mortgage the Egyptian economy to the Soviet Union far into the future. Lastly, it brought the Cold War into Arab-American relations as never before. These arguments failed to impress the Egyptian government, which pointed out both that it had tried unsuccessfully to acquire arms from the West and that it thought the Czech deal was a good swap for Egyptian cotton. Syria and Saudi Arabia indicated their willingness to make similar arrangements. In the United States the fear grew that the "northern tier" had been hurdled.

The Palestine problem remained, as it remains today, a focal point of all the separate problems of the area and, therefore, of American efforts to assist in the achievement of peace and stability there. To the Council on Foreign Relations on August 26, 1955, Secretary of State Dulles had set out one possible approach to this complex issue. Mr. Dulles suggested that an international loan might enable "Israel to pay the compensation which is due and which would enable many of the refugees to find for themselves a better way of life." He further offered American assistance in determining satisfactory frontiers which the United States would then guarantee against aggression.

Eric Johnston had been appointed in 1953 as a special representative of the President to work on the problem of the Jordan River waters and was then in the midst of protracted negotiations with the Arab states and Israel. These did not produce any agreement but did lay the basis of American aid efforts. In effect, the United States indicated that it was willing to assist both the Arab states and Israel to complete projects which were in accord with the Johnston proposal; thus, though the Johnston Plan was not in principle accepted, it was in practice largely implemented.

It was not until the new administration that the next major public effort by the United States was made in the mission of Joseph E. Johnson as Special Representative of the United Nations Palestine Conciliation Commission. Johnson visited the Middle East in September 1961 and again in April and May of 1962 to attempt to find a solution to the refugee problem.

But in the Arab states there was no appreciation of Western attempts to be impartial. Egyptian anti-Western propaganda grew in bitterness, and this propaganda played an important part in creating an atmosphere in which Great Britain lost its control over the Jordan army. In other Arab states responsible political leaders privately expressed their fears that President Nasser had found his model not in Arabi Pasha but in Mehmet Ali Pasha—that his aim was not liberation of Egypt but regency over the Arabs. To the American public and Congress Nasser began to assume the shape of a villain and the possible range of State Department actions in regard to him narrowed.

Meanwhile, the Egyptian government, anxious to secure the necessary hard-currency funds to construct the Aswan High Dam, had approached the International Bank for a loan. The bank had agreed, contingent upon British and American participation to the amount of $70 million, to lend Egypt $200 million. In December the United States had been prepared to agree to this, but Egypt did not at that time accept. When the president of the International Bank went to Cairo the rumor was "leaked" that agreement with the Soviet Union, on much better terms, was near. If this was a ploy to get the same reaction as in the Czech arms deal, the ploy did not work. The grant from the Soviet Union did not, at that time at least, materialize; then, when President Nasser tried to reopen discussions with the United States by sending an ambassador to Washington to close the agreement, he met with a sharp and, in Egyptian eyes, humiliating rebuff. Secretary Dulles, having already found, but not countered, opposition to such a loan in Congress, announced on July 20 that the United States could no longer consider participating. In its statement, more-over, the United States government questioned "the ability of Egypt to devote adequate resources to assure the project's suc-cess" and also indicated its unfavorable view of the increasingly close ties between Egypt and the Soviet Union. Infuriated by the "public insult," President Nasser struck out at the only available large target, the Suez Canal. In his Alexandria speech of July 26, he announced that the Universal Suez Maritime Canal Company had been nationalized.

Reaction to nationalization of the company was swift. The for-eign ministers of the United States, Great Britain, and France met in London on August 2, and the first London Conference of the "user states" was held from August 16 to 23. It was there agreed that a five-man delegation be sent to Cairo to present to President Nasser the proposals agreed to by eighteen of the users. The dele-gation visited Cairo from September 3 to 9 but failed to reach any agreement. The United States froze Egyptian funds in the United States, on the plea that it must be able to indemnify ship-pers who, while paying tolls to the Egyptian government at Suez, might also be sued for tolls by the Canal Company in Europe.

Up to this point, the reaction had been so swift as to startle the Egyptian government. But already a fatal weakness appeared in the Western position. Greece refused to attend the conference, and there was, within the conference, obvious disagreement as to the ways to negotiate a settlement and on the extent of pressure to be applied to Egypt. The attitude of Sir Anthony Eden was unmistakable, but that of Mr. Dulles was overtly, at least, imprecise. The United States would not recommend to its citizens that they continue to serve in the canal, as other Westerners resigned from their posts, but it also would not urge its shipping lines, all highly susceptible to government pressure as the recipients of its subsidies, to boycott Suez. In these circumstances President Nasser made every effort to keep the canal in operation, so as to avoid charges of obstruction or incompetence, and waited for further disagreements to turn the de facto Egyptian control into one recognized as de jure.

On the eve of his departure for the Second London Conference Secretary Dulles took what must have been read in Europe as a threatening tone toward Egypt. He went on to outline his answer to the problem, the Canal Users Association, the precise nature of which was to become the major point of discussion at the Second London Conference. And at this conference Mr. Dulles issued a statement in which the main lines of American policy are clear—but clear in their exact emphasis, it must be admitted, only in restrospect. "Now we are faced here with a problem whereby great nations are faced with a great peril. It is a peril that they could readily remedy if they resorted to the methods which were lawful before this charter was adopted. Then, we wouldn't be sitting around here—perhaps somebody else wouldn't be sitting where he is, either. But those days, we hope, are past. There has been exercised, and is being exercised, a great restraint in the face of great peril. But you cannot expect that to go on indefinitely unless those of us who appreciate the problem, who are sympathetic with it, rally our forces to try to bring about a settlement in conformity with the principles of justice and international law."

On September 21 the United States subscribed to the Co-operative Association of Suez Canal Users which later was called the Suez Canal Users Association. Five days later the United States announced that it would back the United Kingdom and France in the forthcoming United Nations debate. In his press conference on that day Secretary Dulles commented that "the decision of the United States, at least, as I put it, [is] not to shoot its way through the canal." He went on to say that "there are pressures which gradually grow up, not artificially stimulated but as quite natural and inevitable . . . But I do not believe that the situation is such now as to call for any drastic action like going to war."

In the rush of events and in the circumstances, as now known, within the British government and the French government, these remarks did rather less than clarify exactly what the United States would agree to. The position of the United States was, in fact, throughout opposed to the use of force, but each statement, such as that of Secretary Dulles on October 6, was so worded as always to hedge with a "But those who are concerned about peace ought to be equally concerned about justice."

Apparent indecision in the United States government was certainly matched by confusing moves by the British government; only the French and Israeli Governments appear, at the beginning of October, to have had clear plans. On October 10–11, when Israeli forces attacked Qalqilya, the British government reaffirmed its treaty obligations to Jordan despite the fact that Jordan was obviously and rapidly moving in the direction of closer ties with Egypt. (On October 26 a unified military command of Jordan, Egypt, and Syria was established.) The British and French governments certainly did not, however, keep the United States informed of what plans they had. Former Secretary Acheson said bluntly in 1958, in his *Power and Diplomacy*, that "the British Government did not inform ours of its plans to use force. It is fair to go further and say that, at that stage, its conduct was deceitful."

When reports of an Israeli mobilization reached President Eisenhower, he sent a personal message to Prime Minister Ben Gurion "expressing my grave concern and renewing a previous recommendation that no forcible initiative be taken which would endanger the peace." On October 28 the President again wrote to the Prime Minister. It is now known that already at that early date the United States was applying strong pressure on Israel not to act. But the Israeli army struck the next day; the following day came the Anglo-French ultimatum, and on the thirty-first, the Anglo-French invasion.

On the day of the ultimatum the United States took the issue to the Security Council (where its resolution was vetoed by Britain and France) and the President made a national radio and television address on the events in Hungary and the invasion of Egypt. In the course of his talk, Mr. Eisenhower said: "We believe these actions to have been taken in error . . . The actions taken can scarcely be reconciled with the principles and purposes of the United Nations to which we have all subscribed. And beyond this, we are forced to doubt even if resort to war will for long serve the permanent interests of the attacking nations . . . There can be no peace—without law. And there can be no law—if we were to invoke one code of international conduct for those who oppose us and another for our friends."

At the General Assembly, to which the United States had taken its vetoed resolution from the Security Council, Secretary Dulles on November 1 summed up, as perhaps no other statement he had ever made did more truly, the feelings of many Americans: "I doubt that any delegates ever spoke from this forum with as heavy a heart as I have brought here tonight. We speak on a matter of vital importance, where the United States finds itself unable to agree with three nations with whom it has ties, deep friendship, admiration, and respect, and two of whom constitute our oldest, most trusted and reliable allies."

The General Assembly adopted, 64–5, the United States resolution calling for an immediate cease-fire and withdrawal. But on November 3 this was rejected by France, Great Britain, and Israel. Negotiations were conducted by the UN Secretary General with Israel and Egypt, but both the United States and the Soviet Union took strong independent action. On November 4 the Soviet government delivered a note to the British government in which it "emphatically protests against these illegal actions by the United Kingdom and France and declares that the responsibility for all the possible consequences of those actions rests with the Governments of the United Kingdom and France." At the UN the United States supported a draft resolution introduced by Canada, Colombia, and Norway to establish the United Nations

Emergency Force. On the same day Soviet Foreign Minister Shepilov sent a note to the UN Security Council president declaring its readiness to send to Egypt "the air and naval forces necessary to defend Egypt and repulse the aggressors." Soviet Premier Bulganin wrote at the same time to President Eisenhower proposing "joint and immediate use" of the strong naval and air forces of the two powers to end the attack. In a statement from the White House, the United States immediately rejected the proposal saying that "neither Soviet nor any other military forces should now enter the Middle East area except under United Nations mandate . . . The introduction of new forces under these circumstances would violate the United Nations Charter, and it would be the duty of all United Nations members, including the United States, to oppose any such effort." The United States note went on to contrast the Soviet attitude on Egypt with the Soviet intervention in Hungary.

On October 7 Prime Minister Ben Gurion, far from indicating any fear of the Soviet attitude, which had included the withdrawing of the Soviet ambassador to Israel, spoke of the "glorious military operation . . . an unprecedented feat in Jewish history and . . . rare in the world's history." But on the same day the General Assembly once again called upon Israel to withdraw, and President Eisenhower again wrote to express his "deep concern" at the refusal of the Israeli government to withdraw its army from Egyptian territory. In reply, the following day, in the face of strong American pressure, Ben Gurion agreed to comply but indicated that the problem of the Sinai hostilities could not be separated from the context of the whole aftermath of the Palestine War. As Israel saw the steps toward peace, they must include, along with evacuation of Sinai, an end to the economic boycott of Israel, direct negotiations between Israel and the Arab states, and freedom of passage for Israeli ships through the Straits of Tiran and through Suez.

Israeli demands were regarded with sympathy in Washington since it was the opinion of the United States government that Egypt had done much to provoke the attack and that a return to the status quo ante was dangerous. Yet, the United States also was worried about the implications of a solution brought about by the use of force, for if the invasion could be reckoned a success, even indirectly, then the dangers of coups de main were certainly increased. Consequently, both in public and in private, the American government assured Israel that it would do all in its power to settle the outstanding problems of the status quo ante, but that, as Ambassador Lodge said in the General Assembly on several occasions and Secretary Dulles affirmed in dispatches to the Israeli government, the United States agreed with the Secretary General that "withdrawal is a preliminary and essential phase in a development through which a stable basis may be laid for peaceful conditions in the area."

The United States government felt, possibly, less sympathy with the British and French position, in that the actions of such close allies—particularly in the context of NATO—put the United States in a position of acute embarrassment. It was felt also that the Anglo-French invasion had at least mitigated the effects of the brutal Soviet repression of Hungary and was thus not only irresponsible but tragic. Considerable relief was felt in Washington when the last of the Anglo-French force was evacuated on December 23, the United Nations Emergency Force began their forward movement into Sinai. The last Israeli troops left Egyptian territory on March 1, 1957.

It was at this point that the United States had to try to pick up the tangled lines of its various alliances and to reassess the general context of its foreign policy. If the United States was to attempt to hold together a broad and at times mutually hostile coalition of Europe and Asia, it must have firm, clear, and definite policy assumptions and goals by which crises could be controlled. The Eisenhower Doctrine was an attempt to accomplish this purpose.

A part of the justification for the British intervention in Suez was given in Commons on December 3 by Foreign Secretary Lloyd as a response to "Soviet mischief making." "The large supply of Soviet arms to Colonel Nasser," said Mr. Lloyd, "put him very much under Soviet influence. The Baghdad Pact gave a measure of security against direct Soviet penetration from the

North, but the arming of Syria and Egypt, was no doubt intended to turn its flank also." It was this element which rapidly re-emerged from momentary eclipse in American thought as the local crisis became manageable. On January 5, at a time in which the United States was attempting at the United Nations and through direct pressure to bring about a withdrawal of Israeli forces in Egypt, President Eisenhower turned his attention back to the threat of the Soviet Union in the Middle East. In the course of his address to Congress the President said: "All this instability [in the Middle East] has been heightened and, at times, manipulated by International Communism . . . Russia's interest in the Middle East is solely that of power politics. Considering her announced purpose of Communizing the world, it is easy to understand her hope of dominating the Middle East . . . [If this came about] Western Europe would be endangered just as though there had been no Marshall Plan, no North Atlantic Treaty Organization. The free nations of Asia and Africa, too, would be placed in serious jeopardy."

The UN, said President Eisenhower, had shown its abilities when faced by nations with a decent respect for the opinions of mankind, but in Hungary the situation was otherwise. Therefore, "a greater responsibility now devolves upon the United States. We have shown, so that none can doubt, our dedication to the principle that force shall not be used internationally for any aggressive purpose and that the integrity and independence of the nations of the Middle East should be inviolate. Seldom in history has a nation's dedication to principle been tested as severely as ours during recent weeks." The President went on to propose a joint congressional-presidential declaration embodying three features: (1) provision for the United States to cooperate with nations in the area to build up their economic strength; to this end $200 million yearly for the discretionary use of the President was requested; (2) greater flexibility for the President to use funds already allocated to assist any nation or group of nations desiring military assistance and cooperation; and (3) permission to use the "armed forces of the United States to secure and protect the territorial integrity and political independence of such nations, requesting such aid, against overt armed aggression from any nation controlled by International Communism."

Congress passed the Eisenhower Doctrine as a joint resolution on March 9, 1957, and on the same day the President appointed James P. Richards, former chairman of the House Foreign Affairs Committee, as his special assistant to carry the doctrine to the Middle East. Like the doctrine itself, the mission was largely redundant since all that it gained was public endorsement by those states that had already indicated their friendly attitude toward the same policy in a former guise. But upon his return Ambassador Richards spoke glowingly on June 13 to the House Foreign Affairs Committee of his mission. "This new departure, this entirely American line of action, evoked a heart-warming trust from the nations of the area." On his trip, Mr. Richards said, he had managed to give out $120 million of which one half went for economic aid. And his optimism was echoed by other officials. Assistant Secretary Rountree, on May 16, affirmed that American policies were "definitely" achieving their goals. "International Communism," reads the first report of the Richards mission on August 5, 1957, "has been put on notice . . . and the nations of the area are encouraged to help themselves."

The "Syrian crisis" of August and September was a clear test of the assumptions underlying the new doctrine. On August 6 the Soviet government agreed to provide large amounts of economic aid to Syria; on August 15 the Syrian chief of staff was replaced by a man regarded in Washington as pro-Soviet. Then officials of the United States embassy in Damascus were expelled, and in retaliation the Syrian ambassador was asked to leave Washington. United States arms shipments were announced to Jordan (by airlift), Lebanon, Iraq, and Saudi Arabia. These moves were followed by a statement from Secretary Dulles that "Turkey now faces growing military danger from the major build-up of arms in Syria." Nowhere in the Middle East was this taken at face value. Given the facts—the Syrian army contained only about 50,000 men, mostly lacking in battle experience, whose presence on the Israeli frontier was necessary, and whose equipment was new and for which they were poorly trained; the Turkish army of half a million men (the largest field force in NATO) had been armed and trained for a decade by the United States, and, in being able to rely upon NATO guarantees, were able to deploy on the Syrian frontier—it is not surprising that many in the Middle East thought that the United States was looking for an excuse to employ the Eisenhower Doctrine.

It is now clear that the United States was not prepared to take decisive action to block the Soviet Union's offer of aid, but having given the impression that it intended to do so, had both to back down and to be damned for having opposed the good that might result from such aid. As it was, the actions of the United States government were both futile and damaging to its position.

But if the Syrian crisis of the fall showed the shortfalls of the Eisenhower Doctrine, the Lebanese crisis of the spring and summer showed its dangers. On May 8, 1958, the editor of a Beirut newspaper was shot, and this act touched off an already tense and smoldering atmosphere. The contributing causes of the tension were many and deeply rooted in history. A more recent element, of import here, was what many Lebanese regarded as an excessive identification of the government of Lebanon with United States policy to oppose President Nasser of Egypt. The Richards Mission had been interpreted in the Middle East as a demand that the Middle Eastern states leave the neutralist position, which many had found attractive, and "stand up to be counted," a posture for which the United States was prepared to pay cash. Thus, on May 10 the United States Information Service (USIS) library in Tripoli was sacked; on the twelfth Beirut was blockaded. On the fourteenth the United States said it was doubling the marine force with the Sixth Fleet; on the sixteenth announced that it would shortly send further military assistance to Lebanon; and on the seventeenth stated that it was considering sending troops to Lebanon if requested. On the eighteenth the Soviet Union accused the United States of interfering in Lebanese domestic affairs. Great Britain and the United States agreed to joint action if needed and on the twenty-fifth the Royal Air Force delivered arms to Lebanon. By June 3 the last (the fifth) USIS center was closed.

The United States, worried by reports of external espionage activity in Lebanon, maintained its offer to send troops if required but was constantly concerned about the use made of the arms it had supplied for regular military units—these were often given over to partisan forces. On July 3 a United Nations observer group reported "no evidence" of mass infiltration by non-Lebanese agents as charged by the Lebanese government. The situation remained dangerously tense and frightening. Finally, on July 15 some 5000 United States marines landed near the Beirut airport.

The precipitating cause of the American landings had nothing to do with Lebanon directly but was the reflex action following a coup d'etat in Baghdad in the early dawn of July 14.

Like the Lebanese civil war, the coup in Baghdad was the result of many factors. Important also in Iraq was the identification of the Iraqi government with the United States government to such an extent, in the opinion of a large section of the Iraqi population, that the Iraq government was not acting on Iraqi or Arab interests but on behalf of the British and American governments. The attempt to use Iraqi troops outside Iraq to stabilize the Middle Eastern situation was the event which touched off the coup.

In short, the very act of getting the governments in the Middle East to "stand up and be counted" weakened them domestically and so produced results opposite to those expected in Washington.

The coup d'etat in Baghdad clearly caught the United States as much by surprise as it did the senior officials of the Iraq government. Yet, there had been ample warnings from observers both in the United States and in England. The fact that these warnings were not heeded gives rise to the question as to whether or not the assumptions made in the Eisenhower Doctrine prevented it from comprehending Middle Eastern politics. In any event, the United States was clearly left with no reasonable move. It could not seriously maintain that the coup in Iraq was due to Communist subversion, for the Communists initially had almost no part in it. Moreover, having landed a large force in Lebanon with more troops and materials in the "pipe line," and having compromised the Lebanese government by that landing, the United States was faced with the delicate task of extricating itself gently. It is fortunate that the Lebanese gift for compromise quickly enabled General Fuad Shihab to become president. Thus the United States was able gracefully, to the tune of heavy spending in the Beirut markets, to withdraw its troops.

No answer had been found to the new situation in Iraq and indeed it is possible that no meaningful action—and perhaps as important—no meaningful inaction within the framework of the Eisenhower Doctrine was possible. The United States was blamed at least as often for what others assumed it might do as for what it did. Baghdad, from being the center post of the Baghdad Pact, rapidly became one of the most anti-American cities in the Middle East, and the United States was forced passively to watch the new government make firmer and closer alliances with the Soviet Bloc. Ironically, this development frightened other Arab nationalists and so proved as awkward in Soviet-Arab politics as the Baghdad Pact had proved in American-Arab relations.

American policy in the last years of the Eisenhower administration might be summarized as embodying a willingness to assist those governments which want American help in their development efforts (to this end American mission furnished advice and the American government grants and loans); the firm determination to prevent "another round" in the Arab-Israeli hostilities (to this end the United States reaffirmed the tripartite guarantee of frontiers and has granted arms where an imbalance threatened the peace); and a desire to stay out of Arab politics as completely as American commitments and national security interests allow. But the intense preoccupation with the Middle East of the period 1955–58 failed or was eclipsed by other areas of concern from 1959–1961.

XVIII. United States Interest in the Arab World

What is it that the United States wants in the Arab Middle East? Does this clash with what the Arabs want? Is the American position there now better or worse than formerly? Are American interests in danger? How can the United States accomplish its objectives? What are the principal contingencies against which the United States must guard? And what are the major opportunities which lie ahead? There are some of the questions which now must be addressed on the basis of the description and analysis presented in preceding chapters.

First a few words of caution: None of the questions can be answered definitively and finally. Ours is an age of extraordinary fluidity in which our own interests, in the Arab Middle East as elsewhere, must constantly be reassessed and redefined. What we regarded some years ago as critical or even vital to American security may be of secondary interest today, while other interests may have grown more valuable.

Secondly, it is both necessary and difficult to establish a standard by which we can evaluate the seemingly endless succession of crises and alarms. The bulk of this study has been directed to that purpose. We have seen that the Arab Middle East is today caught up in a great social revolution common to the Tropical belt of developing nations in Latin America, Africa, South Asia, and Southeast Asia. Throughout that vast area, whole societies are being transformed and are seeking to catch up with the industrial north of the world. The pace, extent, and violence of change has, in part at least, also involved a reaction against prior Western intrusions and hegemony. This reaction against the West on the one hand and on the other the nature of the revolution have significantly affected American interests in the past and will continue to do so into the future.

To avoid jumping from crisis to crisis without a sense of purpose or direction, we must therefore take both a short-term and a long-term view as well as both a Middle Eastern and a Western view and, finally, both an absolute and a relative view. Only from these multiple perspectives can we see a "real world." No one can deny that this is difficult nor can one deny that it is necessary. Reality is never so simple as representations of it.

It may be of some comfort to know that this feat of multiple vision is neither a new problem nor one confined to the American "newcomers" to Middle Eastern perplexities. This is how one part of the problem was put in an official British report: "It is, indeed, scarcely to be wondered at that, in speaking of Egypt . . . the most opposing statements should have gone forth to the world. Materials enough there are both for praise and blame. Any one who turns with a fixed eye towards the good which exists in Egypt—the increased revenues, the novel productions, the progress of toleration, the spread of education, the introduction of military and naval tactics, the improved communication, the safety of travellers, the respect for authority, the personal character [of the ruler]—may long expatiate on the bright hues of the picture; while he who is willing only to dwell on what is dark and discouraging, may find, in the despotic acts of the governors, in the poverty and exhaustion of the governed, in the oppressions of the few and the sufferings of the many, an interminable theme. Judged by the standard of our own civilization, by the rules of Christian philanthropy, the condition of the people will seem deplorable; but contrasting what has been done in Egypt by the struggle for improvement, with what is presented by any other Mahomedan country, the results will appear in the highest degree interesting and important."

It is sobering to learn that this dispatch was written in 1840 to Parliament by Dr. John Bowring. Both the date and the content are relevant: On the one hand, many of the problems and frustrations we face today and will face in the years to come are or will be troublesome, but they are not unique to our age, and we, like our ancestors in the "good old days," will have to learn to live with many of them. On the other hand, as the dispatch suggests, we must have a standard to judge whether things are now tolerable and are getting better or worse. This standard must be a dual one with a comparison both to the Arabs' own development and to our development.

On the Arab side, we have seen that there is virtually universal agreement that the recent past is a time of misery, poverty, disease, weakness, and national humiliation; such disagreement as exists between Arabs centers on the speed, nature, and control of change, not on the categorical imperative of change. In the eyes of virtually all Arabs there can be no doubt that while the present leaves much to be desired, it is infinitely to be preferred to any period in the last thousand years. But, of course, standards have changed and will change, so that absolute improvement, though necessary, is politically less significant than relative change: yesterday's dream is today's norm and tomorrow's failure.

On the American side, there can be no doubt that there is today much of which we cannot approve in the Arab World. The physical conditions of the peoples are tragically below those even in the poverty areas of America. Ignorance and illiteracy are still prevalent. Governments are still far from public participation and often appear less urgently concerned with the betterment of their peoples than with strident pronouncement of national assertiveness. It would be as unwise as dishonest to pretend otherwise. Bland reassurance that the constitutions and congresses of the 1930's were the real stuff of democracy did not make them any more popular but did discredit the concept of democracy in the Arab countries. A smug satisfaction with today's obviously unsatisfactory state of affairs can only suggest that America is a "status quo" power in a changing world. This is neither true nor realistic. In America as abroad, Americans certainly wish to see and intend to help to bring into being a better world than we have today.

What does the United States want in the Arab Middle East? American interests and objectives are few and can be stated clearly. The ability to retain these will, naturally, constitute the working assessment of the success or failure of United States policy in that area.

The first American interest—one shared with all of the states in the area—is the prevention of an outbreak of hostilities. Hostilities, with their inherent danger of escalation to area-wide or even world war are simply too dangerous for the United States passively to tolerate. The ultimate goal is of course the establishment of a just and lasting peace in the area. But as a practical matter, in the short term, a level of tension *short of* overt, large-scale hostilities can be and is tolerated.

The second objective is to prevent the areas from falling under the control of a great power hostile to the United States. The United States does not, of course, seek such control for itself.

The third interest is in the maintenance of air and sea transit rights for the United States and her allies. The Suez Canal is one of the world's great arteries of commerce and communications, and the Arab countries are athwart the international air routes from Europe to South Asia and Africa. Closure of this area to air and sea traffic would present the United States and the Atlantic Community with serious economic and military problems which, while solvable by sea traffic diversion around the Horn of Africa and air transit through the center of Africa, would be a serious blow to Western interests.

The fourth interest is the maintenance of the flow of oil from the Middle Eastern oil fields to Western markets. United States companies that have profitable investments in Middle Eastern oil production would like to maintain their ownership of these investments; the United States government, responsive to the wishes of its citizens and corporations and aware of the value of these investments to its balance of payments, would like to maintain the present situation. However, it cannot be argued that maintenance of ownership is on the same order of priority as maintenance of the flow of oil, which is vital to the security of the European component of the Atlantic Community. Again, the flow of oil can be and, if prices rise considerably, will be replaced by oil from other sources, and ultimately in part by nuclear power. Middle Eastern oil, indeed, is a declining interest. It is not nearly so vital as it appeared to be a decade ago; a decade, hence its importance may be lowered to a secondary level of American interest.

The second level of United States interests in the Middle East area is, of course, wider. It includes at least the following items. The United States would like to secure for its citizens access to Middle Eastern markets; free and safe entry into the area; progress toward the eventual solution of the Palestine problem, including settlement of the refugees now under the care of the United Nations Relief and Works Agency; a greater concentration on the problems of social growth and improvement; and a lesser concern with arms and military establishments.

The third level of United States interest includes the growth of democratic institutions, popularity of the West, and under-standing and sympathy for the American way of life.

These are things which will be of considerable importance to the United States over the longer run but which the nation is not, in candor, prepared to pay a high price to achieve in the shorter run. Americans believe, because they believe that their way of life is a good approximation to a workable ideal, that as the Arabs acquire a better social base and aspire to a richer, fuller life, they will want a similar way for themselves. If Americans are right, then ultimately the Arabs and others will work for a well-being for themselves which will accord with that of the United States.

Do American objectives clash with those of the Arabs?

The basic Arab objective as we have seen is to build a more modern, richer, healthier, stronger, independent Arab society which the world will respect. If the Arabs are to do this, they must undertake big development programs. To finance development, all of the Arab countries must rent their transport and communications facilities, sell their oil and cotton, and secure loans and aid from abroad. These can only be done in a reasonably peaceful and constructive atmosphere. Denial of the flow of oil, for example, would hurt Arab interests at least as much as American interests. Even nationalization of the oil fields might hurt Arab interests significantly since the thing which gives value to these fields in the current circumstances of a glut of oil is control of markets. The Russians, who are oil exporters, cannot buy this oil. Denial of air and sea routes would, similarly, lose the Arabs significant income not only from the facilities themselves but from the growing tourist trade. Lastly, in an outbreak of hostilities or in the increased diversion of resources to unproductive military expenditure, Arab interests will surely be hurt far more than American. Thus, while the United States government and the several Arab governments will not always put the same priority on each of these various interests, or agree on means to safeguard or enhance them, at base the major interests of both sides coincide to an impressive degree.

Is the American position now better or worse than formerly?

As we have seen, the United States had no real position in the Middle East, as a great power, prior to 1947. America, as the land of the movie cowboy, a place of universal wealth, the source of the colleges, hospitals, and relief efforts that dot the Middle Eastern scene, and the author of ringing pronouncements on the imperative of freedom and morality, occupied a warm spot in the hearts of the Arabs. But it is only realistic to say that the golden respect for America was little tarnished by political contact. When, after 1947, as a world power the United States came to act on the Middle Eastern stage, it naturally disappointed many who had never considered it as a world power.

Since 1947 United States diplomatic relations have undergone a series of changes. America came under severe Arab criticism for her stand on the Palestine partition issue at the United Nations, but efforts to assist the Arab countries were appreciated and welcomed in some. Following the 1952 coup d'etat in Egypt the United States enjoyed very close relations with the new government and, at the same time, wih Nuri Said's government in Iraq, as well as with the Saudi Arabian, Lebanese, and Jordanian governments. But then efforts to induce the Egyptians to join the Middle East Defense Organization failed, and the United States shifted her emphasis to Iraq which joined in the formation of the Baghdad Pact. Nasser regarded this as an attempt to split the Arabs and as a blow to his leadership, so that American relations with those Arabs under Nasser's influence suffered. The United States regarded it as a serious blow to her position in the Middle East when the Egyptians turned to the Soviet Bloc for arms. American refusal to assist in the construction of the Aswan High Dam and Egyptian nationalization of the Suez Canal were the most publicized episodes of this period. There were many others. But this period was ended when the United States acted to halt the invasion of Egypt by Great Britain, France, and Israel in 1956.

The era of the Eisenhower Doctrine was one of cool relations with Egypt and those countries influenced by it and increasingly close ties with Iraq. Then, following the coup d'etat in Baghdad in July 1958, the United States dramatically placed troops in Lebanon and showed that she had the determination and ability to intervene decisively when she thought American interests were in grave jeopardy. The period of 1959–61 was one of relative inactivity in which the United States took no major initiatives and the Middle East was relatively calm.

Following the advent of the new administration in 1961 the United States reassessed its policies in the Middle East and decided to assist more actively in the growth process of the several countries and, diplomatically, to establish much closer contacts with the Arab governments; in some instances, notably in Yemen, the United States attempted to work out a formula to end inter-Arab quarrels and has tried to foster a slow-down of the arms race between the Arab states and Israel.

Thus, *tactically*, the American position appears to swing from one of success to one of near failure and back again. But viewed in a longer perspective, several things can be said. First, as the Arabs achieved real control over their national affairs following World War II, they naturally came to act on their own interpretation, rather than that of their European tutors, of their national interest. It was some time before they could be expected to do so

responsibly. Today the West is dealing with more mature governments than it was twenty years ago; they are, generally, more
powerful, more capable, and better informed. Where the interests
of both sides clash, therefore, they are in greater danger; where
they coincide, they may be more secure. Since the most important
interests do coincide, they are probably in no greater danger today
than formerly.

Conversely, it is clearly true that the Middle East is no longer
a Western preserve in which Western countries can set the rules
of the game. The Soviet Union offers alternatives which, short of
war, invasion, and occupation, cannot now be denied to the Arabs.
Relations are thus more complex and fluid than were those of
Britain and France to the Arab World in the 1920's and 1930's.
Relative to the Soviet Union, however, the Western position in
the Middle East is still very strong. As the Arab governments
have become more sophisticated and have witnessed naked and
ruthless power grabs by the local supporters of the Soviet Union,
such as the Iraqi Communists in 1959, they have taken steps, often
with Western help, to guard against Communist subversion.

And, finally, as they have set about reorganizing their economies the Arabs have picked organizational methods which are
often not to American taste. As we have seen, the role of the
state is large and the sanctity of private property is not deeply
rooted in Arab culture or in Middle Eastern history. Popular
involvement in government, similarly, is far from the Western
conception of democracy. Yet, as a growing proportion of the
Arabs become more educated, healthier, and better fed, they
can afford to aspire to the "good life." Even today, it is evident
that public pressures are exercising a greater influence on governments. As the "new men" of today's schools come forward
power will be diffused amongst them, and some acceptable version of popular participation in government, within an Arab
cultural context, will evolve.

What this analysis has suggested is that in the Arab Middle
East, and possibly in much of the developing world, the short-
term future, like the present and the immediate past, is a period

of readjustment, often noisy, prickly, and painful readjustment, from a period of Western dominance to one of partnership and sharing in which American vital interests—at least those appropriate to a relationship of mutual respect—should be safer than in the past.

Are American interests in danger?

Yes. American interests are always in danger and require vigil, care, energy, commitment, and sophistication on the part of the government and the public to be safe-guarded. Tensions between the Arab states and Israel, setbacks in development programs, excessive violence in the social revolution, and other factors could lead to war, despair, and chaos; small problems can quickly grow into big crises. No one else has evolved a policy which will be self-protecting and self-correcting, and Americans are unlikely to do so. Policies depend upon people, and must be constantly reassessed. Failure to do so results in a policy out of touch with the real—and changing—world. Following such policies can result in losing genuine interests in pursuit of mirages or secondary objectives. Americans have a right to demand the best from their policy-makers but will get it only in proportion to a national standard of commitment and knowledge.

How can the United States accomplish its objectives?

Actions—and inactions—available to the United States as a great power cover a tremendous range from the supplying of technical advice on planting wheat to interdiction of an invasion by nuclear weapons, from the granting of massive economic assistance to economic boycott, from acquiescence to ultimatum. The tools in the kit are impressive, but they can turn out a product only as good as the skill and discrimination of those who use them. It is the carpenter, not the hammer and saw, that builds the house. But the "house" in international relations is a community project—the Americans, the Arabs, and others will build it—and, consequently, both the design and the materials that go into it must be reasonably acceptable to all. Moreover,

over the long run the instruments of any foreign policy must be respected and accepted by those with whom the nation deals in order for the policy to be effective.

A wise policy will, therefore, attempt to accentuate areas of agreement and narrow areas of disagreement, using such instruments as are appropriate to each task. Basically, national self-interest is the bedrock of international relations and such devices as frustrate this interest must ultimately fail or become excessively costly. In general, therefore, the United States will find that major instruments of policy in the Middle East in the years to come will be in supplying advice and aid on the one hand, and on the other the retention of a police force. The one will facilitate a growth of healthier societies in the area, and the other will prevent an outbreak of hostilities.

The principal contingencies against which the United States must guard and the principal opportunities which lie ahead are two sides of the same coin.

The principal danger now discernible is a renewed outbreak of the Arab-Israel war, and the principal opportunity is a settlement of the Arab-Israel hostility. War in the area, even if it did not endanger world peace, would severely disrupt the development programs on which hopes for the future rest. Even short of large-scale, overt hostilities, the present tension is costing the Arabs— and the Israelis—vast amounts of resources which are badly needed elsewhere. Even saving 1 percent of the 10 percent or more of gross national product now diverted to armaments would significantly assist national development. If a settlement became possible, of course, not only would this drain be reduced, but positive contributions of trade and aid would speed up efforts at social improvement.

Failure of development programs and growing population pressure could result in the growth of more radical governments, desperately seeking short cuts and trying to suppress internal urges for a better life. In this circumstance American interests would be threatened. Conversely, with reasonable success development programs will contain pressures for violent and extreme solutions, will achieve a satisfactory rate of improvement in the life of the people, and, gradually, will so broaden the base of public participation as to evolve something like representative government in societies having a vested interest in peace.

Progress will not be easy and the means will often be obscure. But since, at the end, American goals and those of the Arabs are not in conflict, the United States should be able to work out an acceptable degree of accommodation on the means to achieve a future so important to all. However difficult or frustrating, the fact must be faced that the stakes are high and no player can afford to throw in his hand.

In human affairs there are no crystal balls. But the future grows out of the past and is shaped by men. Knowing the past, and devoting ourselves with energy and wisdom to the present, we can create a better future.

SUGGESTED READING

The purpose of the following list is to suggest further reading on the various subjects treated in broad brush strokes in this book. Obviously it cannot be exhaustive in any section. Only reasonably accessible works in European languages are included.

GENERAL WORKS on the Arabs or on the whole Middle Eastern area abound; unfortunately, generality often masks ignorance of the specific. One of several books which may be highly recommended is M. Berger, *The Arab World Today* (New York, 1962). Another is J. Berque: *Les Arabes d'Hier a Demain* (Paris, 1960). An overall view of the modern Arab scene is given in W. R. Polk (ed.), *Perspective of the Arab World*, an *Atlantic Monthly* Supplement, which was also separately published by Intercultural Publications, Inc. (New York, 1956). Included are articles on Arabic culture, social reform, Arabic literature, and Islam, and translations of Arabic short stories, plays, and poetry. Another delightful collection of Arabic literature is H. Howarth and I. Shakrullah, *Images from the Arab World* (London, 1944).

Beginning students will profit by reading J. Sauvaget, *Introduction à l'histoire de l'Orient Musulman*, Eléments de Bibliographie (Paris, 1946) which, although now somewhat out of date, is a valuable guide. More detail is usually to be found in the *Encyclopaedia of Islam*, now being issued in a new edition, in Leiden.

Among the periodicals which deal with Middle Eastern affairs the *Middle East Journal* is probably the most accessible and useful. Published in Washington, D.C., quarterly since 1947, it includes articles, book reviews, surveys of other periodicals, and a chronology which make it particularly valuable to students of the modern period. The *Middle East Forum*, published at the American University of Beirut, and *Middle Eastern Affairs* both often contain useful materials. The *Mid-East Mirror*, published weekly since 1947, is a digest of the Arabic press. The Italian magazine *Oriente Moderno* is most valuable for the period of the 1920's and 1930's as is the English *Journal of the Royal Central Asian Society*. The French journal *Orient*, published three times yearly since 1957, contains, among other useful features, frequent translations of significant treaties and pronouncements from the Arab countries. *Studia Islamica*, dealing less with the modern period, contains many significant articles on the history and culture of the Arabs; it is published in Paris, roughly every six months.

Most of the general studies contain bibliographies. None, obviously, can be kept up to date. Perhaps the best ways to keep reasonably up to date is through the reviews in the *Middle East Journal* and *International Affairs*. The Middle East Institute is revising its bibliography and this should be published in 1965. A. R. C. Bolton, *Soviet Middle East Studies, An Analysis and Bibliography* (London, 1959), is so arranged as to show the evolution of Soviet attitudes at different stages of Soviet policies.

THE PEOPLE ON THE LAND are covered in a wide assortment of works. On the bedouin, Alois Musil, *The Manners and Customs of the Rwala Bedouins* (New York, 1928), G. W. Murray, *Sons of Ishmael* (London, 1935), H. Charles, *La Sédentarisation entre Euphrate et Balik* (Beirut, 1942), H. R. P. Dickson, *The Arab of the Desert* (London, 1949), H. Charles, *Tribus moutonnières du Moyen-Euphrate* (Damascus, n.d.), and J. L. Burckhardt, *Notes on Bedouins and Wahabys* (London, 1831), are all classics of description. Important information is also to be found in J. C. Glubb, "The Bedouin of North Arabia" in the *Journal of the Royal Central Asian Society*, 1935, and, in the same journal in 1938, E. Epstein, "The Bedouin of Transjordan." All considered the most masterful survey of bedouin life is R. Montagne, *La Civilisation du desert* (Paris, 1947).

On the nonbedouin rural Arabs, perhaps the best overall studies are A. Latron, *La Vie rurale en Syrie et au Liban* (Beirut, 1936), and J. Weulersse, *Paysans* (Paris, 1941). The Egyptian peasant is treated in H. Ayrout, *The Egyptian Peasant* (new edition, Boston, 1963), J. Berque, *Histoire sociale d'une village Egyptienne au XXème siècle*, and Hamed Ammar, *Growing up in an Egyptian Village* (New York, 1954). The "marsh Arabs" of Iraq are the subject of S. M. Salim, *Marsh Dwellers of the Euphrates Delta* (London, 1962), and Fulanain (pseud.), *Haji Rikkan, Marsh Arab* (London, 1927). Studies of urban life and the relations of the city to the countryside include three excellent Arabic novels, now available in English, Tawfiq el-Hakim, *The Maze of Justice* (London, 1947), and Taha Hussein, *An Egyptian Childhood* (London, 1932) and *The Stream of Days* (London, 1948). C. Hurgronje, *Mekka* (London, 1931), and J. L. Burckhardt, *Travels in Arabia* (London, 1829), give fascinating pictures of Arabia at the beginning and end of the nineteenth century. E. W. Lane, *The Manners and Customs of the Modern Egyptians* (London, 1836 and many subsequent editions), is one of the great classics of description of all times. It was a by-product of the half a lifetime which Lane spent in Cairo translating a huge lexicon of Arabic. Albert de Boucheman: *Une Petite cité caravanièré: Suhné* (Damascus, n.d.) shows a typical desert outpost.

Special areas are treated in A. Hourani, *Minorities in the Arab World* (London, 1947), H. St. J. Philby, *The Empty Quarter* (London, 1933), H. Ingrams, *Arabia and the Isles* (London, 1942), D. Ingrams, *A Survey of Social and Economic Conditions in the Aden Protectorate* (Eritrea, 1949), and H. Scott, *In the High Yemen* (London, 1942).

Aspects of the geography of the Arab Middle East are discussed in W. Fisher, *The Middle East* (New York, 1950), and the particular importance of water is brought out in N. Moussly, *Le Problem de l'eau en Syrie* (Lyon, 1951).

Emrys Peters, "Aspects of Rank and Status among Muslims in a Lebanese village" in J. Pitt-Rivers, *Mediterranean Countrymen* (Paris, 1936), is the product of one of the most detailed studies ever made of Arab village life. Finally, G. Baer, *Population and Society in the Arab East* (New York, 1964), is a major synthesis of current knowledge.

THE ANCIENT ARABS are best shown in their own literature. Obviously, this is best understood in Arabic, but the non-Arabist will profit from C. J. Lyall, *Ancient Arabian Poetry* (London, 1930), which contains not only a wide sample of translations but a superb introduction. Two other surveys which put the classical literature in perspective are H. A. R. Gibb, *Arabic Literature* (London, 1926), and R. Nicholson, *Literary History of the Arabs* (Cambridge, Eng., 1953). The heart of pre-Islamic literature is translated in *The Seven Golden Odes of Pagan Arabia, Known Also as the Moallakat* by Lady Anne Blunt and Wilfrid Scrawen Blunt (London, 1903). The scene in Arabia of that period is sketched in H. Lammens, *Le Berceau de l'Islam* (Rome, 1914), *La Mecque à la veille de l'Hégire* (Beirut, 1924), and *La Cité Arabe de Taif à la veille de l'Hégire* (Beirut, 1922).

ISLAM is, of course, the subject of a vast literature in many languages. To understand it, however, it is probably unwise to begin with the *Koran*. Even the Arab Muslims read the *Koran* with the help of a teacher and a commentary. The best translation, however, is very good. It is M. Pickthall, *The Glorious Koran* (London, 1930). To begin, one should read one or more of the following, R. Bell, *Introduction to the Qur'ān* (Edinburgh, 1953), H. A. R. Gibb, *Mohammedanism* (New York, 1955), which is possibly the best general introduction to the whole religious system, A. S. Tritton, *Muslim Theology* (London, 1947) and *Islam, Belief and Practices* (London, 1951), and R. Roberts, *The Social Laws of the Qorân* (London, 1925). A more detailed account of the *Koran* itself is given in A. Jeffry, *The Qur'an* as *Scripture* (New York, 1952). The life of Muhammad is treated in detail by M. Watt in his two volumes *Muhammad at Mecca* (Oxford, 1953) and *Muhammad at Medina* (Oxford, 1956). The older study of W. Muir, the *Life of Mahomet* (London, 1894), is still delightful and valuable, but perhaps the best all-round introduction is T. Andrae, *Mohammed, the Man and his Faith* (London, 1936).

M. Gaudefroy-Demombynes, *Muslim Institutions* (London, 1950), is the best introduction to the social elaboration of Islam. G. von Grunebaum, *Islam, Essays in the Nature and Growth of a*

Cultural Tradition (London, 1955) and *Medieval Islam* (Chicago, second ed., 1953), and L. Gardet, *La Cité Musulmane,* Vie sociale et politique (Paris, 1954), are significant contributions to the subject.

Special topics in Islam are treated in R. A. Nicholson, *The Mystics of Islam* (London, 1914), A. J. Arberry, *Sufism* (London, 1950), and D. Donaldson, *The Shi'ite Religion* (London, 1933). Detailed coverage on virtually every conceivable aspect of Islam is given in the *Encyclopaedia of Islam,* and those articles of particular interest on the religion have been separately published in H. A. R. Gibb and J. H. Kramers, *Shorter Encyclopaedia of Islam* (Leiden, 1953). Lastly, G. von Grunebaum, *Muhammadan Festivals* (New York, 1951), is a good companion to have if one is living in a Muslim country.

THE CONQUESTS AND CALIPHATE are introduced concisely in B. Lewis, *The Arabs in History* (London, 1950), which is one of the best books ever written on the Arab Middle East. The conquests are the subject of an excellent essay by C. H. Becker in the *Cambridge Medieval History* (Cambridge, Eng., vol. II, 1936) and of M. J. de Goeje, *Mémoire sur la conquête de la Syrie* (Leiden, 1900). S. Lane-Poole, *A History of Egypt in the Middle Ages* (London, 1914), deals with the Arab invasion and subsequent history; H. A. R. Gibb, *The Arab Conquests in Central Asia* (London, 1923), deals with the invasions in the East. Various articles by Gibb on other aspects of the caliphate are reprinted in S. J. Shaw and W. R. Polk (ed.), *Studies on the Civilization of Islam by Hamilton A. R. Gibb* (Boston, 1962). The cultural aspects of medieval Arabic civilization as they affected medieval Europe are covered in T. Arnold and A. Guillaume, *The Legacy of Islam* (Oxford, 1931). Other general histories of note are C. Brockelmann, *History of the Islamic Peoples* (New York, 1947), which has a somewhat wider scope than B. Lewis (above) and P. Hitti, *History of the Arabs* (London, 1951), which is much more detailed but less critical. The caliphate is the subject of a virtually undiscriminating reading of the Arabic chronicles in W. Muir, *The Caliphate, Its Rise, Decline and Fall* (Edinburgh, 1915). The Umayyad caliphate is the subject of a number of excellent works including H. Lammens, *Etudes sur le règne du Calife Omaiyade Mo'awia i^er* (Leipzig, 1907) and *Etudes sur le siècle des Omayyades* (Beirut, 1930), and, above all, J. Wellhausen, *The Arab Kingdom and Its Fall* (Calcutta, 1927).

The Abbasid caliphate of Baghdad is dealt with in the general studies and in a series of fascinating essays in T. Nöldeke, *Sketches from Eastern History* (Edinburgh, 1892). The bureaucratic breakdown of the empire is the subject of H. Bowen, *Life and Times of 'Ali ibn 'Isa* (Cambridge, 1928). The cultural recovery of Islam in an age of political decline is described in A. Mez, *The Renaissance of Islam* (London, 1937).

THE PERIOD OF THE ALIEN EMPIRES is covered in some of the general studies noted above. S. Runciman, *History of the Crusades* (Cambridge, Eng., 1952–54), is a masterful and well-written account; other articles on the Crusades of relevance are contained in Marshall W. Baldwin (ed.), *The First Hundred Years*, volume I of *A History of the Crusades* (Philadelphia, 1955). H. A. R. Gibb (trans.), *The Damascus Chronicle of the Crusades* (London, 1932), and P. K. Hitti (trans.), *Memoires of an Arab-Syrian Gentleman* (New York, 1929), present Arab views of the Crusades. C. Cahen, *La Syrie Nord à l'époque des Croisades* (Paris, 1940), is one of the best studies available. The Mongols are treated in G. Vernadsky, *The Mongols and Russia* (New Haven, 1953), better though with less detail on the Middle East than elsewhere. H. Lammens, *La Syrie, précis historique* (Beirut, 1921), deals with the whole sweep of Syrian history; the Mamluk period is covered in Gaudefroy-Demombynes, *La Syrie à l'epoque des Mamelouks* (Paris, 1923); and Lebanon is being treated in a series of volumes by Adel Ismail, *Histoire du Liban du XVIIe siècle à nos jours* of which volume I, *Le Liban au temps de Fakhr-ed-Din II*, was published in Paris in 1955. H. A. R. Gibb and H. Bowen, *Islamic Society and the West* (Oxford, 1950, 1957), is a major study of the Arab areas under the Turks. G. Stripling, *The Ottoman Turks and the Arabs* (Urbana, Ill., 1942); S. Longrigg, *Four Centuries of Modern Iraq* (Oxford, 1925); Henri Dehérain, *L'Egypte Turque* (Paris, n.d.); A. N. Poliak, *Feudalism in Egypt, Syria, Palestine and the Lebanon, 1250–1900* (London, 1939);

and W. R. Polk, *The Opening of South Lebanon* (Cambridge, Mass., 1963), deal with Arab affairs under Turkish rule. Life in Cairo is the subject of a separate study in Marcel Colombe, "La Vie au Caire au 18ème siècle," Conferences de l'Institut Français d'Archaéologie Orientale (Cairo, 1951), and more detailed is S. J. Shaw, *Ottoman Egypt in the Age of the French Revolution* (Cambridge, Mass., 1964).

THE IMPACT OF THE WEST is the subject of a large number of studies. My own *Opening of South Lebanon, A Study of the Impact of the West on the Middle East* (Cambridge, Mass., 1963) is directly addressed to this topic and centers on the Levant. H. A. Rivlin, *The Agricultural Policy of Muhammad 'Alī in Egypt* (Cambridge, Mass., 1961), and G. Baer, *History of Land-ownership in Modern Egypt, 1800–1950* (London, 1963), deal with rural problems; Moustafa Fahmy, *La Révolution de l'indus-trie en Egypte et ses conséquences sociales au 19e siècle, 1800–1850* (Leiden, 1954), treats urban changes. J. Heyworth-Dunne, *Introduction to the History of Education in Modern Egypt* (London, 1938), treats cultural affairs, and J. Bowring, *Report on the Commercial Statistics of Egypt and Syria* (London, 1840) is a mine of information on economic affairs. Egypt under the impact of the West is wonderfully described in E. W. Lane, *Manners and Customs of the Modern Egyptians* (above), and A.-B. Clot, *Aperçu général sur l'Egypte* (Paris, 1840). The best general treat-ment of Egypt is F. Charles-Roux, *L'Egypte de 1801–1882* (Paris, n.d.). On the Persian Gulf see A. T. Wilson, *The Persian Gulf* (London, 1928).

ON THE COMING OF THE WEST to the Arab Middle East, David S. Landes, *Bankers and Pashas* (Cambridge, Mass., 1958), is fas-cinating and can be put in a wider Middle Eastern context with H. Feis, *Europe, the World's Banker* (New Haven, 1930), and W. L. Langer, *The Diplomacy of Imperialism* (New York, 1935). Zaki Saleh, *Mesopotamia, 1600–1914* (Baghdad, 1957), gives a good account of Iraq in tandem to the spirit of W. S. Blunt, *The Secret History of the English Occupation of Egypt* (New York, 1922). The Crimean War is dealt with, in its Near Eastern aspects, in H. W. V. Temperley, *The Crimea* (London, 1934).

The English view of imperialism is best set out in Lord Cromer, *Modern Egypt* (London, 1908) and *Abbas II* (London, 1915). The political impact and Egyptian reaction is the subject of N. Safran, *Egypt in Search of Political Community* (Cambridge, Mass., 1961), J. Landau, *Parliaments and Parties in Egypt* (New York, 1954), Jamal Ahmad, *The Intellectual Origins of Egyptian Nationalism* (London, 1960), C. C. Adams, *Islam and Modernism in Egypt* (London, 1933), and A. H. Hourani, *Arabic Thought in the Liberal Age, 1798–1939* (London, 1962). The Egyptian view of the history of the period is in M. Rifaat, *The Awakening of Modern Egypt* (London, 1947).

WORLD WAR I is dealt with in a number of studies and collections of memoirs as well as in official dispatches. On Iraq, the most important work, written by the chief political officer of the British forces, is A. T. Wilson, *Loyalties, Mesopotamia, 1914–1917* and *A Clash of Loyalties, 1917–1920* (London, 1930 and 1931). Edouard Brémond, *Le Hédjaz dans la guerre mondiale* (Paris, 1931), gives a French view of the "reality" behind the Lawrence of Arabia legend. Lawrence's own account, T. E. Lawrence, *Seven Pillars of Wisdom* (New York, 1926), should be read with the critics not far away. Richard Aldington, *Lawrence of Arabia* (London, 1955), is devastating if picky. The diary of the chief political officer of the British forces in the theater, R. Meinertz-hagen, *Middle East Diary* (London, 1959), is conclusive. Sir R. Storrs, *Orientations* (London, 1937), is one of the most fascinating views of the period. Lady Bell (ed.), *The Letters of Gertrude Bell* (London, 1927), gives a view of happenings in Baghdad similar to that of Storrs in Cairo and Jerusalem.

Among the official documents, E. L. Woodward and R. Butler (eds.), *Documents on British Foreign Policy, 1919–1939*, first series, vol. IV, 1919 (London, 1952), is essential for the critical year. The terms on which the Arabs entered the war are set out and discussed in Cmd 5957: *Correspondence between Sir Henry McMahon and the Sharif Hussein of Mecca, July 1915–March 1916* (London, 1939); Cmd 5964: *Statements Made on Behalf of His Majesty's Government during the Year 1918 in Regard to the Future Status of Certain Parts of the Ottoman Empire* (London,

1939); and Cmd 6974: *Report of a Committee Set Up to Consider Certain Correspondence between Sir Henry McMahon and the Sharif of Mecca in 1915 and 1916* (London, 1939). The *Balfour Declaration* is the subject and title of a masterly work by Leonard Stein (London, 1961). A fascinating insight into the critical work of Sir Mark Sykes both on the Balfour Declaration and on the Sykes-Picot Agreement is given in Christopher Sykes, *Two Studies in Virtue* (New York, 1953).

E. Kedourie, *England and the Middle East, The Destruction of the Ottoman Empire, 1914–1921* (London, 1956), is well written but somewhat forced. Perhaps the best work on the English role for this as for later periods is E. Monroe, *Britain's Moment in the Middle East* (Baltimore, 1963), although Sir R. Bullard, *Britain and the Middle East* (London, 1951), is a good introduction. American efforts are the subject of H. N. Howard, *The King-Crane Commission* (Beirut, 1963), and the work at the Peace Conference is ably covered in H. W. V. Temperley, *The Peace Conference of Paris* (vol. VI, London, 1921). The Arabs' efforts are described best in Zeine N. Zeine, *The Struggle for Arab Independence* (Beirut, 1960). A fascinating comment on Arab-Zionist negotiations should be read in M. Perlmann, "Chapters of Arab-Jewish Diplomacy, 1918–1922" in *Jewish Social Studies*, 6 (1944): 123 f. Misunderstandings between the British and the French are sketched in H. H. Cumming, *Franco-British Rivalry in the Post-War Near East* (London, 1938). The immediate postwar period is summed up in A. J. Toynbee, *The Islamic World since the Peace Settlement, Survey of International Affairs, 1925*, vol. I (London, 1927).

THE MANDATES PERIOD is the subject of an ever-growing volume of literature. The yearly reports to the League of Nations on the mandates are a treasure house of information. But a number of first-rate studies on one or more of the mandate countries exist. On Syria and Lebanon, S. H. Longrigg, *Syria and Lebanon under French Mandate* (London, 1958), is exhaustive, but older works by A. H. Hourani, *Syria and Lebanon* (London, 1946), and N. A. Ziadeh, *Syria and Lebanon* (London, 1957), are easier to digest and more pointed. In addition to Z. N. Zeine, *The Struggle for*

Arab Independence (Beirut, 1960), R. de Gontant-Biron, *Comment la France s'est instalée en Syrie* (Paris, 1923), sets out the beginnings of French power. E. Rabbath, *L'Evolution politique de la Syrie sous mandat* (Paris, 1928), and P. Rondot, *Les Institutions politiques du Liban* (Paris, 1947), are very important for an understanding of domestic affairs. An independent view is given in D. Censoni, *Siria e Libano dal Mandato all'indipendenza, 1919–1946* (Bologna, 1948), and the difficulty the French had with the Druze (and others) is described in Général Andréa, *La Révolte Druze et l'Insurrection de Damas, 1925–1926* (Paris, 1937). An overall view, but at something of a distance, from the mandates is given in Quincy Wright, *Mandates under the League of Nations* (Chicago, 1930).

Iraq is the subject of many studies by Englishmen. A basic book is S. H. Longrigg, *'Iraq, 1900–1950, A Political, Social and Economic History* (London, 1953). Still valuable on earlier periods are P. Ireland, *'Iraq* (London, 1937), and M. Khadduri, *Independent Iraq* (London, 1950).

Egypt is dealt with competently in M. Colombe, *L'Evolution de l'Egypte, 1924–1950* (Paris, 1951). However, following the 1952 coup, much of the overt political history of that period seemed to many writers of less consequence than underlying social and economic changes, of which more below. Anglo-Egyptian relations are soberly described in the Royal Institute of International Affairs, *Great Britain and Egypt, 1914–1951* (London, 1952), and, somewhat more vigorously and impartially, in John Marlow, *Anglo-Egyptian Relations, 1800–1953* (London, 1954). The sort of biting satire of Egyptians in the 1930's referred to in the text is C. S. Jarvis, *The Back-Garden of Allah* (London, 1939), which went through nine printings although banned in Egypt, and his *Oriental Spotlight* (London, 1937).

There really is no good book on Arabia during this period, but a beginning can be made with K. S. Twitchell, *Saudi Arabia* (Princeton, 1953), and H. R. P. Dickson, *The Arab of the Desert* (London, 1949).

Neither is there a first-rate book on Jordan. F. G. Peake, *History and Tribes of Jordan* (Miami, 1958), and J. B. Glubb, *The*

Story of the Arab Legion (London, 1948), are the product of the two creators of the military force of Jordan.

THE PALESTINE PROBLEM has received several times the deluge of printer's ink as all the rest of the topics of this book combined. This author has contributed in W. R. Polk, D. Stamler and E. Asfour, *Backdrop to Tragedy, The Struggle for Palestine* (Boston, 1957). For the beginner, the book contains a comprehensive bibliography, a complete set of maps, a concise history, and the assembled viewpoints of an American, an English Zionist, and a Palestine Arab. Perhaps the best study of the political aspects of the Palestine problem is J. C. Hurewitz, *The Struggle for Palestine* (New York, 1950). R. Montagne, "Pour la paix en Palestine," *Politique etrangère*, 1938, is important for the Arab mood of the 1930's, and A. Grannot, *The Land System in Palestine* (London, 1949), is a valuable account of the basis of the problem in the mandate. The many official studies must be read and can be said to be about the best in academic standard and readability of any published. Cmd 5479: *Palestine Royal Commission Report* (London, 1937) and *A Survey of Palestine, Prepared in December 1945 and January 1946 for the Information of the Anglo-American Committee of Inquiry* (Jerusalem, 1946) are extremely valuable. They are followed by the *United Nations Special Committee on Palestine Report* (Lake Success, N.Y., 1947) in utility. G. Kirk, *The Middle East in the War* (London, 1952) and *The Middle East, 1945–1950* (London, 1954), are of great value not only for Palestine but for the whole Middle East.

THE PERIOD OF TURBULENCE FOLLOWING WORLD WAR II, of *formal independence* and *coups*, is covered in a number of works. G. Kirk, just mentioned, is a good beginning. J. Kimche, *Seven Fallen Pillars* (New York, 1953), is a harsh but accurate description, and M. Alami, "The Lesson of Palestine," *Middle East Journal*, 1949, is an Arab indictment of Arab affairs. A Hourani, "The Decline of the West in the Middle East," *International Affairs*, 1953–54, is a sensitive and deep study of Arab-European relations. E. O'Ballance, *The Arab-Israeli War* (London, 1952), sets out the events of the Arab defeat in Palestine.

The Egyptian coup of 1952 and its aftermath is dealt with in a number of books. One of the best is Jean and Simon Lacouture, *Egypt in Transition* (New York, 1958). Nasser and his "team" are described in W. Wynn, *Nasser of Egypt, the Search for Dignity* (Cambridge, Mass., 1959), K. Wheelock, *Nasser's New Egypt* (New York, 1960), P. J. Vatikiotis, *The Egyptian Army in Politics* (Bloomington, Ind., 1961), and T. Little, *Egypt* (New York, 1958). The view from the inside is given in Gamal Abdul Nasser, *The Philosophy of the Revolution* (Washington, 1955), Mohammed Naquib, *Egypt's Destiny* (New York, 1955), and Anwar Sadat, *Revolt on the Nile* (London, 1957).

The situation in Syria is well described in G. Torrey, *Syrian Politics and the Military, 1945–1958* (Columbus, Ohio, 1964). Iraq has yet to receive comparable treatment. M. Ionides, *Divide and Lose* (London, 1960), and "Caractacus" (pseud.), *Revolution in Iraq* (London, 1959), give the best book-length accounts. Also see W. R. Polk, "The Lesson of Iraq," *Atlantic Monthly*, 1958, for the immediate aftermath of the July coup in Baghdad. King Hussein of Jordan, *Uneasy Lies the Head* (New York, 1962), describes this era of turbulence from another angle. Finally, W. R. Brown, "The Yemeni Dilemma," *Middle East Journal*, 1963, is the best account yet available on Yemen.

The Suez crisis is the subject of M. Adams, *Suez and After* (Boston, 1958), and G. Wint and P. Calvocoressi, *Middle East Crisis* (London, 1957). The U.S. Department of State publication *The Suez Canal Problem* (Washington 1956) gives many of the documents.

Social Change is a newer subject than any other. The best book in the field is M. Halpern, *The Politics of Social Change* (Princeton, 1963). Forthcoming is a more comprehensive work called *The New Men* (New York, 1965) edited by William R. Polk. H. el-Saaty, "The Middle Classes in Egypt" (Cairo, 1957), and S. Fisher (ed.), *The Role of the Military in the Middle East* (Columbus, Ohio, 1963) are also valuable. C. Issawi, "Economic and Social Foundations of Democracy in the Middle East," *International Affairs*, 1956, is a sobering account of the lack of a basis in the current scene for democratic institutions.

THE ECONOMY of the Arab countries is a relatively new subject. Though much useful work was done by the Middle East Supply Centre during World War II, the first comprehensive study was the Clapp Commission Report, United Nations Conciliation Commission for Palestine, *U.N. Economic Survey Mission for the Middle East* (Lake Success, N.Y., 1949). The rural base of the economy is the subject of D. Warriner's shocking and powerful books, *Land and Poverty in the Middle East* (London, 1948) and *Land Reform and Development in the Middle East* (London, 1957). On industry see A. A. I. El-Gritly, *The Structure of Modern Industry in Egypt* (Cairo, 1948), K. M. Langley, *The Industrialization of Iraq* (Cambridge, Mass., 1961), and A. D. Little, Inc., *A Plan for Industrial Development in Iraq* (Cambridge, Mass., 1956). On development efforts see W. R. Polk (ed.), *The Developmental Revolution* (Washington, 1963). The International Bank studies on *Iraq* (Baltimore, 1952), *Syria* (Baltimore, 1955), and *Jordan* (Baltimore, 1957) are comprehensive. E. Asfour, *Syria, Development and Monetary Policy* (Cambridge, Mass., 1959) is about the best on Syria. C. Issawi, *Egypt in Revolution* (London, 1963), the third edition of a book first published in 1947, is in a class by itself. Oil is the subject of a number of studies of which perhaps the best is S. H. Longrigg, *Oil in the Middle East* (London, 1954), and labor is studied in F. Harbison and I. Ibrahim, *Human Resources for Egyptian Enterprize* (New York, 1958). Surveys are available from the United Nations Department of Economic and Social Affairs, *Economic Development of the Middle East, 1945–54* (New York, 1955), with supplements in later years. Finally, the economic research center at the American University of Beirut publishes occasional papers on the economy of the Middle East.

ON THE ARABS IN THE WORLD one should be able to consult the Arabic literature. The American Council of Learned Societies started to make that possible, some years ago, when it began to publish a series of translations of significant Arabic political studies, in its Near Eastern translation program, Washington, 1953 and subsequently. N. Ziadeh, "Recent Arabic Literature on Arabism," *Middle East Journal*, 1952, provides a now-dated but useful survey. H. Z. Nuseibeh, *The Ideas of Arab Nationalism* (Ithaca, N.Y., 1956), is disappointing. W. R. Polk, *What the Arabs Think* (New York, 1952), is based on the thought of the "new men" of Iraq. A. Hourani, *Arabic Thought in the Liberal Age* (London, 1962), G. Antonius, *The Arab Awakening* (London, 1938), C. C. Adams, *Islam and Modernism in Egypt* (London, 1933), H. A. R. Gibb, *Modern Trends in Islam* (Chicago, 1947), and S. G. Haim (ed.), *Arab Nationalism* (Los Angeles, 1962), all deal with aspects of the background to contemporary developments. W. Z. Laqueur, *Communism and Nationalism in the Middle East* (London, 1956), and Laqueur (ed.), *The Middle East in Transition* (New York, 1958), bring the account more up to date. L. Binder, "Radical Reform Nationalism in Syria and Egypt," *Muslim World*, 1959, pushes an analysis of ideology about as far as it can go. The best account of the foreign policy of the Arabs is C. D. Cremeans, *The Arabs and the World* (New York, 1963).

UNITED STATES INTERESTS IN THE MIDDLE EAST are the subject of a large number of works. John C. Campbell, *Defense of the Middle East* (New York, 1960), and G. Stevens (ed.), *The United States and the Middle East* (Englewood Cliffs, N.J., 1964), are good beginnings. J. C. Hurewitz, *Middle East Dilemmas* (New York, 1953), discusses problems that are still with us. Official publications on United States policy include a series by H. N. Howard, *Development of U.S. Policy in the Near East, 1945–51* (Washington, 1952), *U.S. Policy in the Near East, South Asia and Africa, 1951–1952* (Washington, 1953), *U.S. Policy in the Near East during 1953* (Washington, 1954), *U.S. Policy in the Near East during 1954* (Washington, 1955), and *U.S. Policy in the Near East during 1955* (Washington, 1956). An essay by R. H. Nolte and W. R. Polk, "Toward a Policy for the Middle East," *Foreign Affairs Quarterly*, July 1958, may still have interest.

Periodic collections of documents, as in *United States Policy in the Middle East, September 1956–June 1957* (Washington, 1957), hearings before congressional committees, and speeches printed in the State Department *Bulletin* provide source materials.

THE SOVIET ROLE IN THE MIDDLE EAST is described, historically, by Ivar Spector, *The Soviet Union and the Muslim World, 1917–1958* (Seattle, 1959), and W. Z. Laqueur, *The Soviet Union and the Middle East* (New York, 1959).

BRITISH INTERESTS are set out in The Royal Institute of International Affairs, *Britsh Interests in the Mediterranean and the Middle East* (London, 1958).

INDEX